ORGANC
ART Or rlEALING

by
SAMUEL HAHNEMANN

First Edition

TRANSLATED IN ENGLISH

by

DR. MAHENDRA SINGH
DR. SUBHAS SINGH

FOREWORD for this SPECIALCOMMEMORATIVE ISSUE BY
DR. ESWARA DAS
Director, National Institute of Homoeopathy, Kolkata

SPECIAL COMEMMORATIVE ISSUE

B. Jain Publishers (P) Ltd.
An ISO 9001 : 2000 Certified Company
USA—EUROPE—INDIA

Organon

der rationellen

Heilkunde

von

Samuel Hahnemann.

Die Wahrheit, die wir alle nöthig haben,
die uns als Menschen glücklich macht,
ward von der weisen Hand, die sie uns zugedacht,
nur leicht verdeckt, nicht ales vergraben.

GELLERT.

Dresden, 1810.

in der Arnoldischen Buchhandlung.

ORGANON OF RATIONAL
ART OF HEALING
by
SAMUEL HAHNEMANN

The Truth which human beings do need,
For their survival and welfare,
With a purpose of it being found, not buried
deep but lightly covered,
By the Wise Hand that blesses us with care.

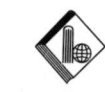

B. Jain Publishers (P) Ltd.
An ISO 9001 : 2000 Certified Company
USA—EUROPE—INDIA

Original Page Missing

ORGANON OF RATIONAL ART OF HEALING BY SAUMUEL HAHNEMANN

First Edition: 2010
1st Impression: 2010

Published by Kuldeep Jain for
B. JAIN PUBLISHERS (P) LTD.
An ISO 9001 : 2000 Certified Company
1921/10, Chuna Mandi, Paharganj, New Delhi 110 055 (INDIA)
Tel.: +91-11-4567 1000 • Fax: +91-11-4567 1010
Email: info@bjain.com • Website: www.bjainbooks.com

Printed in India by
J.J. Offset Printers

ISBN: 978-81-319-0988-1

Our Expected and Respected readers are

Those unknown, unidentified and silent sections of the homoeopathic students, teachers and practitioners who appear dormant and voiceless today but possess the courage, potential and purity of purpose in them to stand as pillars of tomorrow; who will defend Homoeopathy against the perverts who try to undermine the merit of Homoeopathy, try all weapons against Homoeopathy or use every pervert expressions and explanations as shields to cover their own incompetence crimes, failures, follies and commercial intents;

Those whom people may misunderstand as lifeless and insignificant today but who have the wisdom to distinguish between external pretensions and internal purpose of the managers of Homoeopathy;

Those who are determined to survive by their own merit, by the strength of Homoeopathy and will be the ideals whom these managers will avoid, neglect, suppress and yet will be afraid to confront, will criticize but not dare to face;

Those who will remain a minority in the crowd and mob of medical profession and Homoeopathy,

but will remain a glorious minority, a brilliantly shining minority in an ignoramus crowd of dark ignominy, *and*

Those who will read this writing and will try to rectify its errors, point out its anomalies and identify its faults

Dr. Mahendra Singh
Dr. Subhas Singh

Dedicated to

My father, Sri Suraj Singh,

&

My mother, Smt. Anarkali Devi,

For it was their wisdom, which was beyond their background,
their forbearance, which was beyond their sufferings, and
the universality of their thoughts, *which is reflected
in all my brothers and sisters and other family members,*
For their spirit to accept life as it is,
and for making all of us believe in *putting our efforts
to change the things which can be changed,
Accepting the things, which cannot be changed, and
striving for the wisdom to know the
difference between the two.*
I am, what I am for they made me so.

Mahendra Singh

FOREWORD

(To this Special Commemorative Issue)

Homoeopaths around the world are celebrating the bicentenary of the publication of the First Edition of Organon of Medicine, the *Magnum Opus* by Dr. Christian Frederick Samuel Hahnemann. The book has undergone six editions and the present day homoeopaths are masters of the concept and principles propounded by Master Hahnemann though they might have seen only the last edition.

Organon of Medicine is the codification of the basic principles in medicine, which a practitioner of any discipline of any of medicine needs to know. As such it need not be confined to homoeopaths only. It contains in most of the parts such concepts which are true for any discipline of medicine. Except for some aphorisms where specific instructions for homoeopathy is given, it contains matters which are applicable to the medical science in general. In fact, the book was written with this idea that it would be read by anybody, preferably a medical person and by its sheer rational and logical approach will convince the reader about the benefits and advantages of homoeopathy over other system of medicine. We should not confine the book to homoeopaths only, rather we should show respect and express our confidence in Hahnemann and homoeopathy by inviting all the medical profession as a whole to read and express views on Organon of Medicine, which I

am sure will open new avenues of understanding the system in a more rational manner.

The importance of the first edition of this epic is tremendous as it gives the original idea of Hahnemann in formulating new concepts, principles and theories of homoeopathy, many of these remain quite unconventional even today. When other medical disciplines are searching for explanations for the cause and cure of diseases, Hahnemann in the simplest language describes diseases as simple derangement of life force and the highest responsibility of the physician is to restore the same. I am sure the profession will like to read and enrich itself by reading the First Edition of Organon and knowing the whole process of evolution of Homoeopathic system of medicine.

Many Homoeopaths adore the Organon of Medicine as their religious scripture and consider Hahnemann as their prophet. Though this may not be the appropriate way in which the master-piece on the basic principles of homoeopathy and its founder should be considered but this depicts the highest esteem the followers of the system extend to the book and its author, more so in the Indian subcontinent. I am informed that there has been no complete translation of the First Edition of Organon in English. I am sure the profession needs to know the original thought of Hahnemann when he was giving shape to a new medical discipline which he called 'Homoeopathy'. The first edition gives the original unedited thought process of the medical revolutionary. The later editions have gone into modifications with revision and reviews of the original thoughts. This is the beauty and originality of the first edition which would always remain a subject matter of deep research for all times to come. This translation, I am told is the first complete translation done by Dr. Mahendra Singh and Dr. Subhas Singh, is a befitting tribute to Master Hahnemann. The importance is

that this is being published after 200 years of the publication of first edition containing the basic principles propounded by Hahnemann which still baffles the world of science, but the benefit of this system marvels any other medical discipline.

As regards the translation, it is done by the most authentic and acclaimed teachers, the father and son duo, who are very committed to the subject. The long experience of Dr. Mahendra Singh as a teacher of Organon, his knowledge of German language, his commitment to bring the work to perfection and the legacy inherited by Dr. Subhas Singh have all added in bringing out such a marvellous work to the profession. I am sure that they must have put long hours of labour and meticulous efforts to make this translation perfect. It is a great contribution of Indian homoeopaths to homoeopathic literature.

I hope the book will get the acceptance and appreciation that it deserves from the profession. The efforts made by the translators are lauded for their efforts.

February, 2010   **Dr. Eswara Das**
Kolkata   *Director*, National Institute of Homoeopathy

WHY THIS BOOK?

When I was a student, I was asked to cram - up the year of publications of different editions of Organon. At that time I did not realise that most of our teachers have not seen the German editions of Organon, nor the different English translations excepting those of R.E. Dudgeon and some had copies of C. Wesselhoeft. B.K. Sarkar's Commentary on the Organon of Medicine was the text book and not until 3rd year of my student days I was able to procure a copy of Boericke and Tafel's print of Dudgeon's translation of the 5th edition. On going through the Appendix of the book, Dudgeon's chart of comparison of aphorisms of different editions of the Organon, it proved to be an eye - opener. For the first time few aphorisms of different editions of the Organon was seen carefully. My teachers were not of much help in the search of different editions of Organon. I hoped that some day the German editions of the book which moulded our destiny will be in my hands. I did a short course in German language at Max Mueller Bhavan, Kolkata. The wait was really big. The Fortune smiled at last. In 1998 Dr. Krishna Saha of C.L. Chouksey Homoeopathic Medical College and Hospital, Bilaspur went to Germany for a short course in Anesthesia. She brought for me all the five German editions of the book. By the time Dr. R.K. Joardar, the teacher - of Organon in M. Bhattacharya Homoeopathic Medical College who had graduated in German language and was the main strength of German knowing homoeopaths of West Bengal became totally

blind. Our whole plan of translation was postponed for some time but not wound up.

In the meantime, Dr. Subhas Singh passed his B.H.M.S. from The Calcutta Homoeopathic Medical College and learned rudiments of German. We bought the different varities of German - English dictionaries of both medical and non medical. We were surprised that R.E. Dudgeon, the best translator of Homoeopathic books from German to English has committed errors, had taken liberties and in order to keep the frame of the German sentences intact had made the sentences difficult.

C.E. Wheeler translated the First edition. It was published in 1913. His translation had an aura of literary fluency but he neither translated the whole of 1st edition nor tried to keep the parity of the words or sentences of different editions.

We deserve credit that despite our lack of fluency in German language, despite the words being 200 years old and not available in current German English dictionaries and despite the differences in the content and style of Dudgeon and Wheeler we have brought forth in a plain language as near as possible to Hahnemann's intentions in using a words and sentence and the demand of the scientific spirit.

We have struck to the original but have also used the current English. We have maintained the parity of Hahnemann's words in different editions.

We will wait for response of the profession to give us an impetus to finalise the English translation of the 4th edition of Organon of Medicine which we have completed.

Mahendra Singh
February 2010   **Subhas Singh**

PROLOGUE

An earlier attempt was made to translate the 1st edition of Organon of Medicine, by **Dr. C. E. Wheeler**. It must have been a tough and well thought of decision of Wheeler to attempt to translate the First Edition when already the later editions were available in original and in their English translations. His reason for selecting the 1st Edition was that he considered it less controversial. He wrote –

"The Organon is put forward here as a piece of history rather than as a contribution to polemics. For this reason the original edition of 1810 was selected for presentation as it both constitutes a landmark in medical history and is less controversial than the later editions."

Being a Organon teacher for nearly 50 years in the oldest existing homoeopathic college of world, I had referred to Wheelers translation of 1st edition on many occasions. I found shortcomings in his translation which I jotted down in my personal copy.

It must be clearly understood that the intention is not to undermine Dr. Wheeler's contribution. In fact his work – *Knaves or Fools?* is the book from which we refer frequently before teachers, students and in presentations. This work of Wheeler is compulsory for all newcomers to homoeopathy and for those who are in double mind about homoeopathy.

In the critical analysis of Wheeler's translation of 1st edition, I am aware of my responsibility and the scientific spirit and I

hope that one day my work will also have the honour to be read so seriously and scrutinized in the same spirit. In words of our medical prophet *'my vanity does not go far'*.

Here I give details of sturucture of translation given be Dr. C.E. Wheeler.

ORGANON OF MEDICINE
First Edition
English translation
By Dr. C.E. Wheeler

Title : Organon of the Rational Art of Healing

Year of Publication : 1913 (March 13)

Publisher : The Homoeopathic Publishing Co. Ltd., 24 st., George Street, Hanover Square: London (W)

Reprint : Its copy for Everyman's *Library* edited by Ernest Rhys was published by J.M. Dent. & Sons Ltd.; London and by E.P. Dutton & Co., New York. The contents remained exactly same. (But there was a Reprint in or after 1945 as can be seen from a footnote of 13 lines on p. XXIII which says 'In this year of Grace (1945) the profession abounds in enthusiasm for the ....). Year of publication not mentioned.

a. *Contents :* p. VII

b. *Translator's Preface :* pp. IX-X

c. *Introduction :* pp. XI-XXVI

d. *Author's Preface :* Hahnemann's Preface to the First Edition p. XXVII-XXVIII

   Lower half of p. XXVIII - *Translator's note.*

e. *Bibliography :* pp. XXIX - XXX :

   a. Wheeler gives a list of 12 of the writings of S. Hahnemann and its translation.

Part – II
Hahnemann's Essays

A Review

Dr. Wheeler did a good job of providing the English Version of the first edition of the greatest medical classic which divided the medical profession of Europe and then world in the distinct groups from the prevailing and predominant school.

Comments

In his Translator's Preface Dr. Wheeler begins '*The Organon is put forward here as a piece of history rather than as a contribution to polemics. For this reason the original edition of 1810 was selected for presentation, as it both constitutes a land mark in medical history and is less controversial than the later editions.*'

It is surprising that a homoeopath of the height and calibre of Dr. Wheeler could say it.

He says : '........*and is less controversial than the later editions.*' Each

edition of the Organon is an improvement, both in style and content, than its preceding edition. The storm in medical world was unleashed by the first edition of the book and no other edition or publication of Hahnemann brought so instant, such wide and intense reaction in the European World of Medicine as did the first edition of the Organon. It can be said without any fear of being contradicted or qualm of consciousness that the first edition started the biggest controversy and divide in the medical profession.

Secondly the so called controversy came, when Hahnemann propounded his Theory of Chronic Diseases and Chronic Miasms (incorporated in 4th edition, 1829 of Organon of Medicine) and when his Theory of Potentization and Vital Force was published (in the 5th edition of Organon of Medicine printed in 1833).

Even if it is assumed that later editions of the Organon were controversial, why a confirmed and convinced homoeopath like Dr. C.E. Wheeler should worry and use it as an execuse by explanation for the publication.

Dr. C.E. Wheeler's *Introduction* of (pp – xi – xxvi) of 12 lengthy paragraphs and 2 footnotes deals lightly with Hahnemann, Organon, Vaccination, etc.

Translator's note : Total 16 lines published on the lower part of the page-XXVIII, where Hahnemann's *Preface* to first editions ends.

Dr. Wheeler says *'In the original edition, between the Preface and the body of the work, Hahnemann inserted an introduction, devoted mainly to a record of applications of the homoeopathic law made unconsciously by other physicians and recorded by them. This Introduction is therefore mainly of a technical interest and is here omitted.'*

Comments

1. The example of intentional or unintentional cures by which Wheeler calls '*made unconsciously*' contemporary and ancient

physicians is certified important and dropping it out on the grounds of a technical interest is odd and unacceptable.

Besides, a translator is not the judge to decide what part of a book is to be included and what omitted.

Thus, Dr. Wheeler's translation is incomplete by his own admission.

Dr. Wheeler contradicts himself in the very first line of his *Translator's Preface*. He says, '*The Organon is put forward here as a piece of history rather than a contribution to polemics.*' How the aphorisms become a piece of history and Introduction a contribution to polemics? *Polemics* means: *A speech, piece of writing, etc., containing very forceful arguments for or against.* (*Oxford's Advanced Learner's Dictionary*). The first edition of the book that identified homoeopathy as a separate school of medical can not be anything other than a polemic.

2. Hahnemann quotes nearly two hundred and fifty instances of unconscious Homoeopathy, most of them not isolated cases but records of repeated experiences, and support them by the evidence of no fewer than four hundred and forty physicians mentioned by name, with a reference to the source from which each opinion is derived.

   a. It is not a correct statement. Dr. Dudgeon in reference to paragraph-83 of *Introduction* (**Boeriske & Tafel, 6ᵗʰ American edition,** 1916); on p. 207 of the APPENDIX in Economic Homoeo Pharmacy print; p. 203 in B. Jain Publishers' print, 1988; p. 159 IBPP print, 2003; p. 190 of Pratap Medical Publishers print, p. 183, wrote -

   'In the first edition very few references to the source of these cases are given, but they are mostly carefully indicated by footnotes in the second, third and fourth editions.'

b. The fact is that the **Enleitung** (*Introduction*) of the First edition of Organon of Medicine has 64 paragraph and only one footnote of 4 lines on p. XLIII to paragraph – 57.

Aphorism Section

Hahnemann's First edition has a total of 222 pages, containing 271 aphorisms and 76 footnotes.

In Dr. Wheeler's book the aphorisms occupy 113 pages and contains Translator's Notes under the aphorisms.

1. It itself is a proof that all the footnotes have not been translated.

2. He gives a total of 16 translator's note in Aphorisms.

3. Last sentence of aphorism 36 in Wheeler's translation is actually a separate footnote in Hahnemann's original book.

4. Aphorism 158 totally wrongly translated. Actually it is the aphorism 159 which is given by Wheeler as 158. He did not translate § 158 and printed Hahnemann's § 159 as 158, § 160 as 159 and omitted §160 completely.

5. The reference of aphorism 14 given in bracket is also out of context.

6. No aphorism 160 in Wheeler.

7. Among the footnotes of the aphorisms he translated only a few.

Dr. Mahendra Singh
Dr. Subhas Singh

ORGANON OF MEDICINE
First Edition[1] (1810)

THE PRECURSORS[2] OF ORGANON

1796 : *An Essay on a New Principle for Ascertaining the Curative Powers of Drugs and a Review of the Previous Principles*

[In Hufeland's Journal, vol. ii, parts 3 – 4, pp. 391-439 & 465-561]

Dr. Denis Demarque [in Chronological Biography of Hahnemann in **The Hahnemannian Gleanings**, Sept., 1977] translated the title as: **Essay on a New Principle for Discovering the Curative Values of** *Medicinal Substances Followed by Some Opinions on the Principles Accepted upto our Time.*

[1.] The present chronology in view of the time of publication of the 1st edition is only a concise form of a larger and complete chronology included in **Organon of Medicine**, 6th & 5th editions, Corrected, Retranslated & Redacted by Drs. Mahendra Singh & Subhas Singh, published by M/s Homoeopathic Publications, Kolkata-9.

[2.] Although R. E. Dudgeon in his Translator's Preface to the Fifth Edition of the Organon names Hahnemann's **Essay on a New Principle.......** and **Medicine of Experience** as the *Precursor of Organon of Medicine* but after the publication of An Essay.......(1796) and before the publication of **The Organon** (1810), Hahnemann's following 12 articles related to Homoeopathy and his arguments in favour of Homoeopathy were published:

: **Richard Haehl** (S. Hahnemann: Life & Work, vol. i, p. 65, vol. ii, p. 513) uses the word **'some examinations'** in place of **'Review'**.

1806 : *Medicine of Experience*

Reprinted in Hufeland's Journal, vol., 22, part 3, pp. 5 – 99.

1. 1797: Are the Obstacles to the Attainment of Simplicity and Certainty in the Practice of Medicine insurmountable? [Hufeland's Journal, vol. 4, part 4. Its English translation in British Journal of Homoeopathy, vol. 2, p. 172].

2. 1800: A Preface to the Thesaurus Medicaminum.

3. 1801: Observations on the Three Current Methods of Treatment.

   (in Hufeland's Journal, vol. ii, part 4).

4. An Essay on Small Doses of Medicine and of Belladonna in Particular.

   (in Hufeland's Journal, vol. 13, part 2, January 1801)

5. View of the Professional Liberality at the Commencement of the Nineteenth Century (in Allgemeine Reichs Anzeiger, no. 32).

6. 1805: Preface to Fragmenta de Viribus Medicamentorum Positivis Sive in Sano Corpore Humano Observatis, pp. 269 & 470.

7. Aesculapius in Balance, Dresden, M/s Arnold, pp. 70.

8. 1806: What are Poisons? What are Medicine?[1]

   (in Hufeland's Journal, vol. 17, part- 3, old series, vol. 24).

   This writing is not available in Hahnemann's The Lesser Writings. Its First Indian print in book form edited by Dr. Mahendra Singh, published by M/s Homoeopathic Publications, Kolkata-9

9. 1808: Extract from a Letter to a Physician of High Standing on the great Necessity of a Regeneration of Medicine.

(in Allegemeine Anzeiger d. Deustschland, no. 343).

10. On the Value of Speculative Systems of Medicine, especially as viewed in Connection with the Usual Methods of Practice with which they have been Associated. [in Allgemeine Reichs-Anzeiger d. D., p. 263; 2nd English translation in British Journal of Homoeopathy, vol. 2, p. 233 & American Journal of Homoeopathy, February, 1835].

11. Indication of the Homoeopathic Employment of Medicines in Ordinary Practice.[2] (in Hufeland's Journal, vol. 26, part 2). It appeared as The Introduction to the First, Second & Third Editions of the Organon. It is available in short form in Dudgeon's Appendix to the Organon. In this book, it has been corrected, completed and the references to the concerned editions properly marked.

2. 1809: Signs of the Times in the Ordinary System of Medicine.

(in Allgemeine Arzeiger d. Deutschland, no. 326)

: **R. Haehl** (S. Hahnemann: Life & Work, vol. i, p.74) translates it as: *The Therapy of Experience.*

: **Denis Demarque** translates it as: *Experimental Medicine.*

: **T.L. Bradford** (Bibliography, p. 113) translated it as: *A New System of Medicine Based on Experience.*

: These two writings are available in:

E. Stapf 's *Kleine Medicinische Schriften* published by, M/s *Arnold*, 1829, Dresden & Leipsic, 2 vols, pp. 250 & 284.

: *Its English translation* by *Dr. R.E. Dudgeon*:

: **1843** : British Journal of Homoeopathy,Vol.,1, p. 330.

: **1851** : The Lesser Writings of Samuel Hahnemann, published by M/s Headlands, London, 8 vol., pp. 881.

Reprints by :

: M/s Swaran Publishing House, New Delhi, pp. 438-476

: M/s B. Jain Publishers, New Delhi, pp. 438 – 476.

: **Second German Edition** in book form, pp. 75, published by M/s Karl F. Haug Verlag, Heidelberg, Germany.

: **First Indian print & Re-translation in book form** 2003 by Dr. Mahendra Singh

: **Index** to **Medicine of Experience**: Dr. Mahendra Singh. Published by Homoeopathic Publications, Kolkata-9.

Background

Dr. Samuel Hahnemann, born in a poor family, in a very small town, at the young age of 21 years, knew 7 languages in which he could translate. He passed his M. D. from Erlangen University on 10th of August, 1779, and started practising medicine. The uncertainties of the principles and palliative nature of Allopathy soon frustrated him. He abandoned medical practice and started to earn his livelihood by translating books on medicine and other branches of science.

In 1790, while he was at Sttotteritz, a suburb 4 kilometers south–east of Leipsic, he undertook the translation of **Dr. William**[3]

[3.] **Dr. William Cullen** (1710-1790) was an accepted authority on Materia Medica, an able chemist and an experienced and beloved teacher in Edinburgh, England. The first edition of his work appeared in London in 1773, the second edition in 1789 in 2 volumes was the titled: **A Treatise of the Materia Medica**. Hahnemann used this edition for his translation.

Cullen's *A Treatise of Materia Medica,* in 2 vols. on the request of a publisher.

In the second volume of his book **Dr. Cullen** had devoted 20 pages to the Peruvian bark or Cinchona officinalis or Peruvian bark or Cortex peruvianus, the drug which is commonly called China.

Dr. Cullen explained the curative properties of this medicine in Ague (Intermittent Fever) of which it was and is an allopathic specific. He wrote, "that the bark acts in these cases by means of its strengthening power exerted on the stomach........"

This remark of Cullen appeared to be unscientific and incorrect to Hahnemann and induced him to make experiments upon himself with this remedy. He wanted to find out what effects it would produce on a perfectly healthy person.

To test the veracity of Cullen's remarks he took '4 drachms of good Cinchona bark juice twice daily for several days,' and as a result 'all the symptoms usually associated with Intermittent fever appeared in succession, yet without the actual rigor'. Hahnemann's experiments with the juice of the bark of Cinchona officinalis lead him to the discovery of homoeopathic system of treatment.

HAHNEMANN'S HOMOEOPATHIC WRITINGS BEFORE ORGANON OF MEDICINE

After six years, i.e., in 1796, he published *An Essay on a New Principle for Ascertaining the Curative Powers of Drugs and a Review of the Previous Principles² in Hufeland's Journal of Practical Medicine* (Vol. II, Parts 3, pp. 391-439 & 465-561). About the importance of this writing Dudgeon wrote that it was this Essay 'in which he propounded the Homoeopathic Therapeutic Rule..........."

In 1805, Hahnemann published, in Latin language, the first materia medica compiled on the basis of experiments on human beings. He named it Fragmenta de viribus medicamentorum positivis sive in sano corpore humano observatis. The book was of two volumes. The 1ˢᵗ volume contained the symptomatic Materia Medica of 27 medicines and 2ⁿᵈ volume of 476 pages had an Index or Repertory of the symptoms.

In 1805, Medicine of Experience (Heilkunde der Ehrfahrung), pp. 99, was published in the form of a book by M/s *Wittig,* Berlin. In 1806, it was subsequently published in *Hufeland's Journal* (Vol. 22, Part-3, pp. 5-99). About this book, Dudgeon wrote "In the Medicine of Experience, he enunciated the rule with no such limitations of its applicability. The Essay contains much of what we find in the first and later editions of the Organon. .... both of which essays *[An Essays on a New Principle.............and Medicine of Experience]* may be regarded as the *Precursor of Organon.* "

These two essays were in the form of a continuous writing and the paragraphs were not numbered. These writings were included by **Dr. E. Stapf** in his collection of **S. Hahnemann**'s **Kleine Medicinesche Schriften** published in 1829. This

collection was translated by **R.E. Dudgeon** into English in 1851 as: **S. Hahnemann's** *The Lesser Writings*. In this collection An Essay on a New Principle had 170 paragraphs and 29 footnotes and Medicine of Experience had 176 paragraphs and 47 footnotes.

In 1805, Hahnemann shifted to Torgau, a town 30 miles north–east of Leipsic.

In 1810, was published the book which established homoeopathy as a separate system of treatment, gave the logic of its superiority and the principles and methods of its practice. Hahnemenn named it *Organon der Rationellen Heilkunde*, i.e., Organon of the Rational Art of Healing or *Organon of Rational Medical Science*. This was the first complete book on the logic, philosophy, principles and methods of practice of homoeopathy. It was neither an overnight work nor a book about the thoughts and experiences of an individual.

Richard Haehl says, "In his Essay on a New Principle for Ascertaining the Curative Powers of Drugs......, he had merely shown the external frame work, or, shall we say, the corner stone of his convictions. In his Fragmenta de viribus medicamentorum .... he had collated a number of experimental proving of medicines. In his Medicine of Experience and in the smaller and larger treatises just mentioned he had carried his investigations further. But in his Organon this organically constructed work on rational healing or on the healing art in general, he brought all this to completion."

Hahnemann gives his explanations in the *Preface* of the book. He says, "I count it to my credit, that, in recent days, I have been alone in subjecting it (i.e. the practice of medical art) to a serious impartial investigation, and that I have laid before the world in signed or anonymous publications the convictions which have resulted therefrom.

Through this enquiry I found the road to truth, upon which I have to tread alone, a road far removed from the common highway of medical routine. The further I advanced from truth to truth the further did my conclusions move from that ancient structure, which, having been built out of opinion, was upheld only by opinions, although I allowed no single one of my conclusions to stand unless fully confirmed by experiment. The results of these convictions are stated in this book."

Title or Name of the Book

Dr. Samuel Hahnemann, the great medical thinker, translator, research scholar, master of languages and an authority on the ancient history of European Medicine named his great work, Organon der Rationellen Heilkunde. This word *Organon* has originated from Latin ORGANUM which means: An instrument. A method of scientific investigation. It was used by ancient Greek philosopher *Aristotle*[4] as a title for his treatise on philosophy and then in the 16th century, the renowned philosopher and statesman *Francis Bacon*[5] named the second volume of his work on logic as NOVUM ORGANUM.

---

[4] **ARIISTOTLE** (384-322 B.C.): Aristotle was the son of the physician to king Philip and he was the tutor of Alexander, the great. He was the greatest scientific name after Hippocrates. Aristotle of Stagira in Thrace, Macedonia is 'the master of those who know', who correlated the utility of Botany, Zoology, Comparative Anatomy, Embryology, Teratology and Physiology and the use of formal logic as an instrument of precision to the science of the medicine. His six writings on logic were collected in one volume titled ORGANON, which means, instrument.

[5] **FRANCIS BACON** (1561-1626): He was the younger son of Sir Nicholas Bacon, English statesman, philosopher and scientist. His emphasis on the observation and classification of the natural world, became the basis of the Inductive method in scientific research. His works were Advancement of learning (1605), Novum Organun (1620), De Aigmentis scientiarum (1623), etc. The preliminary write-up of the book had appeared as Cogita et Visa in 1607. Novum Organum translated in English by Ellis and Spedding was published by Routledge, London.

On the cover page of the book, the name Organon der Rationellen Heilkunde was printed, but after a *Voreinnerung* (Foreword) of 4 pages and an *Einleitung* (Introduction) of 44 pages, on p. 1, i.e., the beginning of the text the title was printed as: **Organon der Rationellen Heilkunde nach homoeopathischen Gesetzen** (Organon of Rational Healing Art on Homoeopathic Principles.)

This book was published with the financial help of a grateful patient.

English translations of the title

The original German title of the book was 'Organon der Rationellen Heilkunde' has been translated differently by various authors, translators and commentators but the correct translation can only be: *Organon of Rational Medical Science.*

Richard Hughes (Principles and Practice of Homoeopathy, p. 14) translated it as: Organon of the Rational Medical Science. Hughes says "In my Hahnemannian Lecture, I rendered **Kunde,** by **doctrine.** A consideration of the discussion on the subjects carried on in the **Homoeopathic World** of 1881 suggests that I shall be more closely adhering to the German, while not weakening my argument, if I now translate it as: Science".

Hughes[6] explains further and says "Hahnemann first called

---

6. The long list of CAUSATIONS in **footnote** to **paragraph 29** of **Medicine of Experience** - and in **footnote to aphorism 59 of the First Edition** were omitted in the Second and Third editions. It was an exhaustive list of the causes including pollutions of different kinds that can derange health and cause disease. Similarly, the pages after pages of examples of accidental cures by allopaths through homoeopathic principles in the INTRODUCTION of **First to Fourth** editions of the Organon were dropped by him in the Fifth Edition. The details of the difficulties caused by the local removal of symptoms by local application given in the aphorisms and especially the **footnotes to aphorism 214** of the Third edition were also not included by him in the Fourth edition. The details of Potentization and Dilutions in footnote to aphorism 269 of the Fourth Edition were not improved or enlarged but dropped altogether. There are other examples.

his work *Organon of the Rational Medical Science* (Heilkunde), but from the Second Edition onwards the title was changed to *Organon of the Healing Art* (Heilkunst) - the rational being here, and in all other places of its occurrence, either dropped or replaced by true or genuine (**Wahre**). Why this alteration? The elimination of the term "**rational**" has been supposed to "imply that his followers were required to accept his doctrines as though they were the revelations of a new Gospel, to be received as such, and not to be subject to rational criticism. I cannot think so. To me the clue of it seems to be afforded (and the Preface to the Second Edition bears out my view) by the coincident change from Heilkunde to Heilkunst. The name "science," the epithet "rational", were in continual use for the hypothetical system of the day. The promulgation of his views had arrayed the advocates of all these in bitter opposition against him. Hahnemann was accordingly anxious to make it clear that, in entering the lists of conflict, he came armed with quite other weapons. He was seeking, not the consistency of a theory, but the success of a practical art to him it mattered little whether a thing commanded itself or not to the speculative reason, his one concern was that it should be true."

The word **Medicine** has two meanings. It means a drug or a substance used to cure, palliate or prevent a disease. It also means "A System of treatment". So, the meaning of the title of the book is, Organon of a Rational Healing Art or Organon of Rational System of Medicine.

Year of Publication

It was published in April, 1810, while Hahnemann was at Torgau.

Publisher

This book was published with the financial help of a grateful patient. Its publisher was M/s **Arnoldishen Buchhandlung**, a famous book Publisher of Dresden in Germany.

Title Page

On the first title page the name Organon der Rationellen Heilkunde was published and below it Von Samuel Hahnemann was printed. Then on the lower part of the title page, there were 4 lines from a poem of the renowned German poet **Christian Gellert** (1715-1769) :

Die Wahrheit, die wir alle nothig haben,

Die uns als Menschen gluchlich macht,

Ward von der wisen Hand, die sie uns zugedacht,

Nur leicht verdecht, nicht tief vevgranen.

It has been translated as:

The Truth which human beings do need,

For their survival and welfare,

With a purpose of it being found, not buried deep but lightly covered,

By the Wise Hand that blesses us with care.

Some other authors have translated it as authors:

The Truth we mortals need

Us blest to make and keep,

The All wise slightly covered o'er

But did not bury deep. (Dudgeon)

Truth for which all the eager world is fain,
which makes us happy, lies for evermore
Not buried deep but lightly covered over,
By the wise Hand that destined it for men.

(Marie L. Wheeler)

Truth, which men have sought, and sought in vain,
Their undiscovered treasure, yet has lain
Buried not deep, but just below the ground
By the wise Hand that wished it to be found.

(Dr. Pierre Schimidt)

Hahnemann, in **Medicine of Experience** (1806), had written,

The Sagacious and Benevolent Creator of the Universe has allowed those limitless states (conditions) of the human body different from health, which we call diseases, he simultaneously must have communicated to us a definite method by which we may acquire a knowledge of diseases which will be seen sufficient to help us to use the remedies capable of eradicating them. He must have shown to us an equally definite method we may find out in medicines those properties which does not make them suitable for the cure of diseases—if His intention was not meant to leave his children helpless, or to demand from them what was beyond their power. So this art, so indispensable for suffering humanity, cannot remain concealed in the unreachable depths of indistinct speculation, or be scattered in the limitless empty conjecture; it must be accessible, READILY ACCESSIBLE to us within the scope of our external and internal powers of knowledge.

Contents

The **First Edition** of *Organon of Rational Art of Healing* was published in 1810. It had 2 + XLVIII + 222 + 1, a total of 272 pages consisting of Title pages, a **Preface** of 6 paragraphs in 4 pages, an **Introduction** of XLVIII pages containing 64 paragraphs and 1 footnote, **271** *Aphorisms* and 73 footnotes in p. 1 to p. 222 and a page for Verbesserungen (Errata).

The original book has the following contents:

i. **PREFACE** (Vorerinnerung): It consisted of 4 pages, (p. I to p. IV) and had 6 paragraphs, consisting of a total of 48 lines. It had no date or year mentioned at the end of the Preface.

ii. **INTRODUCTION** (Einleitung): The first edition had an Introduction of 44 pages, from p. V to p. XLVIII. It had *64 paragraphs* and *1 footnote* (attached to paragraph 57). The paragraphs of the *Introduction* were not numbered.

The **Introduction** had 4 chapters. These chapters had no heading or title but the difference between two chapters was indicated by a bigger space in between two paragraphs. The first chapter was from paragraph 1 to paragraph 8, the second from paragraph 9 to paragraph 17, the third from paragraph 18 to 54 and the fourth chapter was from paragraph 55 to 64.

Subject Matter of Introduction:

About the Introduction, Richard Haehl (S. Hahnemann: His life & Work, Vol. 1, p. 80) wrote, "In the smaller first part of the book – the so-called 'Introduction'–he set his newly discovered rules of healing over against the traditional treatments, and accompanied his axioms with numerous examples."

The lengthy *Introduction* of 44 pages contained the example of cures performed, unknowingly, by the practitioners of ancient and contemporary allopathic medicine and in the practice of folk medicine, traditional medicines, etc. Hahnemann quoted the name of the physicians but very occasionally the name and page number of the books, journals on Domestic Medicines etc. By these examples Hahnemann tried to establish that many cures were performed by practitioners of different systems of medicine because in the treatment, accidentally, incidentally or intentionally, the *relationship between the symptoms of the patient and symptoms of medicine (produced on healthy persons) were similar.*

Richard Hughes says,

"Hahnemann, set forth his new doctrine in this writing and quoted many examples of the cures performed or homoeopathic law applied or similar action of the medicines observed by ancient and contemporary medical men. About his discovery, he wrote on page V of the Introduction:

"Hitherto, diseases of man were not healed in a rational way or according to fixed principles, but rather according to very varied curative purpose, amongst others, according to the palliative rule; contraria contrariis curentur. In contrast to this lay the truth, the real way of healing, which I am pointing out in this volume. In order to cure gently, quickly and lastingly, choose in every case of illness a remedy which can itself arouse a similar malady, to that which it is to cure (similia similibus curentur)."

Hitherto nobody has taught this homoeopathic method of healing. But if it is the Truth behind and as the basis of the prescriptions then even if this truth has been disregarded for thousands of years, it is to be expected that traces of its Immortal influence can be discovered in all epochs. And so it is.

Importance of the Introduction :

Richard Hughes explains the importance of Hahnemann's **Introduction** to Organon in the following words:

"If we were going through the **Introduction** in detail, there would be many points on which criticism and correction would be necessary; but the general soundness of its attitude must be sufficient for us to-day. It bears to the body of the work the same relation as Bacon's 'De Augmentis' to his Novum Organum and the treatise on Ancient Medicine to the Aphorisms of Hippocrates."

iii. **APHORISMS** : The main content or substance of homoeopathy is in the aphorisms. This is the main part of the book. The Aphorisms are in 222 pages, from p.1 to p.222.

The first edition had 271 aphorisms and 76 footnotes.

About the aphorisms, **Dr. Hughes** said : "While each aphorism is complete in itself, and might be made the text of a medical discourse, the work they collectively constitute has a definite outline and structure."

Errata

In the end of the book, on page 223, there was an Errata of 5 lines.

Style of Writing :

Hahnemann had two earlier writings on the principles and methods of Homoeopathy. In 1796, he wrote An Essay on a New Principle for Ascertaining the Curative Powers of Drugs and a Review of the Previous Principles. It was published in Hufeland's Journal of Practical Medicine. In 1806, he published his Medicine of Experience. These were written as essays and a continuous writing. But Organon of Medicine was written in a

different style. It is called *aphoristic style*. Here the paragraphs were serially numbered. These numbered paragraphs are known as aphorisms or sections or paragraphs. There was a total of 271 **aphorisms** or sections and 76 *footnotes*. Hahnemann followed this style in all the later editions of the Organon. Because of these serially numbered aphorisms it is easy to discuss, give reference or compare the contents.

About this style of writing followed in the Organon, **Dr. Hughes** wrote, "This is a form of composition eminently suggestive and stimulating. It is endeared to many of us by Coleridge's Aids to Reflection but Hahnemann must have taken it from the Novum Organum, perhaps also with a recollection of the father of medicine which derives its name therefrom."

Footnotes

For footnotes, Hahnamann followed a simple style in First Edition. He added the footnote just underneath the aphorism. The next aphorism began only after the end of the previous aphorism and its footnotes. The letters or types used for the aphorisms were bigger and those for the footnotes were smaller. The footnotes were marked with the letters ANM which is an abbreviation of the German word Anmerung, which means **Annotation** or **Note**.

Subject Matter

It was an enlargement, improvement and addition to the ideas contained in Hahnemann's An Essay on a New Principle ...... (1796) and in Medicine of Experience ......(1806). **In this book :**

i.   Hahnemann explained the demerits of the dissimilar and opposite principles of drug application.

ii. He explained the logic and advantages of homoeopathic principle.

iii. Hahnemann classified diseases according to their clinical characters.

iv. He explained the necessity and method of Human Proving of Drug.

Translations

: **1810: Organon der Rationellen Heilkunde** von **Samuel Hahnemann,** Dresden, 8vo., pp. 222; M/s Arnold.

: **1878:** Review of 50 pages of the first edition, in British journal of Homoeopathy, vol. 36, January, 1878.

: **1913: Ist English translation** by **Dr. C. E. Wheeler,** a noted homoeopath of England as **S. Hahnemann's Organon of the Rational Art of Healing,** Pp. XXX + 109, M/s *The Homoeopathic Publishing Co. Ltd.,* London. There were complaints and dissatisfaction about the errors in translation. He did not translate Hahnemann's Introduction. He translated few footnotes but most of it he did not translate.

: **1927:** Another print of the book by **Everyman's Library** published by M/s *J.M. Dent & Sons, Ltd.,* London and *E.P. Dutton & Co.,* New York.

: **2009: 2nd English translation:** by **Drs. Mahendra Singh & Subhas Singh,** M/s Homoeopathic Publications, Kolkata.

Importance of First Edition

This book : Organon of Rational Medical Science

i.   Established homoeopathy as a completely separate system of treatment, quite different from Allopathy.

ii. It divided the medical practitioners of Germany, Europe and then the whole world into two classes, viz. **The homoeopaths** and **the rest**.

iii. **Wheeler** who had witnessed the publication of so many translations and reprints of the fourth and fifth editions, went back and translated the first edition in 1917 because there was always a demand by English reading people for the English version of the first, second, third and fourth editions especially the First edition, because of the storm in the medical world unleashed by the First edition and the tirade against Hahnemann and Homoeopathy which began only two months after its publication. The venom against Homoeopathy was poured in the July issue of **Heinroth's** monthly journal named *'Anti-Oranon'*. What a name to express the hatred, hostility and enmity!

iv. **Wheeler** wrote, "This is put here as a piece of history rather than as a contribution to polemics. For this reason the original edition of 1810 was selected as it both constitutes a landmark in medical history and is less controversial than the later editions".

v.   Hahnemann kept on improving the exactitude of language and adding new theories and principles for practice of homoeopathy in every edition. The fifth edition has been claimed and accepted by all as the most perfect of all

editions. But many important things and ideas published in different editions were dropped[6] in later editions.

vi. The persons interested in the literary research or standardization of homoeopathic principles, uniformity and cohesion of all the principles of homoeopathy and in the study of Evolution of Homoeopathy are not able to make desired progress because the English translations of the Organon from first edition to the fourth edition are not available.

vii. For the proper assessment and understanding of Homoeopathy, its logic, its gradual development and evolution, the reading and understanding of the First edition is essential. To properly understand and, to some extent, for evaluating the authority and the strength of its initiator and its author, Dr. Hahnemann, First edition of Organon of Medicine has no alternative. It is the solid foundation formed with future areas of research defined with glimpses of the contemporary practice of Medicine.

Thus, although Fifth and Sixth Editions of the Organon are the text books and last editions of the Great Master, but the First edition of the Organon has its own importance for understanding Hannemann's Homoeopathy, its development, its evolution, its different aspects and Hahnemann's hard work and views on many topics.

---

6. The long list of CAUSATIONS in **footnote** to **paragraph 29** of **Medicine of Experience** - and in **footnote to aphorism 59 of the First Edition** were omitted in the Second and Third editions. It was an exhaustive list of the causes including pollutions of different kinds that can derange health and cause disease. Similarly, the pages after pages of examples of accidental cures by allopaths through homoeopathic principles in the INTRODUCTION of **First to Fourth** editions of the Organon were dropped by him in the Fifth Edition. The details of the difficulties caused by the local removal of symptoms by local application given in the aphorisms and especially the **footnotes to aphorism 214** of the Third edition were also not included by him in the Fourth edition. The details of Potentization and Dilutions in footnote to aphorism 269 of the Fourth Edition were not improved or enlarged but dropped altogether. There are other examples.

Organon of Medicine: FIRST EDITION: *The Frame*

Year of Publication	Title	Preface	Text	Introduction	Aphorisms
• The First edition was *published in 1810.* • Hahnemann was at **orgau.** • He was *55 years old.*	• Its title was: **Organon der Rationellen Heilkunde** (*Organon of Rational Healing Art* or *Art of Healing*). • On the cover page, a stanza of 4 lines from the German poet Christian Gellert (1715-1769) was quoted. • Another title: **Organon of Rational Healing Art according to Homoeopathic principles** was printed on page 1 (from where the aphorisms starts), after the end of Introduction on p. XLVIII	Its *Preface* had 4 pages, from p. I to IV, consisting of 6 paragraphs and a total of 48 lines.	It nad no **INHALT,** i.e. *Content* or *Text*	• First edition had an **Introduction** of 43 pages, from p. V to XLVII. • It consisted of 64 paragraphs and 1 *footnote* (to paragraph 57). • The paragraphs were not numbered. It was a continuous writing. • It contained the examples of unintentional cures on the basis of homoeopathic principles by prominent physicians. This writing had appeared as an article (in Hufeland's Journal, Vol. 26, Part 2, pp. 5 – 43; titled *Indication of the Homoeopathic Employment of Medicines in Ordinary Practice.*	• The **Aphorisms** occupied, 222 pages, i.e. from p. 1 to p. 222. • The **Aphorisms** were numbered. There were 271 aphorisms and 76 footnotes. • The footnotes were not numbered. They appeared not at the bottom of the page but just at the end of the aphorism and were denoted by *ANM,* which stands for *Anmerkung* which means *note, footnote or remark.*

FIRST EDITION : The Frame

Novelties in First Edition	Comparison with the Preceding writing	Translations
• Its *Introduction* contained 42 pages of examples of unintentional or accidental application of drugs on homoeopathic principles by ancient or contemporary allopathic physicians. • The Antipathic axiom **Contraria Contrariis** given in paragraph 47 of his *An Essay on a New Principle* was given in complete as: **Contraria Contrariis Curentur** in paragraph 1 of the **Introduction** of this edition. The homoeopathic axiom used by Hahnemann in paragraph 64 of his *Essay on a New Principle* as **Similia Similibus** was made complete as **Similia Similibus Curentur** in paragraph 2 of the **Introduction** of the First Edition of the Organon.	• Its preceding writing was *Medicine of Experience* (1805). • The first edition retained some portion of *Medicine of Experience* but this was an essay type of writing without number of paragraphs while Organon had numbered aphorisms. Some portions of *Medicine of Experience* remain important even to-day, such as footnote no.1 to paragraph no. 29. Hahnemann's prevision about the hazards of pollution, adulteration, fast food, occupation, etc. are summed up in this footnote. A part of it only has been retained in §§ 223 - 226 of 1st, § 285 of 2nd & 3rd, § 261 of 4th and § 261 of 5th-6th editions	• Its **First English translation** was done by **Dr. C.E. Wheeler** in 1917 and published from London. Two different prints of this translation were published. This is the Second *English Translation first COMPLETE ranslation* of First Edition done by **Dr. Mahendra Singh & Dr. Subhas Singh** of Kolkata – 9 (India) in 2009. The errors in Wheeler's translation and editing have been corrected in this edition.

PREFACE

Preface in the original German edition was of 4 pages (from p. I to p. IV), had 6 paragraphs, consisting of a total of 48 lines. No date or year was mentioned at the end of the Preface.

Vorerinnerung.

Kein Geschäft ist nach dem Geständnis-
se aller Zeitalter einmüthiger für eine Vermuthungskunst (ars conjecturalis) erklärt
worden, als die Arzneikunst; keine k...
sich daher einer prüfenden Untersuchung,
ob sie Grund habe, weniger entziehen,
als sie, auf welcher das theuerste Gut

Preface

1. All the generations have unanimously admitted and explained that the art of medicine and no other trade can be the art of speculation (conjecture) (*ars conjecturalis*); consequently it has least ground to refuse an investigation to test whether it is well founded than it (art of medicine), on which man's prime possession on earth, his health, depends.

im Erdenleben, Menschengesundheit sich stützt.

Ich rechne mirs zur Ehre, in neuern Zeiten der einzige gewesen zu seyn, welcher eine ernstliche, redliche Revision derselben angestellt, und die Folgen seiner Ueberzeugung theils in namenlosen, theils in namentlichen Schriften dem Auge der Welt vorgelegt hat.

Bei diesen Untersuchungen fand ich den Weg zur Wahrheit, den ich allein gehen mußte, sehr weit von der allgemeinen Heerstraße der ärztlichen Observanz abgelegen. Je weiter ich von Wahrheit zu Wahrheit vorschritt, destomehr entfernten sich meine Sätze, deren keinen ich ohne Erfahrungsüberzeugung gelten ließ, von

2. I reckon, honour goes to me in these recent innovative times, I am the only one subjecting the same to an earnest and honest revision and have submitted before the eyes of the world, in named or in unnamed (anonymous) writings, the beliefs which have resulted subsequently

3. During this investigation I found the way to the truth on which I must walk alone, very remote from the usual highway of medical routine. The further I advanced from truth to truth, the further did my impressions move from that old architecture which, having a conceptual whole built out of opinion, is now only maintained by opinion, although I allowed no single one of my impressions to stand unless fully confirmed by practical knowledge.

dem alten Gebäude, was aus Meinungen
zusammengesetzt, sich nur noch durch
Meinungen erhielt.

Die Resultate meiner Ueberzeugungen
liegen in diesem Buche.

Es wird sich zeigen, ob Aerzte, die
es redlich mit ihrem Gewissen und der
Menschheit meinen, nun noch ferner dem
heillosen Gewebe der Vermuthungen und
Willkürlichkeiten anhangen, oder der heil-
bringenden Wahrheit die Augen öfnen
können.

Soviel warne ich im Voraus, dafs Indolenz, Gemächlichkeit und Starrsinn vom
Dienste am Altare der Wahrheit ausschliefst, und nur Unbefangenheit und
unermüdeter Eifer zur heiligsten aller

4. The results of my impressions are stated in this book.

5. It is to be proved whether physicians, who mean to act honestly with their conscience and feel for humanity, will continue to be further affixed with the unholy web of presumptions and arbitrariness, or be able to open their eyes to the salutary truth.

6. *I must warn beforehand* that indolence, leisureliness and stubbornness make effective service at the altar of truth

menschlichen Arbeiten fähigt, zur Ausübung der wahren Heilkunde. Der Heilkünstler in diesem Geiste aber schliefst sich
unmittelbar an die Gottheit, an den Wel-
tenschöpfer an, dessen Menschen er erhalten hilft, und dessen Beifall sein Herz
dreimahl beseligt.

impossible, and only from impartiality and untiring zeal, one can qualify for the holiest of all human tasks, the practice of the true system of healing. The physician who enters on his work in this spirit becomes immediately assimilated to the Deity, whose human creatures he helps to preserve, and whose acclamation renders his soul thrice blessed.

Samuel Hahnemann

INTRODUCTION

The Introduction to the First Edition had appeared as an article (in Hufeland's Journal, vol. 26, part 2, pp. 5 to 43 titled *Indication of the Homoeopathic Employment of Medicines in Ordinary Practice.*

The **Introduction** (*Einleitung*) in the First Edition began on p. V and ended on p. XLVII. **It had 64 paragraphs** and **1 footnote** (attached to paragraph 57). It was a continuous writing and the paragraphs were not numbered and had no division of the chapters.

The references of the article, book, journal or its year of publication were very few and incomplete. Hahnemann set forth his new doctrine in this writing and quoted many examples of the cures performed by application of Homoeopathic law or similar action of the medicines observed by ancient and contemporary medical men.

About the content of this Introduction, **Richard Haehl** in *S. Hahnemann: His life & Work,* vol. 1, wrote, *"In the smaller first part of the book – the so-called "Introduction" – he set his newly discovered rules of healing over and against the traditional treatments, and accompanied his axioms with numerous examples."*

About the importance of Introduction, **Richard Hughes** in *The Principles & Practice of Homoeopathy* says: *"It bears to the body of the work the same relation as **Bacon's De Augmentis** to his **Novum Organum** and the treatise on **Ancient Medicine** to the **Aphorisms of Hippocrates**."*

Einleitung.

Man kurirte bisher die Krankheiten der Menschen nicht rationell, nicht nach feststehenden Gründen, sondern nach sehr verschiednen Heilzwecken, unter andern auch nach der palliativen Regel: contraria contrariis curentur.

Im Gegentheile hievon lag die Wahrheit, der ächte Heilweg, zu welchem ich in diesem Werke die Anleitung gebe: wähle, um sanft, schnell und dauerhaft zu heilen, in jedem Krankheitsfalle eine Arznei, welche ein ähnliches Leiden (ὅμοιος πάθος) vor sich erregen kann, als sie heilen soll (similia similibus curentur)! Diesen homœopathischen Heilweg lehrte bisher niemand. Ist es aber die Wahrheit, die diesen Weg vorschreibt, so läfst sich erwarten, dafs

INTRODUCTION[1]

1. Upto now, the diseases of human beings were treated not in a *rational way,* nor according to fixed principles, but according to many means and with different therapeutic purposes, and among them according to the palliative rule: *contraria contrariis curentur*[2].

2. The truth stands exactly opposite to this, the real path to healing, for which I am giving the guidelines in this work. To cure truly and mildly, permanently and rapidly, it is essential to select, in every case of disease, a medicine which can of itself produce an affection *similar* (μὅιυ πχθοσ) to that which it intends to cure *(similia similibus curentur*[3]*)!* Till now no one has ever taught this homoeopathic method of healing. But if it is the Truth which is guiding this method, then even if it has been neglected for thousands of years, it

---

[1] **Translator's note:** This writing was published in *Hufeland's Journal der Praktischen Arzneikunde (Journal of Practical Medicine),* commonly called *Hufeland's Journal, vol. 26, part 2, pp.* 5-43 under the title of *Indications of the Homoeopathic Employment of Medicines in Ordinary Practice.* It was first published in 1807 (vide Clarke's Homoeopathy Explained, p.-28, 29) and interestingly, it was the first article of Hahnemann in whose title he has used the word – Homoeopathy. This writing was subsequently reprinted with little alteration as **Introduction** to the *First Edition* (1810), then enlarged, modified and printed as **Introduction** to the *Second Edition* (1819), *Third Edition* (1824) and *Fourth Edition* (1829) of Organon of Medicine.

[2] **Translator's note:** Let opposites be cured by opposites.

[3] **Translator's note:** Let similars be cured by similar.

gesetzt sie wäre auch Jahrtausende nicht geachtet worden, sich dennoch Spuren von ihr, der Unsterblichen, in allen Zeitaltern werden auffinden lassen. Und so ist es auch. (In allen Zeitaltern sind die Kranken, welche wirklich, schnell, dauerhaft und sichtbar durch Arzneien, — nicht durch ein grofses andres Ereignifs, nicht durch den Selbstverlauf der akuten Krankheit, nicht durch die Länge der Zeit, nicht durch das allmählige Uebergewicht der Energie des Körpers, u. s. w. gesünd wurden, blos durch die homöopathische Wirkung eines Arzneimittels genesen, obgleich ohne Wissen des Arztes.)

Selbst bei den (— seltnen —) wirklichen Heilungen mit vielerlei zusammen gemischten Arzneien, findet man hie und da, dafs das stark vorwirkende Mittel von der homöopathischen Art war.

Doch noch auffallend überzeugender findet man diefs, wo die Aerzte, wider die Observanz, zuweilen mit einem einfachen Mittel die Heilung schnell zu Stande brachten. Da siehet man, zum Erstaunen, dafs es durch eine Arznei (nach Art der in die-

should be expected that traces of its immortal influence can be discovered in all epochs. And so it is. In all ages, the patients *who were cured truly, rapidly, permanently and definitely by medicines, and they did not recover* only due to some important factor, or because the acute disease had finished its course, or were cured simply because of the length of the time or because the energy of the organism which gradually attained supremacy, and so on but the health were recovered, only by means of the homoeopathic action of a remedy which possessed the power of producing a similar morbid state, although without the knowledge of the physicians.

3. Even in true cures (rarely), here and there, by means of *mixtures of medicines* it will be found that the remedy whose action was predominating over other medicines was always of a homoeopathic nature.

4. But this fact is observed, much more clearly in those cases where physicians sometimes performed a rapid cure with one simple medicine in the form of a prescription. With surprise we see that this always occurred by means of a medicine that in *itself* was capable of producing an affection similar to the case of disease though the physician did not know what he was doing, and acted, forgetting the opposite teaching of his own school.

I shall give some examples here :-

sem Werke vorgetragenen homöopathischen Heilgesetze) geschah, die geeignet war, ein ähnliches Leiden zu erzeugen; ob sie gleich was sie da thaten, selbst nicht wußten, und es in einem Anfalle von Vergessenheit der gegentheiligen Lehren ihrer Schule thaten.)

Hier einige Beispiele:

Schon *Hippocrates* heilte (*hodaxuris*, lib. 4.) die *Cholera*, die sich durch nichts stillen lassen wollte, einzig durch Weiss-nieswurzel, welche doch vor sich Cholera erregt, wie *Forestus, Lentilius, Rei-mann, Ettmüller* und mehrere Andre sahen.

Das englische *Schweissfieber*, was im Jahre 1485 zuerst erschien, und anfänglich, wie *Willis* versichert, von 100 Personen 99 tödtete, konnte nicht eher gebändigt werden, bis man den Kranken *Schweiss* erregende Mittel zu geben lernte. Von der Zeit an starben nur Wenige, wie *Sennert* bemerkt.

Darmsaiten in die gesunde Harnröhre gelegt, erregen allemal einen *Schleimab-fluss*; und eben deshalb heilen sie so oft alte *Nachtripper*.

5. Hippocrates *(επιδημιων*[4], lib. 4*)* mentions a case of *cholera* which did not respond to any remedy, but which he cured by means of *Veratrum album*[5] (**Translator's note:** the German common name as used by Hahnemann is *Weifsnieswurzel*) alone, which, however, itself produces *cholera*, as was seen by **Forestus, Lentilius, Reimann, Ettmüller** and many others.

6. The English *sweating sickness*[6], which first appeared in the year 1485, and which, was a greater killer than the *Plague* itself, killed at its beginning, as **Willis** observed, 99 patients out of every 100, could not be controlled until physicians learned to administer *sudorifics*[7] to their patients. After that time, according to the observations of **Sennert** few persons died of it.

7. There is always increased discharge of mucus caused by the introduction of Catgut[8] bougies[9] in urethra of healthy persons and it is because of this reason that it often cures old gleet[10].

---

[4] **Translator's note:** *The Epidemics*, a writing of Hippocrates.

[5] **Translator's note:** Hahnemann, sometimes, used German common names of medicines for plants and chemicals. Dudgeon and other translators of Hahnemann's works have wisely used the English Common names but we have included the German name considering the fact that Common names are often mistranslated.

[6] **Translator's note:** Interestingly, Hahnemann uses the German word *Schweifs* with this spelling which means 'trail, to wander' where as the correct spelling should have been *Schweiß* which means sweating or perspiration.

[7] **Translator's note:** *Sudorific* - A drug or other agent that causes sweating.

[8] **Translator's note:** *Catgut* - An absorbable surgical suture material made from the collagenous fibers of the submucosa of certain animals, usually from sheep or cows; misnamed catgut.

[9] **Translator's note:** *Bougie* - A hollow or solid cylindrical instrument, usually somewhat flexible and yielding, used for calibrating or dilating constricted areas in tubular organs, such as the urethra or esophagus; sometimes containing a medication for locaapplication.

[10] **Translator's note:** *Gleet* - A discharge of purulent mucus from the penis or vagina resulting from chronic gonorrhoea.

Ein jahrelanger, den Tod drohender *Bauchfluß*, wo alle andre Arzneien ganz ohne Erfolg waren, ward, wie *Fischer* zu seiner (nicht meiner) Verwunderung wahrnahm, von einem ungelehrten Kurirer mit einem *Purgirmittel* schnell und dauerhaft gehoben.

Murray, statt aller andern Zeugen, und die tägliche Erfahrung zählt unter die Symptomen, welche der Gebrauch des *Tabaks* hervorbringt, vorzüglich *Schwindel*, *Uebelkeit* und *Aengstlichkeit*. Und gerade *Schwindel*, *Uebelkeit* und *Aengstlichkeit* waren es, von denen sich *Diemerbrock* durch Tabakrauchen befreite, wenn er unter der ärztlichen Behandlung der epidemischen Krankheiten in Holland von diesen Beschwerden befallen ward. — *Chomel*, *Grant* und *Marriguet* sahen vom starken Gebrauche des Tabaks Konvulsionen entstehen, und lange vor ihnen hatte *Zacutus* der Portugiese in dem aus dem Safte des Tabakskrautes bereiteten Sirupe ein sehr heilbringendes Mittel in vielen Fällen von Epilepsie gefunden.

8. A case of *diarrhoea* which had continued for many years and in which death of the patient appeared to be inevitable, and for which different medicines were used but without success, was, to the great surprise of **Fischer**, (but not mine) cured in a rapid and lasting manner by a *purgative*[11] medicine administered by an ill-educated medical quack.

9. Murray (whom I am quoting out of many other authorities) lets us know, and so also does our daily experience that the chief symptoms among the symptoms produced by the use of *tobacco,* are: *vertigo, nausea* and *anxiety*. Now **Diemerbroek**, when attacked with those very symptoms of *vertigo, nausea and anxiety* during his medical treatment of epidemic diseases in Holland, got rid of it by smoking *tobacco*. **Chomel**, **Grant** and **Marrigues** observed that the excessive smoking of *tobacco* produced *convulsions;* but long before them **Zacutus, the Portuguese**, discovered a salutary blessings in the form of a syrup prepared from the juice of *tobacco* to be a very beneficial remedy in several patients of epilepsy.

---

[11] **Translator's note:** *Purgative* – A drug or other substance that causes evacuation of the bowels.

Die schädlichen Wirkungen, welche
einige Schriftsteller, und unter ihnen *Georgi* vom Genusse des Fliegenschwammes bei den Kamtschadalen anmerken,
Zittern, Konvulsionen, Fallsucht,
wurden wohlthätig unter den Händen
Whistling's, der sich des Fliegenschwammes
mit Erfolge gegen *Konvulsionen mit Zittern* begleitet, und unter *Bernhardt's* Händen, der sich desselben hülfreich in *Fallsuchten* bediente.

Die bei *Murray* zu findende Wahrnehmung, daß Anies - Oel von Purganzen
erregtes *Leibweh* stillt, setzt uns nicht in
Verwunderung, wenn wir wissen, daß *J.
B. Albrecht Magenschmerzen* und *P.
Forest* heftige *Koliken* vom Anies - Oele beobachtet hatten.

Wenn *Fr. Hoffmann* die Schafgarbe
in mehrern *Blutflüssen* rühmte, *Stahl,
Buchwald,* und *Löseke* sie im übermäßigen
Flusse der Goldader sehr dienlich fanden, die *Breslauer Sammlungen* Heilungen
des *Blutspeiens* durch Schafgarbe anführen, und *Thomasius* bei *Haller* sie mit Glück
in *Mutterblutflüssen* anwendete, so be-

10. Georgi, among many other authors, attributed the harmful effects consisting of *tremors, convulsions* and *epilepsy,* to the use of the *toad-stool* (**Translator's note:** the German common name of *Agaricus muscarius* as used by Hahnemann is *Fliegenschwammes*) by the inhabitants of Kamtschadalen[12], yet it acted as a remedy in the hands of **Whistling,** who successfully used this *mushroom* in cases of *convulsions accompanied with tremor,* similarly **Bernhardt** used it with success in a type of *epilepsy.*

11. Murray's observation that the *oil of anise-seed* (**Translator's note:** the German common name as used by Hahnemann is *Anies-oel*) relieves *pains in the stomach* caused by purgatives, is not surprising to us because we find that **J.B. Albrecht**[13] observed *pains in the stomach,* and **P. Forest** found *violent colic* caused by oil of *anise-seed.*

12. Fr. Hoffmann praises the usefulness of *yarrow,* i.e., *Achilea millefolium* (**Translator's note:** the German common name as used by Hahnemann is *schafgarbe*) in different kinds of *haemorrhage,* **Stahl, Buchwald** and **Löseke** find this plant useful in extensive *haemorrhage from haemorrhoidal vein,* the editors of the *Breslauer Sammlungen*[14] talk of its curative effects

---

[12] **Translator's note:** Dudgeon named it Kamtschatka, which is a peninsula of Siberia, situated between the sea of Okhotsk and the Bering Sea and was under Russian dominance since 1706. Its capital was Petropavlovsk. The severe climate did not allow agriculture and a very thin population survived by hunting and fishing.

[13] **Translator's note:** This name (in the *First Edition* and *Second Edition* part II) is J. B. Albrecht whereas in *Second Edition* (Paragraph 10), *Third Edition* (Paragraph 10) and *Fourth Edition* (Paragraph 79) is given as J. P. Albrecht.

[14] **Translator's note:** Breslauer's collections or collected works.

ziehen sich diese Heilungen offenbar auf die ursprüngliche Neigung dieses Krautes, vor sich *Blutflüsse* und *Blutharnen*, wie *Fr. Hoffmann* beobachtete, und eigenthümlich *Nasenbluten* zu erzeugen, wie *Boecler* von demselben wahrnahm.

Scovola, nächst Andern, heilte *schmerzhaften Abgang eiterigen Harns* mit der Bärentraube, welche dieses nicht vermocht hätte, wenn sie nicht vor sich schon *Harnbrennen mit Abgang eines schleimigen Urins* erzeugen könnte, wie wirklich *Sauvages* von der Bärentraube entstehen sah.

Der jezt so sehr vernachlässigte Fleckenschierling hat homöopathisch nicht selten schwierige Krankheiten geheilt, wie die Schriften der besten Aerzte bezeugen. Wenn er nun, wie *Baylies* erfuhr, vor sich *Engbrüstigkeit*, nach *Stoerek verkürztes, keuchendes Athemholen*, nach *Lange heftigen Husten*, abermahl nach *Stoerck* einen *trocknen Husten*, nach einer andern Beobachtung von ihm *sehr gewaltsamen Husten*, und nach noch einer andern, einen *nächtlichen Husten*, nach *Landeutte* aber *Kurzäthmigkeit* und eine

in *haemoptysis,* and, lastly, **Thomasius**, according to **Haller,** used it with success in *uterine haemorrhages,*—these cures are obviously because of the power possessed by this plant to cause *haemorrhages* and *haematuria,* as was observed by **Fr. Hoffmann**, and very particularly in *epistaxis* as observed by **Boecler.**

13. Scovolo, in addition to others, cured a case of *painful discharge of purulent urine* by *bearberry,* i.e., *Arbutus uva ursi* (**Translator's note:** the German common name as used by Hahnemann is *bärentraube*) which never could have happened if the plant did not possess the property of producing *scalding during urination with discharge of slimy urine,* as was actually found by **Sauvages.**

14. The writings of the best physicians are testimony to the frequent homoeopathic cures of many serious diseases by *spotted hemlock,* i.e., *Conium maculatum* (**Translator's note:** the German common name as used by Hahnemann is *fleckenschierling*) which is much neglected now. If it can cause *shortness of breath* (as was observed by **Baylies**), *short and wheezy respiration* (as was observed by **Stoerck**), *violent cough* (as was

Art *nächtlichen Keuchhusten* vor sich
erzeugen kann, so wird es leicht begreiflich, wie er unter *Boulard's* Augen ein
nächtliches Asthma, und bei *Stoerck* einen *konvulsivischen Husten* nach unter-
drückter Krätze, bei *Florentius* einen *har-
näckigen Husten*, und eine Art *Keuchhusten* unter *Butter's*, *Armstrong's*, *Lentin's* und *Ranoe's* Erfahrungen hat glücklich
heilen können. — Die Heilung einer
Harnwinde durch Schierling bei *Stoerck*
wird erklärlich aus der *Strangurie*, welche
Lange und *Ehrhardt* von eben diesem Kraute haben entstehen sehen. — Hat *Stoerck*
einen *schwarzen Staar* damit bezwungen,
so ward diefs durch die natürliche Eigenschaft des Schierlings möglich, vermöge
welcher er (nach *Amatus* dem Portugiesen)
plötzliche Blindheit, (nach *Bayles* und
Andree) *Gesichtsverdunkelung* und
(nach *Gataker*) *Gesichtsschwäche* schon
von selbst zu erzeugen pflegt.

Wenn es auch die vielen Erfahrungen
von *Stoerck*, *Marger*, *Planchon*, *du Monceau*,
F. Ch. Juncker, *Schinz*, *Ehrmann* und Ande-
rer nicht versicherten, dafs die Herbst-

observed by **Lange**), *dry cough, very severe cough* and *nocturnal cough* (as was observed by **Stoerck**) and, *dyspnoea* and a type of *nocturnal whooping cough* (as was observed by **Landeutte**), then it can easily be understood how the same hemlock (by virtue of its homoeopathicity) was able to cure a *nocturnal asthma* (as was observed by **Boulard**), a case of a *convulsive cough produced after suppressed scabies* (as was observed by **Stoerck**), a case of *obstinate cough* (as was observed by **Viventius**), and a kind of *whooping cough* (as was observed by **Butter, Armstrong, Lentin** and **Ranoe**). **Stoerck's** cure of a *dysuria* by *hemlock* is justified by the *strangury* which **Lange** and **Ehrhardt** found it producing. **Stoerck** could cure a case of *amaurosis* (blindness) by *hemlock* because of its power to produce *sudden blindness* (according to **Amatus, the Portuguese)**, *dimness of vision* (according to **Baylies** and **Andree**), and *weakness of sight* (according to **Gatacker**).

15. Although the repeated experiences of **Stoerck, Marges, Planchon, du Monceau, F.Ch. Juncker, Schinz, Ehrmann,** and others had not previously established the truth that *Colchicum autumnale* (**Translator's note:** the German

zeitlose eine Art *Wassersucht* geheilt
habe, so würde diese Kraft schon aus ihrer
Eigenschaft, *verminderte Absonderung*
eines feuerreichen Urins mit stetem
Harndrange vor sich zu erregen (wie
nächst *Stoerck* auch *de Berge* sah) leicht zu
erwarten seyn — Sehr sichtbar aber ist
das von *Göritz* durch die Zeitlose geheilte
hypochondrische Asthma, und die von
Stoerck durch sie gehobene *Engbrüstig-*
keit mit einer *Brustwassersucht* (wie es
schien) verbutten, in der Tendenz dieser
Wurzel, *Schwer-äthmigkeit* und *Asthma*
vor sich hervorzubringen, gegründet, dergleichen *de Berge* von ihr wahrnahm.

Muralto sah was man noch täglich sehen kann, dafs die Ialappe aufser
Bauchweh auch eine *grofse Unruhe* und
Umherwerfen zuwege bringt und, ganz
begreiflich für jeden denkenden Arzt, fliefst
aus dieser ihrer Tendenz, jene wohlthätige
Kraft derselber, kleinen Kindern in *Leib-*
weh, *Unruhe* und *Schreien* oft zu helfen
und ihnen einen ruhigen Schlaf zu ver-
schaffen, wie *G. W. Wedel* ihr mit Recht
nachrühmt.

common name as used by Hahnemann is *herbstzeitlose*) cures a kind of *dropsy*, this quality was expected from it, because of its characteristic peculiarity to *diminish the urinary secretion with constant desire to urinate* and *scanty discharge of fiery red urine (haematuria)*, and *burning during micturition* as was observed by **Stoerck** and **de Berge**. The cure of *hypochondriacal asthma* by **Göritz** by means of *herbstzeitlose* and that of *shortness of breath* complicated with an apparent *hydrothorax* by **Stoerck** with the same plant, were definitely due to the tendency which this root possesses of exciting *dyspnoea* and *asthma*, as was observed by **de Berge**.

16. Muralto has found what we observe every day, that *Jalapa*, *i.e. Exogonium purga* (**Translator's note:** the German common name as used by Hahnemann is *Ialappe*) in addition to causing *stomach-ache*, also produces *great uneasiness and distressing mental restlessness*. **G.W. Wedel** has justly praised this property of *Jalapa*, which every reasonable physician who is familiar with truth on which homoeopathy is based, can easily understand, for by virtue of these beneficial power to help young children affected with *colic, restlessness* and *screaming* it accords them restful sleep.

Bekanntlich (wie auch *Murray*, *Hillary* und *Spielmann* zum Ueberflusse bezeugen) machen die Sens blätter eine Art *Leitschmerzen* und bringen das Blut in *Wallung* (die gewöhnliche Ursache der *Schlaflosigkeit*) und eben dieser ihrer natürlichen Eigenschaft wegen, konnte *Detharding heftige Kolikschmerzen* mit ihnen heben und den Kranken die *unruhigen Nächte* benehmen.

Ganz nahe lag es dem sonst scharfsinnigen *Stoerck*, einzusehen, daſs der beim Gebrauch der Diptamwurzel von ihm selbst bemerkte Nachtheil, zuweilen eine *Leukorrhöe zähen Schleims* mit Blutstriemen vermischt, zu erzeugen, eben die Kraft sei, wodurch er mit dieser Wurzel einen *langwierigen weiſsen Fluſs* bezwang.

Eben so wenig durfte es *Stoerck* auffallen, wenn er mit der Brenn-Waldrebe eine Art langwierigen, feuchten, fressenden, allgemeinen *Krätzausschlags* heilte, da er selbst von diesem Kraute wahrgenommen hatte, daſs es *tratzigt*

17. As everybody knows and also been very strongly testified by **Murray, Hillary** and **Spielmann**), that *Senna leaves, i.e. Senna acutifolia* (**Translator's note:** the German common name as used by Hahnemann is *Sensblätter*) produce a type of *colic,* and cause *flatulence* and *turmoil of the blood* (the usual cause of *sleeplessness*), and because of this natural property *Senna* helped **Detharding** to cure, with its help, sick persons suffering from *violent colicky pain,* and enabled him to relieve them from their *restless nights.*

18. Stoerck, usually an acute observer, might have discovered that the property of *Dictamnus root, i.e. Dictamnus albus* (**Translator's note:** the German common name as used by Hahnemann is *Diptamwurzel*) to cause, sometimes, *leucorrhoea of sticky mucus mixed with streaks of blood from the vagina* was the very same power of this root which helped him to cure a *leucorrhoea of long standing.*

19. Furthermore, **Stoerck** should not have been surprised when he cured a *general, discharging (humid), eroding, scabies-like eruption* of long standing with *Clematis erecta* (**Translator's note:** the German common name as used by Hahnemann is *Brenn-Waldrebe*) because he himself had described that this plant had the power to produce a *pustular scabies like eruption over the whole body.*

Pusteln über den ganzen Körper vor
sich schon erzeugen könne.

Aus eben dem Grunde, aus welchem
von Auflegung der Wolfsmilch blos auf
den Unterleib unter *Scopoli's* Augen *Wassergeschwulst des ganzen Körpers* erfolgte, konnten auch in den ältern Zeiten
eine Menge Aerzte und gemeine Leute eine
Art *Wassersucht* mit Wolfsmilch heilen,
wie *Herrmann* und *Boecler* anführen.

Wenn nach *Murray* die Euphrasie
das *Triefauge* und *Augenentzündung*
geheilet hat, wodurch vermochte sie diefs
sonst, als durch ihre (von *Lobelius, Bonnet*
und *S. Paulli* beobachtete) Eigenschaft, vor
sich schon eine Art *Augenentzündung*
erzeugen zu können?

Nach *Lange's* braunschweigischer Hausmittelpraxis hat sich die Muskatnuss
sehr hülfreich in *hysterischer Ohnmacht*
erwiesen: doch wohl aus keinem natürlichern Grunde, als weil sie in grofser Gabe
(bei *Cullen*) ein *Verschwinden der Sinne*
und *allgemeine Unempfindlichkeit* bei
gesunden Personen zu erregen fähig ist!

20. As was observed by **Scopoli** that only an application of *Euphorbia corollata*. (**Translator's note:** the German common name as used by Hahnemann is *Wolfsmilch*) to the abdomen caused *oedematous swelling of the whole body* which was the reason of a large number of physicians and common persons being able to cure a kind of *dropsy* by the use of *Wolfsmilch*, as was stated by **Herrmann** and **Boecler**.

21. Murray has claimed that *Euphrasia, i.e. Euphrasia officinalis* (**Translator's note:** the German common name as used by Hahnemann is *Euphrasie*) cures *bleary-eyes* and a certain type of *inflammation of eyes*. But how could *Euphrasie* have produced such an effect except by the power it possesses of causing a kind of *inflammation of the eyes* (as was observed by **Lobelius, Bonnet** and **S. Paulli**)?

22. According to **Lange's**[15] in his *Observations in Domestic Practice, Nutmeg, i.e. Nux moschata* (**Translator's note:** the when it is given in large doses (as has been stated by **Cullen**) to healthy persons, it is capable of producing *a loss of the senses and general insensibility*.

Roettler und *Linné* bezeugen, daſs der Faulbeer - Kreuzdorn beim innern Gebrauche eine Art *Wassersucht* heile. Der Grund hievon liegt ganz nahe; *Schwenckfeld* sah durch äuſsere Auflegung der innern Rinde dieses Strauchs von selbst eine Art *Wassersucht* entstehen.

Die uralte Wahl des Rosenwassers zum äuſserlichen Gebrauche bei *Augenentzündungen* scheint stillschweigend eine Heilkraft dieser Blumenblätter in Ophthalmien anzuerkennen. Es könnte aber doch vielleicht nur Aberglaube seyn, wenn sie nicht auch ihrer eigenthümlichen Natur nach die Eigenschaft besäſsen, vor sich eine Art *Augenentzündung* bei gesunden Menschen zu erzeugen; und diese Kraft besitzen sie wirklich, wie *Echtius* und *Leitlius* bezeugen, von ihnen wahrgenommen zu haben.

Wenn der *Rhus radicans* nach *Rossi* geneigt ist, den Körper *allmählig mit Pusteln zu überziehn*, so sieht ein verständiger Mann leicht ein, wie er homöopathisch den *Herpes* bei *Dufresnoy* und *van Mons* heilen konnte

23. Boecler and **Linne** have testified that Ripe-seed of *Buckthorn*, [**Translator's note:** *Buckthorn (Kreuzdorn)* being the common name of *Rhamnus catharticus*, the German common name as used by Hahnemann is *Faulbeer-Kreuzdorn*] when given internally causes a type of *dropsy*. Its reason being most obvious as **Schwenckfeld** observed that a kind of *dropsy* was caused by application of the inner bark of this shrub.

24. The very old practice of applying *rose water of Rosa damascena* (**Translator's note:** the German common name as used by Hahnemann is *Rosenwassers*) externally in *inflammations of eyes* is a tactful acceptance of the healing powers of these (Rose) petals in *ophthalmia*. It is not because of some superstition but only because the rose-petals have a natural property to produce a kind of *inflammation of eyes* in healthy persons and this fact was testified by **Echtius** and **Ledelius**.

25. If the claim of **Rossi** that the *Rhus radicans*[16] (**Translator's note:** the Scientific name of *Poison Sumach*) has

---

[15] **Translator's note:** In the First edition of the Organon this name was given as LANGE but in subsequent editions as **J.H. Lange**.

[16] **Translator's note:** Hahnemann in this paragraph 25 uses the Botanical or Scientific name *Rhus radicans* and also in the next paragraph (Para 26) of this Introduction uses the Scientific name *Rhus toxicodendron*. In the subsequent editions he changed back to German common name *Wurzel-Sumach* and mixed these two paragraphs (25 and 26) into one and published the matter in paragraph 23 of 2nd and 3rd editions and paragraph 24 of IInd part of *Introduction* of 4th edition. Hahnemann probably understood the error. The information about these two medicines is pathetically contradictory and confusing. *Rhus radicans* has been stated as a synonym of *Rhus toxicodendron* in *The Homoeopathic Pharmacopoeia of the United States, 6th (1941), 7th (1964)* and *8th (1979)* editions, in the *Homoeopathic Pharmacopoeia of India, vol. 1, 1971, p. 166, M. Bhattacharya's The Pharmacopoeia, 12th (1962), 13th (1970)* and *14th (1980)*

Was zwingt den *Rhus toxicodendron*, bei *Alderson* und *Darwin*, *Lähmung der untern Gliedmasen mit Verstandesschwäche* begleitet, zu heilen, wenn es nicht die deutlich zu Tage liegende, eigenthümliche Kraft dieses Strauchs thut, *gänzliche Abspannung der Muskelkräfte mit einer zu sterben fürchtenden Verstandesverwirrung* vor sich erzeugen zu können, wie *Zadig* sah?

Hat das Bittersüfs, wie *Haller* bei *Vicat* versichert, *von Verkältung entstandnen Husten* geheilt, so kam es einzig daher, weil es bei feucht kalter Luft vorzüglich geneigt ist, mancherlei *Verkältungsbeschwerden* hervorzubringen, wie *Carrere* und *de Haen* beobachteten. — Ersterer Arzt sah beim Gebrauche des Bittersüfses eine *Rauhheit der Zunge* entstehen, und eben dieser Eigenschaft wegen war es vermögend, *Schrunden der Zunge* zu heilen, wie *Haller* bei *Vicat* anführt. — Dem *Carrere* verdanken wir die Beobachtung, dafs Bittersüfs eine Art *Leucorrhöe* vor sich erregt. Hieraus hätte man schon im voraus schliefsen können, dafs dieses

the power to produce *pustular eruptions which gradually cover the whole body* is correct then a sensible man easily understands why this plant is capable of curing, homoeopathically, many types of *herpes*, as was witnessed by **Dufresnoy** and **van Mons**.

26. What else could have given *Rhus toxicodendron* (**Translator's note:** the Scientific name of *Poison Ivy*) (according to **Alderson** and **Darwin**) the power to cure a *paralysis of the lower limbs* accompanying with *weakness* except its definite power to cause *complete muscular exhaustion, with mental confusion leading to fear of impending death*, which was observed by **Zadig?**

27. The *Bittersweet*, i.e. *Solanum dulcamara* (**Translator's note:** the German common name as used by Hahnemann is *Bittersüß*) assures **Haller**, on the basis of **Vicat**'s, observations that has cured the *most violent cough caused by a chill*, which could not have resulted by any other reason than because this herb, is absolutely capable to produce various *affections like those which arise from a chill*, in cold and damp weather, as **Carrere** and **de Haen** observed. The early physician used *Bittersweet* in *roughness of the tongue* and because of this property **Haller** on the guide-lines given by **Vicat** cured the *fissure of tongue* by its use. It is to the credit of **Carrere** who observed that *Bittersweet* can cause *leucorrhoea*. It helped people to cure *leucorrhoea* with

editions, in *Willmar Schwabe's Pharmacopoeia Homoeopathica Polyglotta, p. 302* and in *Carrol Dunham's Lectures on Homoeopathic Materia Medica, vol. 1, p. 121, Robin Murphy's Homoeopathic Remedy Guide,* IBPP, *First Indian Edition, Nov. 2001, p. 1481,* in *Kent's Final General Repertory, Rev. edition,* New Delhi, *p. xxix,* in *Kent's Repertory of Homoeopathic Materia Medica,* New Delhi, *p. xv.* Strangely, however, in the *American Homoeopathic Dispnesatory, p. 571,* it is both mentioned as a separate medicine as well as the synonym of *Rhus toxicodendron.* However in most of other books, they are mentioned as **2 separate medicines.**

Kraut eine ähnliche Art *Leucorrhöe* mit
Gewißheit heilen müsse; die Bestätigung
aber hievon, daß es dergleichen auch wirklich heile, haben die Erfahrungen von *Rohn*,
Carrere und *Durande* gelehrt. — Vergeblich würde man den innern Grund, warum
gerade Bittersüß so wirksam eine Art
Flechten und *Herpes* (unter den Augen
eines *Carrere*, *Fouquet* und *Poupart*) geheilt
hat, in dem Reiche der Vermuthungen auf-
suchen, da er uns von der einfachen Natur
so nahe gelegt worden ist, nämlich: das
Bittersüß erregt von selbst eine Art *Flechten*, und *Carrere* sah von seinem Gebrauche
einen *Herpes* zwei Wochen hindurch sich
über den ganzen Körper verbreiten, und
bei andrer Gelegenheit *Flechten auf den
Händen* davon entstehen.

Vom Schwarznachtschatten sah
Rucker eine *Geschwulst des ganzen Körpers* entstehen und *Gataker* konnte deshalb
eine Art *Wassersucht* mit diesem Kraute
(homöopathisch) heilen.

Eine andre Art *Wassersucht* konn-
ten *Beerhaave*, *Sydenham* und *Radcliff* mit
Schwarzholder heilen, eben weil, wie

36

certainty and its curative property was confirmed by the experiences of **Rahn, Carrere** and **Durande**. It is of no use searching in the field of hypothesis (or guess or speculation the reason why *Bittersweet* is so effective in a type of *lichen*[17] and *herpes*, as observed by **Carrere, Fouquet** and **Poupart**) since it is shown to us by nature, that *Bittersweet* of itself produce a kind of *lichen*, and **Carrere** observed that the use of this plant caused *herpetic eruption which covered the whole body* for a fortnight; at another time it produced *lichen over the hands*.

28. **Rucker** observed that the *Black Nightshade*, i.e. *Solanum nigrum* (**Translator's note:** the German common name as used by Hahnemann is *Schwarznachtschatten*) produces *swelling of the whole body* and this was the reason that **Gatacker,** with its help, successfully (homoeopathically) cured a type of *dropsy*.

29. **Boerhaave, Sydenham** and **Radcliff** cured another variety of *dropsy* with *Elder*, i.e. *Sambucus nigra*[18] (**Translator's note:** the German common name as used by Hahnemann is *Schwarzholder*) because according to **Haller**'s information, its external application causes *oedema*.

---

[17] **Translator's note:** A flat papule or an aggregate of papules giving a patterned configuration resembling lichens growing on rocks.

[18] **Translator's note:** *Hahnemann* in his *Materia Medica Pura* (*First edition*, p. xvii & Fourth edition, p. 62, para 3, or para 93) uses its *common name* in German language as *Schwarzholder* but its more accurate German name is *Schwarzer Hollunder* (*The Homoeopathic Pharmacopoeia of United States, 1981*, p. 510). In some of the homoeopathic books it is written wrongly as *Sambucus niger*. It should be *Sambucus nigra*.

Haller berichtet, der Schwarzholder schon bei äußerer Auflegung *Oedem* erzeugt.

De Haen, *Sarcone* und *Pringle* huldigten der Wahrheit und Erfahrung, da sie freimüthig gestanden, den *Seitenstich* mit Squille geheilt zu haben, mit einer Wurzel, die das, hier blos schneidigende, abspannende und kühlende Mittel verlangende System ihrer großen Schärfe wegen durchaus widerrathen mußte; er wich dennoch der Squille und zwar nach dem homöopathischen Naturgesetze, indem schon *J. C. Wagner* (obs. cliu. Lub. 1737.) von der freien Wirkung der Meerzwiebel eine Art *Pleuritis* entstehen sah.

Nach. *Gaterau's* Beobachtung hat der Gebrauch des *Taxus* einen *heftigen Husten* verursacht, und blos deshalb konnte er bei *Perry* (Journ. de Med. 1790.) *Husten* heilen.

Die Eigenschaft des **Terbenthin-Oels** (nach *Stedman*), eine *Harnverhaltung*, eine Art *Wassersucht* und *Nierenschmerzen* erzeugen zu können, gab diesem ätherischen Oele die homöopathische Heilkraft, hie und da eine *Wassersucht*,

30. De Haen, Sarcone and **Pringle** paid proper respect to the fact and practical experience by stating openly that they cured *stitching pain on sides of the chest* with *Squill*, i.e. *Scilla maritime* (**Translator's note:** the German common name as used by Hahnemann is *Squille*), a root which, because of its excessive acrid properties, should be forbidden in a disease of this nature, where, according to the present methods, only sedative, relaxing and cooling remedies are permitted. But the disease, mentioned above subsided, due to the effect of *Squill* in accordance with the *homoeopathic law of nature*, as **J.C. Wagner** (*Observationes Clinicae*, Lubeck, 1737[19]) observed a *pleuritis* being caused by the action of the plant.

31. Gaterau observed that the use of *Taxus baccata*[20] (**Translator's note:** the German common name as used by Hahnemann is *Taxus*) produced *severe cough*, and that is why **Perry** (*Journal de Medecine*, 1790[21]) succeeded in curing a *cough* with it.

32. The *Oil of Turpentine, i.e. Terebinthina oleum* (**Translator's note:** the German common name as used by Hahnemann is *Terbenthin-Oels*), according to **Stedman** has the property to cause *strangury*, a type of *dropsy* and *renal colic* and this power has given this ethereal oil the homoeopathic curative

---

[19] **Translator's note:** Clinical Observations, Lubeck, 1737.

[20] **Translator's note:** Hahnemann uses another German common name *Meerzwiebel* in the same paragraph. Hahnemann's use of this name for (European) *Elder* in 1st edition, p. xviii, 2nd edition, p. 42, 3rd edition, p. 12 and in 4th edition, p. 63 is different in the *Homoeopathic Pharmacopoeia of United States*, 1981, p. 516.

[21] **Translator's note:** *Journal of Medicine*, 1790.

und hie und da eine Art *Hüftweh* zu heben, worüber uns *Home*, *Herz*, *Thilenius*, *Cheyne* und Andre die Belege liefern.

Der chinesische Thee ist seiner Natur nach nichts als ein Arzneimittel. Man findet in den Nov. Act. N. C. und bei *Lettsom* *zusammenziehenden Magenkrampf* von Thee erzeugt, auch erwähnt letzterer eines *drückenden Magenschmerzes* davon, eine Tendenz die das Lob, welches *Buchan* dem Thee bei Hebung der *Cardialgie* der Schwangern ertheilt, hinlänglich motivirt. — Nach mehrern Beobachtungen (von *Geoffroy*, von *Tode* und von *James* bei *Lettsom*) hat er nicht selten *Zuckungen* und *Fallsucht* hervorgebracht und in dieser Eigenschaft stillt er die bei Masern und Pocken gewöhnlichen *Konvulsionen* (Eph. N. C. dec. III. a. I. obs. 1618.) —; so wie er auch ein vorzügliches homöopathisches Heilmittel in der *Ermüdung* von Strappazen (*Lettsom*) abgiebt, ebenfalls einzig durch seine, *allgemeine Schwäche* erzeugende Kraft, welche von *Lettsom*, *Whytt* und *Murray* beobachtet worden ist — und eben dahin scheint auch seine von *Lettsom* be-

property of curing some types of *dropsy* and *pain in the legs*, as has been confirmed by **Home, Herz, Thilenius, Cheyne** and others.

33. The *Chinese tea, i.e. Thea chinensis* (**Translator's note:** the German common name as used by Hahnemann is *Chinesische Thee*), in reality is nothing but a natural medicine. We can find this in the *Nov. Act. N. C.* and **Lettsom**'s *cramping spasm of the stomach* produced by *Chinese tea*; **Lettsom** also mentions a *pressive stomach pain* caused by *Chinese tea*, which was sufficient explanation to the reason of the cure of *cardialgia* in a pregnant women by **Buchan**. The innumerable observations (by **von Geoffroy, von Tode** and **von James** in **Lettsom**'s work) prove that it has frequently produced *convulsions* and *epilepsy*, and because of this power it relieves the *convulsions in measles* and *small-pox* (*Eph. N. C. dec. 3, ann. i, obs. 1618*); it is also an important homoeopathic remedy for the *exhaustion caused by over-exertion* (**Lettsom**) which is only due to its power to cause *general weakness*, which was seen by **Lettsom, Whytt** and **Murray**; and its power to cause *sleepiness*, which was observed by **Lettsom**, enables the Chinese people to cure the *sleepiness in diseases* (**Herrmann**).

merkte, *Schläfrigkeit e*... ...n-
schaft zu gehören, vermöge d... ...i-
nesen die *Schlafsucht in Krankheiten*
(*Herrmann*) mit Thee heilen. ⟶

Die durch Viele (*Dan. Crüger, Ray,
Kellner, Kaaw, Boerhave* u. s. w.) vom Ge-
nusse des Stechapfels beobachtete
Wirkung, *wunderliche Phantasien* und
Konvulsionen zu erregen, setzte die Aerz-
te in Stand, die *Dämonie* (monströse
Phantasien in Begleitung von krampfhaften
Gliederbewegungen) mit Stechapfel (Veckoskrift, IV.) zu heilen, — so wie eine von
Quecksilberdampf und eine andre von
Schreck entstandne Art *Veitstanz* von *Si-
drèn* mit diesem Kraute geheilt ward, oder
eigentlich mittelst seiner Eigenschaft, schon
vor sich dergleichen *unwillkührliche
Gliederbewegungen* erzeugen zu können, wie man von *Kaaw, Boerhave* und *Lobstein* beobachtet findet. — Weil auch der
Stechapfel nach vielen Wahrnehmungen
(auch denen von *P. Schenck*) sehr schnell *alle
Besinnung und Rückerinnerung weg-
nimmt*, so ist er auch fähig, *Gedächt-
nissschwäche* (nach *Sauvages* und *Schinz*) zu

34. A large number of practitioners (**Dan. Crüger, Ray, Kellner, Kaaw, Boerhaave** and some others) have observed that *Thornapple, i.e. Datura stramonium* (**Translator's note:** the German common name as used by Hahnemann is *Stechapfels*) produces *peculiar delusions* and *convulsions*. It is exactly this power which helped the physicians to cure, with its help, *daemonia*[22], *monstrous delusions attended with spasmodic movements of the limbs* and other *convulsions* (Veckoskrift, iv)[23]. If through the hands of **Sidren** it cured two cases of *chorea (St. Vitus Dance)*, one of which was *caused by fright* and the other by *Mercurial vapour* (**Translator's note:** *Quecksilberdampf)*, it did so because it (*Thornapple*) had the power of causing similar *involuntary movements of the limbs,* as was found by **Kaaw, Boerhaave** and **Lobstein.** Many observations (made by **P. Schenck,** in additions to others) have shown us that it can destroy *recollection and memory* in a very short time; it can also, (as was observed by **Sauvages** and **Schinz**), cure *weakness of memory.* On the same principle, **Schmalz,** with this plant was able to cure a case of *melancholia alternating with mania,* because, according to the description of **A. Costa,** the plant has the inherent property to produce similar *alternating mental and emotional abnormalities.*

---

[22] **Translator's note:** abnormal behaviour marked by berserkness and amok in a murderous frenzy as if possessed by a demon.

[23] **Translator's note:** *Veckoskrift for Lakare*, iv, p. 40.

heben, — und eben so [...]
eine *mit Man[...]*
lie mit diesem Krau[...] w[...]
a Costa erzählt, *solche alterni[...]* *Ge-*
müthsverwirrungen auch vor sich zu erzeugen im Stande ist.

Percival, *Stahl* und *Quarin* beobachteten *Magendrücken*, *Morton*, *Friborg*,
Bauer und *Quarin Erbrechen* und *Durch-*
fall, *Morton* und *Dan. Crüger* Ohnmachten,
und viele Andre einen *grofsen Schwäche-*
zustand, *Thomson*, *Richard*, *Stahl* und *C. E.*
Fischer eine Art *Gelbsucht*, *Quarin* und *Fi-*
scher Bitterkeit des Mundes, und mehrere Andre *harte Anspannung des Unter-*
leibes vom Gebrauche der Chinarinde,
und eben diese vereinigten Zustände sind
es, bei deren ursprünglichen Gegenwart in
Wechselfiebern Torti und *Cleghorn* so an-
gelegentlich auf den alleinigen Gebrauch
der Chinarinde dringen, — so wie die ge-
segnete Anwendung derselben in dem *er-*
schöpften Zustande, der *Unverdaulich-*
keit und *Anorexie* nach akuten, besonders mit Blutlassen und erschöpfenden Aus-
leerungsmitteln behandelten Fiebern blos

35. Percival, Stahl and Quarin have observed that *China bark, i.e. Cinchona officinalis* (**Translator's note:** the German common name as used by Hahnemann is *Chinarinde*) causes *pressive pain in the stomach;* **Morton, Friborg, Bauer** and **Quarin** have observed it causing *vomiting* and *diarrhoea;* **Morton** and **Dan. Crüger** have seen it causing *fainting* and many others saw it producing *great debility;* **Thomson, Richard, Stahl** and **C.E. Fischer** saw it in a kind of *jaundice;* **Quarin** and **Fischer** in *bitterness of the mouth;* and, furthermore, others observed it in *bloatedness of the abdomen.* It is exactly when all these symptoms or morbid states occur in *Intermittent Fevers* that **Torti** and **Cleghorn** recommend the use of *China bark,* the curative effects of this bark only in cases of *fagged-state (exhaustion), indigestion* and *anorexia after acute fevers* specially when these have been treated by blood-letting and debilitating purgatives, and they depend on the power which it possesses of causing *severe sinking of the powers of life, producing bodily and mental exhaustion, indigestion and anorexia,* as has been observed by many (**von Cleghorn, Friborg, Crüger, Romberg, Stahl, Thomson** and others).

auf der (von *Cleghorn, Friborg, Crüger, Romberg, Stahl, Thomson* u. A.) beobachteten Eigenschaft dieser Rinde, *ein ungemeines Sinken der Kräfte, erschlafften Zustand Leibes und der Seele, Unverdaulichkeit* und *Anorexie* zu erregen, beruhet.

Aufser *Piso, Huck* und *Meyer* haben noch eine Menge andrer Ärzte die *Durchfall* stillende Kraft der *Ipecacuanhe* anerkannt. Wie könnte sie aber einige Arten Durchfall so kräftig stillen, wenn sie nicht selbst, wie bekannt (*Murray*) vor sich *Purgiren* zu erregen geeignet wäre? — Wie könnte sie mehrere *Blutflüsse* stillen (*Bagliv, Barbeirac, Gianella, Dalberg, Bergius* u. A.), wenn sie nicht selbst *Blutflüsse* zu erzeugen (*Murray, Geoffroy*) im Stande wäre? — Wie könnte sie in *Engbrüstigkeit* und besonders in der *krampfhaften Engbrüstigkeit* (*Akenside, Meyer, Bang*) so hülfreich seyn, wenn sie nicht, auch ohne Ausleerungen zu erregen, schon vor sich die Tendenz besäfse, *Engbrüstigkeit* überhaupt, und *krampfhafte Engbrüstigkeit* insbesondre zu verursachen?

36. **Piso, Huck** and **Meyer,** and many other physicians affirm the power of *Ipecacuanha, i.e. Ipecacuanha officinalis* (**Translator's note:** the German common name as used by Hahnemann is *Ipecacuanhe*) to relieve *diarrhoea.* But how could it do this if it did not have the power to cause *purging*[24] (**Murray**)? How would it have been possible to stop various kinds of *haemorrhage* with *Ipecacuanha* (as was done by **Bagliv, Barbeirac, Gianella, Dalberg, Bergius** and others), if this medicine did not in itself possess the power of producing *haemorrhages* (**Murray, Geoffroy**) ? How could it be so effective in *shortness of breath,* and particularly those *shortness of breath* occurring *spasmodically,* (**Akenside, Meyer, Bang**), if *Ipecacuanha* does not possess the tendency to produce *shortness of breath* in general and *spasmodic shortness of breath* in particular, as **Murray** [*Pract. Bibl. III*], **Geoffroy** and **Scott** have observed it to do? Can any more distinct indications be required that medicines should be applied for the cure of diseases on the basis of the disease effects which they produce?

---

[24] **Translator's note:** vomiting and diarrhoea.

dergleichen *Murray* (pract. Bibl. III.), *Geoffroy* und *Scott* von dieser Wurzel beobachteten. Kann es deutlichere Winke geben, dafs wir die Arzneien nach ihren krankmachenden Wirkungen zur Heilung der Krankheiten anwenden sollen?

Eben so würde es nicht einzusehen seyn, wie die Ignatzbohne in einer Art Konvulsionen (Acta Berolin. *Herrmann*, *Valentin*) so wohlthätig hätte seyn können, wenn nicht bekannt wäre (*Bergius*, *Camelli*, *Durius* in Misc. N. C. Dec. III. ann. 9, 10.), dafs sie selbst dergleichen hervorzubringen im Stande wäre.

Durch *Stofs* und *Quetschungen* beschädigte Personen bekommen Seitenstiche, Brechreitz, krampfhafte, stechende und brennende Schmerzen in den Hypochondern mit Aengstlichkeit und Zittern begleitet, ein unwillkührliches Zusammenfahren wie von elektrischen Stöfsen wachend und im Schlafe, ein Kriebeln in den beschädigten Theilen, u. s. w. Da nun das Wohlverleih eben diese Zustände erregen kann (*de Meza*, *Vicat*, *Crichton*, *Collin*, *Aaskow*, *Stoll* und *J. Chr. Lange*), so wird es leicht

37. It is not easy to conceive how *Ignatia bean, i.e. Ignatia amara* (**Translator's note:** the German common name as used by Hahnemann is *Ignatzbohne*) could be so effective in a certain kind of *convulsions* (in *Acta Berolin,* **Herrmann, Valentin**), if it did not possess the power of producing similar *convulsions* (observed by **Bergius, Camelli, Durius**, in *Miscell. N. at Cur. Dec.* III, *ann.* 9, 10.).

38. Those persons who have been injured by a *blow* or *contusion* feel *pains in the side, nausea, spasmodic lancinating* and *burning pains in the hypochondria, accompanied by anxiety, tremors and involuntary starts when waking and in sleep*, similar to those produced by an electric shock, formication in the injured parts, etc. as *Wolf's bane, i.e. Arnica Montana* (**Translator's note:** the German common name as used by Hahnemann is *Wohlverleih*) produces similar **Aaskow, Stoll** and **J. Chr. Lange**; so it can be easily understood that this plant will cure the *effects of accidents due to a blow, fall or bruise,* as is common in the experiences of a lot of physicians and even of whole nations for past centuries.

begreiflich, wie dieses Kraut die *Zufälle von Quetschung und Fall*, folglich die *Quetschung selbst* heilen kann, wie eine namenlose Menge von Aerzten und ganze Völkerschaften in Erfahrung gebracht haben.

Wenn es mehrere Stufen und Arten von *Hundswuth* giebt, wie mehr als wahrscheinlich ist, so wird man wohl behaupten können, daſs die Belladonne eine Art *Wasserscheu* zu heilen vermögend sei, wie denn wirklich *Münch*, *Buchholz* und *Neimeke* dergleichen mit ihr geheilt haben; auch leuchtet diese Heilkraft aus der eigenthümlichen Wirkungsart dieses Krautes hervor, *mehrere Zufälle von Wasserscheu* schon selbst erzeugen zu können, z. B. das vergebliche Haschen nach Schlaf, das ängstliche Athemholen, der ängstliche brennende Durst nach Getränke, das die Person kaum erhält, als sie es schon wieder von sich stöſst, mit rothem Gesichte, stieren und funkelnden Augen (von welcher Arzneikrankheit durch Belladonne uns *J. F. C. Grimm* das Bild entwirft), während die einzelnen Züge die-

39. Among the range of effects which *Belladonna, i.e. Atropa belladonna* (**Translator's note:** the German common name as used by Hahnemann is *Belladonne*) produces when administered to healthy persons, are symptoms which, when taken in totality, present a portrait very similar to that of *rabies* and a kind *of hydrophobia* which were really cured by **Münch, Buchholz** and **Neimeke**[25] with this plant. *The ineffective attempt to sleep, the hurried respiration, completely anxious burning thirst for liquids which when presented to the patient is rejected by him with violence; the flushed face, fixed and sparkling eyes* (as was observed from the use of *Belladonna* by **J.F.C. Grimm**[26]); *the suffocation caused by drinking with uncontrolled thirst* according to **El. Camerarius** and **Sauter**; the *general inability to swallow anything* as testified by **von May, Lottinger, Sicelius, Buchave, d'Hermont, Manetti, Vicat** and **Cullen,** *the desire to bite those around him alternating with terror* (as was witnessed by **Sauter, Dumoulin, Buchave** and **Mardorf**), *the inclination to spit all around him* (**Sauter**); *and to run away* (**Dumoulin, Eb. Gmelin** and **Buc'hoz**), and *the continuous movement of the body* (**von Boucher, Eb. Gmelin**

---

[25] **Translator's note:** The *spelling* of the name **Neimeke** *in the first edition* (P. XXIV, 13th line) was NEIMEKE, but afterwards in *second edition* (P. 48, 13th line), *third edition* (P. 17, 9th line), and *fourth edition* (p. 68, 4th line) it was written as NEIMIKE

[26] **Translator's note:** In *Ist edition,* P. XXVI, 9th line, *Hahnemann* wrongly wrote Grimm as Glimm.

51

ses Zustandes von mehrern Beobachtern, namentlich das, Ersticken erregende Niederschlingen des Getränks bei übermäßigem Durste von *El. Camerarius* und *Sauter*, und überhaupt das Unvermögen zu schlucken von *May, Lottinger, Sicelius, Buchave, d' Hermont, Manetti, Vicat* und *Cullen* wiederholet, von Andern aber die von diesem Kraute entstandne, mit Furchtsamkeit abwechselnde Begierde, nach den Umstehenden zu schnappen (*Sauter, Dumoulin, Buchave, Mardorf*) und umher zu spucken (*Sauter*), auch wohl zu entfliehen (*Dumoulin, Eb. Gmelin, Buc'hoz*) und die beständige Regsamkeit des Körpers (von *Boucher, Eb. Gmelin, Sauter*) noch hinzugesetzt werden, — alles Zufälle von Belladonne, welche vereinigt ein ziemlich treffendes Bild von der durch sie heilbaren Art *Hydrophobie* darstellen. Ob aber die Behandler der Wasserscheu mit Belladonne auf der einen Seite nicht oft die Gabe übertrieben, auf der andern Seite aber die der Belladonne entsprechende Art von Wasserscheu immer getroffen haben, will ich hier nicht entscheiden — da die häufigsten Arten von Hundswuth mehr den durch

and **Sauter**). All the effects that *Belladonna* produces give a proper image of the different types of *hydrophobia* which are curable by it. Only if those who handle and treat *hydrophobia* would have known its similar relation with *Belladonna* and the correlativity with *Henbane, i.e. Hyoscyamus niger* (**Translator's note:** the German common name as used by Hahnemann is *Bilsenkraut*), then I am sure *rabies* and *types of hydrophobia* would have settled as more frequently curable. *Belladonna* has also cured different kinds of *mania* and *melancholia* (as noticed by **Evers, Schmucker, Schmalz, Münch**, both father and son, and others) because it possesses the power to produce peculiar types of *insanity;* such *Belladonna mental diseases* are recorded by **Rau, Grimm, Hasenest, May, Mardorf, Hoyer, Dillenius** and others. **Henning,** after trying uselessly for three months to cure a case of *amaurosis with coloured spots before the eyes* by a variety of medicines, at last whimsically adopted the idea

Bilsenkraut erzeugbaren Zufällen ähneln, und daher öfterer durch lezteres heilbar seyn müssen. — — Die Belladonne heilte auch Arten von *Manie* und *Melancholie* (*Evers, Schmucker, Schmalz* und *Müsch* Vater und Sohn) das ist, mittelst ihrer Kraft, besondre Arten von *Wahnsinn* eigenthümlich zu erzeugen, dergleichen *Rau, Glimm, Hasenest, May, Mardorf, Hoyer, Dillenius,* u. A. aufgezeichnet haben. — *Henning* brauchte eine Menge vergeblicher Mittel gegen eine *Amaurosis mit vielfarbigen Flecken vor den Augen* drei Monate lang, bis er aus Verdacht gegen etwanige Gicht, die der Kranke doch nicht hatte, endlich Belladonne gab und ihn damit schnell und ohne Beschwerde heilte. Er würde es wohl gleich Anfangs gethan haben, wenn er gewußt hätte, daß Belladonne dies homöopathisch thun muß, da sie selbst *Amaurosis mit vielfarbigen Flecken vor den Augen* erzeugt, wie *Sauter* sah.

Die von einigen Beobachtern (*Blom, Planchon*) zu Anfange der Wirkung des Bilsenkrautes bemerkte *Schlaflosig-*

that this malady might perhaps be excited by gout, which the patient had never suffered; and upon this supposition he was, by chance as it were, induced to prescribe *Belladonna* which effected a speedy cure without any inconvenience. He would certainly have made choice of this medicine at first had he known that it was not possible to perform a rapid and easy cure except by the help of a remedy which produces symptoms similar to those of the disease itself; and that, according to this infallible law of nature, *Belladonna* could not fail to cure this case homoeopathically, because, as **Sauter** observed, it excites a variety of *amaurosis with coloured spots before the eyes.*

40. The *insomnia commonly maintained by anxiety,* as mentioned by some observers (**Blom** and **Planchon**), occurs in the beginning of the action of *Henbane, i.e. Hyoscyamus niger* (**Translator's note:** the German common name as used by Hahnemann is *Bilsenkrautes*) is clearly the only basis of its great power to cause *sleep in similar idiopathic insomnia* and in this palliative hypnotic (sleep producing) action, according

keit, welche gewöhnlich von *Aengstlich-*
keit unterhalten wird, ist auffallend der
einzige Grund der so grofsen Schlaf bringenden Wirkung desselben in *ähnlichen*
idiopathischen *Agrypnien*, die, nach
Stoerck, jene (palliative) hypnotische Wirkung des Opiums weit übertrifft. — Das
Bilsenkraut hat Krämpfe, welche viel Aehnlichkeit mit der *Fallsucht* hatten, auch
wohl dafür gehalten worden sind (nach
Stoerck, Collin und A.), gehoben, weil es
der *Fallsucht* sehr ähnliche Zuckungen
erregen kann (nach *El. Camerarius, Chch.*
Seliger, Hünerwolf, A. Hamilton, Planchon,
a Cotta u. A.) Nicht umsonst hat *Greding*
von diesem Kraute einen *trocknen krampf-*
haften Husten entstehen sehen; diefs
sollte uns zeigen, dafs er ein kräftiges Heilmittel in einem *ähnlichen Husten* sei,
wie auch *Friccius, Rosenstein, Dubb* und
Stoerck wirklich erfahren haben. — In gewissen Arten von *Wahnsinn* hat *Stoerck,*
Fothergill, Herwig und *Ofterdinger* das Bilsenkraut mit Erfolge gebraucht; doch würden noch weit mehrere Aerzte hierin glücklich gewesen seyn, wenn sie keinen an-

to **Stoerck**, is much superior to *Opium* (**Translator's note:** *Papaver somniferum*). *Henbane* has cured *convulsions* which looked very similar and, indeed, were considered as *epilepsy* (as witnessed by **Stoerck, Collin** and others). This it did because it causes *convulsions very similar to those of epilepsy* (according to the writings of **El. Camerarius, Chph. Seliger, Hünerwolf, A. Hamilton, Planchon, A. Costa** and others). **Greding** saw a *spasmodic dry cough* produced by this plant, and this should teach us that it is a powerful remedy for similar cough, as, indeed, was observed by **Friccius, Rosenstein, Dubb** and **Stoerck.** *Henbane* was used by **Stoerck, Fothergill, Herwig** and **Ofterdinger** with success in some varieties of insanity. But many more physicians could have used it successfully in such affections if they limited its use only to the cure of that kind of mental derangement which *Henbane is* capable of producing in its primary action, *viz.,* a kind of *idiotic mental derangement,* which was produced by this plant as was seen by **Helmont, Wedel, J.G. Gmelin, la Serre, Hünerwolf, A. Hamilton, Kiernander, J. Stedman**[27], **Toppetti**[28]**, J. Faber**

---

[27] **Translator's note:** This *spelling* in the name as **J. Stedman** has been wrongly used by Hahnemann in first edition (p. xxviii, 7th line), but as STEDMANN in the 2nd edition (p. 53, 5th line), in 2nd edition (p. 52, 12th line), in 3rd edition (p. 20, 13th line & p. 21, 1st line), in 4th edition (p. 71, 9th line, & 22th line, as STEDMAN (II ed., p. 53, 5th line).

[28] **Translator's note:** Hahnemann printed the name as **Toppetti** in the 1st edition (p. XXVII, 7th line) but subsequently corrected it as **Tozzetti** in 2nd edition (p. 52, 12th line; p. 53, 12th line); 3rd edition (p. 20, 13th line & p. 22, 4th line) and in 4th edition (p. 71, 9th line & p. 72, last line).

dern Wahnsinn damit zu heilen unternommen hätten, als das Bilsenkraut in seinen Primärwirkungen zu erzeugen vermag, nämlich jene Art *stupider Sinnlosigkeit*, wie sie *Helmont*, *Wedel*, *J. G. Gmelin*, *la Serre*, *Hünerwolf*, *A. Hamilton*, *Kiernander*, *J. Stedman*, *Toppetti*, *J. Faber* und *Wendt* vom Bilsenkraute haben erfolgen sehen. — Aus den von diesem Kraute erfahrnen Wirkungen, die man bei obigen Beobachtern nachsehen kann, läfst sich das Bild des höchsten Grades von einer Art *Hysterie* zusammensetzen, und eben diese wird von ihm geheilt (*J. A. P. Gesner*, *Stoerck*). — Unmöglich hätte *Schenckbecher* einen zwanzigjährigen *Schwindel* damit heben können, wenn das Bilsenkraut nicht so allgemein und in so hohem Grade einen ähnlichen *Schwindel* zu erzeugen, von Natur geeignet wäre, wie *Hünerwolf*, *Blom*, *Navier*, *Planchon*, *Sloane*, *Stedman*, *Greding*, *Wepfer*, *Vicat*, *Bernigau* bezeugen. — Die sechs gemischten Arzneistoffe, die *Hecker* in einer *krampfhaften Verschliefsung der Augenlieder* mit dem sichtbarsten Erfolge brauchte, wären vergeblich gewesen,

and **Wendt**. Through the effects of *Henbane* observed by the just-named authors a portrait of *hysteria* of severe character may be constructed; and a very similar one would be cured by this plant, as was observed by **J.A.P. Gessner**[29], **Stoerck** and **Schenckbecher** who would never have succeeded in curing a *vertigo of twenty years' duration* with *Henbane* if this plant did not have the natural power of producing, so commonly and in such an intensity, a *similar vertigo,* as was confirmed by **Hünerwolf, Blom, Navier, Planchon, Sloane, Stedmann, Greding, Wepfer, Vicat,** and **Bernigau**. The mixture of medicines which was employed with the greatest success by **Hecker** in a case of *spasmodic closure of the eyelids,* would have proved useless if by a pleasant coincidence, he had not included *Bilsenkrautes,* which according to **Wepfer,** causes a similar affection in healthy organisms.

---

[29] **Translator's note:** Hahnemann's spelling of this name was **J.A.P. Gesner** in 1st edition (p. XXVIII, 14th line), 2nd edition (p. 52, 20th line), and as **Gessner** in 3rd edition (p. 20, 19th line), and in 4th edition (p. 71, 15th line).

war nicht das hier homöopathische Bilsenkraut glücklicherweise drunter, welches
nach *Wepfer* dasselbe Symptom am gesunden Körper zu erregen pflegt.

Die *Glieder*- und *Gelenkschmerzen*,
welche *A. Richard* (bei *P. Schenk*) vom
Sturmhute in Erfahrung gebracht hat,
sind von der Art, wie sie von vielen Aerzten, deren Namen *Murray* verzeichnet, mit
Sturmhut geheilt worden sind; so daſs der
homöopathische Grund seiner Heilkraft
deutlich in die Augen fällt.

Wie wäre es möglich, daſs der Kampher in den sogenannten schleichenden
*Nervenfiebern mit verminderter Kör-
perwärme, verminderter Empfindung
und gesunkenen Kräften* so ausnehmen-
de Dienste leisten konnte, wie uns der
Wahrheit liebende *Huxham* versichert, wenn
der Kampher nicht in seiner Primarwirkung
gerade einen solchen Zustand erzeugte, wie *Alexander, Cullen* und *Fr. Hoffmann*
von ihm sahen? — Die bis zur höchsten
Schmerzhaftigkeit erhöhete Empfindlichkeit des Organismus mit Hitze verbunden
in der Influenza hebt er deshalb zwar

41. The *pains in the extremities and arthralgia* experienced from *Monk's Hood, i.e. Aconitum napellus* (**Translator's note:** the German common name as used by Hahnemann is *Sturmhute*) by **A. Richard** (according to **P. Schenck***)* were of the same type as those which were cured, with the help of the plant, by many physicians mentioned by **Murray**. Thus is evident the homoeopathic basis of its curative power.

42. How could *Camphor, i.e. Camphora monobromata* (**Translator's note:** the German common name as used by Hahnemann is *Kampher*) produce such extraordinary beneficial effects as the truthful **Huxham** says it does, in the so-called *sneaking nervous fevers*, where *the body-heat is lowered, sensibility diminished* and the *strength sunken*, if, *Camphor* in its primary action upon the body, was not able to produce a *condition perfectly similar*, to that observed by **Alexander, Cullen** and **Fr. Hoffmann?** The *increased sensibility of the body* and the *most intense pain associated with heat in influenza*, is quickly removed by *Camphor*, but only *palliatively*, hence its doses must be constantly increased and repeated so that it shall gain the supremacy over this acute disease (§ 266).

schwerden und Krankheitszufälle den ganz
ähnlichen Körperbeschwerden und Krankheiten entsprechen, welche sie mit Glück
und dauerhaft durch Homöopathie geheilt
hat. Ich sage hier nichts von den Heilungen die sie schon als entgegengesetzt wirkendes Arzneimittel,[*] bei neu entstandnen Fällen von Gefühlsverlust, Schlagfluss,
Lähmungen und schwarzem Staare bei vollkräftigen Körpern zuweilen vollführte —
da sie dergleichen auf diese opponirte Weise in chronischen alten Lähmungen und
Amaurosen der Natur der Sache nach, nie
auszurichten im Stande ist, so wenig als
irgend ein andres Palliativ. Ich erwähne
blos ihrer homöopathischen Wirkungen.
Unzählig sind die Schriftsteller, welche in
der Primärwirkung Beschleunigung
des Pulses von der positiven Elektrisität
wahrnahmen, vollständig *feberhafte Anfälle* aber, blos durch Elektrisität erzeugt,
sahen *Sauvages*, *Delas* und *Barillon* bei *Bertholon*. Diese ihre febrilische Tendenz war
Ursache, dass *Gardini*, *Wilkinson*, *Syme*, und
Wesley eine Art *Tertianfieber* einzig mit

---

[*] Blos in der Nachwirkung sehr heftiger und ungeheurer elektrischen Schläge sind Anwandlung von
Lähmung der Glieder, Gefühlsverlust, und Lähmung der Gehör - und Seh - Nerven enthalten.

43. Murray has confirmed that *Strong wine* (**Translator's note:** the German word used by Hahnemann is *feuriger wein*), often, diminishes a *nagging heat of the body* and the *violent excitation of the pulse*—apparently homoeopathically! A case of *fever with delirium like intoxication without senses, with stertorous breathing,* similar to *the drunken state* caused by wine, was cured by **Rademacher** in a single night by *wine.* Can anyone fail to see the power of an analogous medicinal stimulation *(similia similibus)* in this case?

44. An agony of *convulsions without consciousness,* very similar to the agony of death, alternating with *attacks of spasmodic and jerky, sometimes also difficult and rattling respiration,* with *death-like coldness of the face and body, (blueness of the feet and hands)* and *feebleness of the pulse* (exactly similar to the symptoms of *Poppy seeds-opium, i.e. Papaver somniferum* (**Translator's note:** the German common name as used by Hahnemann is *Mohnsafte*) observed by **Schweickert** and others), was, at first, treated unsuccessfully by **Stütz** with Alkaline-salt (**Translator's note:** the German common name as used by Hahnemann is *Laugensalz*), but was subsequently successfully cured in a pleasant, speedy and permanent manner by *opium. Opium* produces *an extreme and almost irresistible tendency to sleep, accompanied by profuse perspiration and delirium* (as was observed by

ward von *Stütz* vergeblich mit Laugensalz, nachgehends glücklich und schnell und dauerhaft durch Mohnsaft gehoben. Wer erkennt hier nicht das, unwissender Weise ausgeübte homöopathische Verfahren? — Eben diesen, so grofse Neigung zum fast unüberwindlichen Schlafe mit heftigem Schweifse und Delirien (nach *Vicat, J. C. Grimm* und Andern) erregenden Mohnsaft fürchtete sich *Osthoff* in einem epidemischen Fieber, was *dieselben Symptomen* hatte, anzuwenden, weil das System (!) in dieser direkten Schwäche ihn zu geben verbiete. Nur da er nach vergeblichem Gebrauch aller bekannten Arzneien den Tod vor Augen sah, entschlofs er sich, ihn auf gut Glück zu probiren, und, siehe! er war allgemein hülfreich (mufste es seyn, nach dem ewigen homöopathischen Heilgesetze!) — In einem Fieber, wo die Kranken sprachlos waren, die Augen offen, die Glieder starr, der Puls klein und aussetzend, der Athem schwer mit Schnarchen und Röcheln und in Schlafsucht versunken — Zuständen, die der Mohnsaft ganz ähnlich zu bewirken vor sich vermag (wie

Vicat, J.C. Grimm and others). For this reason **Osthoff** was afraid to administer it in an *epidemic of fever* which manifested *similar symptoms,* because the system (!) he practised did not direct the use of *opium* on such cases. After he had used, without success, all the known medicines and saw the death approaching that he decided to try it at all risks on the same people, and see! It was highly beneficial, (as it *must be,* in conformity with the eternal Law of Homoeopathy!). In a fever where the patient had *lost speech, eyes were open, limbs were stiff, pulse small* and *intermittent, respiration difficult, breathing snoring* and *stertorous,* and *deep comatose sleep,* - all of these symptoms are *perfectly similar* to those which *opium* produces, (as was observed by **de la Croix, Rademacher, Crumpe, Pyl, Vicat, Sauvages** and many others) this was the only substance which **Hoffmann** found capable of producing any good effects, (*which was quite natural*). As it (*opium*) produces *lethargy,* **C.C. Matthäi,** in an obstinate case of *nervous disease,* where the main symptoms were *insensibility* and *numbness of the arms, legs and belly,* after treating it for a long time with inappropriate, that is to say, non-homoeopathic remedies, at length brought

de la Croix, Rademacher, Crumpe, Pyl, Vicat, Sauvages und viele Andre beobachtet haben) — da sah Hoffmann in Münster blos den Mohnsaft helfen (wie ganz natürlich!) — Nach langer Quaal mit einer Menge nicht passender Arzneien hob C. C. Matthäi eine hartnäckige Nervenkrankheit, deren Hauptzeichen Unempfindlichkeit, Taubheit und Eingeschlafenheit in Armen, Schenkeln und am Unterleibe waren, mit Mohnsaft (der nach Stütz, J. Young und Andern, dergleichen in vorzüglichem Grade vor sich erregen kann), wie jeder Nachdenkende sieht, blos homöopathisch. — Hufeland's Heilung einer tagelangen Lethargie mit Mohnsaft, nach welchem andern Gesetze erfolgte sie, als nach dem bisher verkannten homöopathischen?

Rave und Wedekind heilten schlimme Mutter - Blutflüsse mit Sadebaum, welcher wie jede freche Dirne weiss, Bärmutter - Blutflüsse bei Gesunden erzwingt. Wer will hier das Heilgesetz der Natur durch Aehnlichkeit, verkennen?

Wie könnte der Biesam im Millarischen Asthma fast specifisch helfen, wenn

a cure by *opium,* which, (according to **Stütz, J. Young** and others,) causes similar *conditions* in a great degree, consequently, as every one must understand, only cures homoeopathically. **Hufeland** performed the cure of a case of *lethargy,* by the use of *opium* – by what other principle could this have been done, except than by the homoeopathic?

45. Rave and **Wedekind** cured severe *uterine haemorrhages* with *Savine, i.e. Sabina officinalis* (**Translator's note:** the German word used by Hahnemann is *Sadebaum)* which every insolent girl is aware of, causes *uterine haemorrhage* in pregnant women. Can anyone, in this case, fail to understand the curative law of similarity in nature?

46. How could *musk, i.e. Moschus moschiferus* (**Translator's note:** the German word used by Hahnemann is *Biesam)* cure, almost specifically, *Millary asthma* if it did not, have its own power to produce *fits of spasmodic, suffocating constriction of the chest without cough* and which was so observed by **Fr. Hoffmann.**

er nicht vor sich selbst *Paroxysmen von
hustenloser, erstickender, krampfhaf-
ter Zusammenschnürung der Brust*
zuwege bringen könnte? und diefs kann
er, wie *Fr. Hoffmann* beobachtete.

Kann die Kuhpocke anders gegen
Kindblattern schützen, als homöopathisch?
sie, welche aufser andern grofsen Aehnlichkeiten mit ihnen, und insbesondre ihrem im
Ganzen nur einmahl möglichen Erscheinen
am menschlichen Körper und der Tiere ihrer Narben, sogar auch Achseldrüsenge-
schwülste, Augenentzündung und Konvulsionen, wie die Menschenblattern erregt hat.

Bekanntlich ist *Harnverhaltung mit
Harnzwang* eins der häufigsten und be-
schwerlichsten Symptome der spanischen Fliegen, wie zum Ueberflusse
*Joa, Camerarius, Baccius, van Hilden, Forest,
J. Lanzoni, van der Wiel* und *Werlhoff* bestätigen. Ein behutsamer innerer Gebrauch
der Kanthariden mufste daher in *äänlichen
schmerzhaften Dysurien* durchaus ein
hülfreiches und homöopathisches Hauptmittel seyn. Und so ist es auch. Aufser fast
allen griechischen Aerzten (deren Kantharide

47. Can the *Kuhpocke* (**Translator's note:** German for *Cow-pox*) protect us against *Kindblattern* (**Translator's note:** German for *Small-pox*) in any other way than homoeopathic? Without mentioning any other character of close similarity existing between these different diseases, this is common in both that they generally *appear only once during the course of life of a person,* leave behind similar deep pock marks on the body, both cause *tumefaction of the axillary glands, an inflamed areola round each pock* and even *inflammation of the eyes* and *convulsions.*

48. It is known to all that *retention of urine with strangury* is one of the most common and troublesome symptoms that the *Spanishfly, i.e. Cantharides, Cantharis vesicatoria* (**Translator's note:** the German word used by Hahnemann is *Spanischen Fliege)* produces and it has been sufficiently established by **Joa**[30], **Camerarius, Baccius, van Hilden, Forest, J. Lanzoni, van der Wiel** and **Werlhoff.** Consequently *Cantharides, i.e., Cantharis vesicatoria* (**Translator's note:** the German word used by Hahnemann is *Kanthariden),* carefully administered internally should have been and in reality this is indeed a very useful homoeopathic remedy in similar conditions of *painful dysuria.* Without making a list of all the Greek physicians who, instead

---

[30] **Translator's note:** Hahnemann wrote this name as Joa in 1st edition (p. xxxiii) but as Joh in 4th edition, p. 81, para. 4, 4th line.

die sehr ähnliche Meloe des Wegwarts war) haben *Fabr. ab Aquapendente*, *Capivaccius*, *Th. Bartholin*, *Riedlin* und Andre *die schmerzhaftesten*, ohne mechanische Hinderung entstandenen *Ischurien* mit Kanthariden geheilt. Selbst *Huxham* sah die vortrefflichsten Wirkungen davon in solchen Fällen; er rühmt sie sehr, und hätte sie gar gern gebraucht. Aber das System hielt ihn ab, wider seine Ueberzeugung! — *Van Hilden* hat in zwei verschiedenen Fällen *Hüftweh* von Kanthariden erfolgen sehn, und dieser ihnen eigenthümlichen krankmachenden Kraft hat man die vielen dauerhaften Heilungen von *Hüftweh* zu danken, welche *Hollerius*, *Riedlin*, *Boerhaave*, *Trallet*, *Tissot*, *Medicus*, *Tode* und Andre aus ihren Erfahrungen anführen, —/Doch kann wohl schwerlich ein stärkeres Beispiel von der Kraft der Arzneien, durch die Tendenz, ähnlich krank machen, und so homöopathisch Krankheiten heilen zu können, gefunden werden, als die Heilsamkeit (ganz kleiner Gaben) der Kanthariden *im frischen entzündlichen Tripper* selbst, wo sie *Sachs von Lewenheim*, *Hannaeus*, *Bartholin*, *Lister*,

of our *Kanthariden,* used *Meloe des Wegwarts* (**Translator's note:** the German common name of *Cichorium intybus*). **Fabr. ab Aquapendente, Capivaccius, Th. Bartholin, Riedlin** and others, completely cured, with *Cantharides, very painful ischuria* which was not due to any mechanical obstruction. **Huxham** witnessed this remedy producing the best effects in such cases; he praises it highly, and would have used it with happiness only if the traditional conceptions of the Old School of Medicine, had not prevented him! **Van Hilden** had seen that *Cantharides* produced *sciatica* in two cases and on the basis of those characteristics it was used for many long lasting cures as the experiences of **Hollerius, Riedlin, Boerhaave, Tralles, Tissot, Medicus, Tode** and others confirm. In cases of recent *inflammatory gonorrhoea,* in which **Sachs von Lewenheim, Hannaeus, Bartholin, Lister, Mead** and, above all, **Werlhoff** administered *Cantharides* in very small doses with complete success, and cured *painful ischuria, burning urine, inflammation of the urethra* **(Wendt),** and even when applied only externally, cured a type of *inflammatory gonorrhoea* **(Wichmann).**

Mead und vor allen *Werlhoff* mit dem auffallendsten Erfolge anwendeten —, eine Heilkraft, die die Kantharide dem Umstande verdankt, dafs sie fast nach allen Beobachtern *schmerzhafte Ischurie, Harnbrennen*, ja selbst *Entzündung der Harnröhre* (*Wendt*) und sogar bei blos äufserlicher Anwendung einen *entzündungsartigen Tripper* (*Wichmann*) vor sich selbst schon, zu erzeugen vermag.

Bei empfindlichen Personen erregt der innere Gebrauch des S c h w e f e l s nicht selten *Stuhlzwang*, zuweilen sogar *Erbrechen, Leibweh* und *Stuhlzwang* (*Walther*) und aus eben diesem Grunde hat man (Med. N. z.) *ruhrartige Zufälle* und nach *Werlhoff Stuhlzwang* bei blinden Hämorrhoiden, und nach *Rave Hämorrhoidalkoliken* mit demselben heilen können. — Bekanntlich erzeugt das Töplitzer Bad, so wie alle lauen und warmen Bäder, welche *Schwefel in Wasserstoffgas aufgelöst* enthalten, oft einen sogenannten *Badeausschlag*, welcher grofse Aehnlichkeit mit der *Krätze* hat, und eben deswegen heilen auch diese Bäder (homöopathisch), so wie

49. The internal administration of *Sulphur* (**Translator's note:** the German word used by Hahnemann is *Schwefels*), in persons of a sensitive tendency, often causes *tenesmus,* sometimes the *tenesmus* is associated with *vomiting* and *colic,* [**Walther**]. It is because of this power of *sulphur* that physicians (Med. N.Z.)[31] have been able to cure by its use *dysentery with tenesmus* and *blind haemorrhoids,* as was observed by **Werlhoff,** and *haemorrhoidal colic* as observed by **Rave.** It is well known that the *Toeplitz-baths,* like all other warm baths contains *sulphurous hydrogen gas,* usually causes a so-called *bath-rash* which is strongly similar to the *scabies like eruptions of wool workers.* It is exactly because of presence of *Sulphur* in these baths and the power (homoeopathic) it gets therefore power to remove permanently the true *scabies* which affects the wool worker.

---

[31] **Translator's note:** *Medecine National Zeitung,* National Medical Journal.

der Schwefel selbst, die wahre *Krätze* der Wollarbeiter dauerhaft.

Die englischen Aerzte haben in den neuern Zeiten, in den Beddoesschen Schriften und anderwärts, die Salpetersäure als ein sehr dienliches Mittel in dem *Speichelflusse* von Quecksilber und den daher entstandnen *Mundgeschwüren* befunden, welches diese Säure nicht hätte ausrichten können, wenn sie nicht schon vor sich, selbst wo sie auch nicht örtlich auf den Mund wirken konnte, und schon als Bad (*Scott*) gebraucht, die Eigenschaft besäfse, *Speichelflufs* und *Rachengeschwüre* zu erzeugen, wie auch *Aloyn, Kellie, Blair, Luks* und *Ferriar* von ihr gesehen haben.

Fritze hat von einem Bade mit *kaustischem Kali* geschwängert, eine Art *Tetanus* erfolgen sehn, und *Humbold* hat die Reitzbarkeit der Muskeln durch zerflossenes Weinsteinsalz bis zum *Tetanus* zu erregen vermocht; kann eine einfachere und wahrere Quelle für die Heilkraft des (ätzenden) *Laugensalzes* in jener Art von *Tetanus*, wo es *Stütz* nebst Andern hülfreich fanden, nachgewiesen werden?

50. We learn from the writing of **Beddoes** and others that the physicians of England found *Nitric acid* (**Translator's note:** the German word used by Hahnemann is *Salpetersäure)* of great utility in *increased flow of saliva* and *ulceration of the mouth* caused by the use of *mercury.* This acid could never prove to be useful in such cases if it, itself, did not excite *increased flow of saliva* and *ulceration of the mouth* caused by the use of *Quick-silver, i.e., Mercury* (**Translator's note:** the German word used by Hahnemann is *Quecksilber).* This acid could never prove to be useful in such cases if it itself did not produce *salivation* and *ulceration of the fauces.* For producing these effects, it is not necessary to administer it through the mouth, simply bathing the surface of the body with it is enough, (**Scott**). The same results have also been observed through its internal administration by **Aloyn, Kellie**[32], **Blair, Luke** and **Ferriar**[33].

51. Fritze saw a type of *tetanus* produced by a bath containing *Caustic potash*, i.e. *Kalium caustic* (**Translator's note:** the German word used by Hahnemann is *Kaustischem Kali)* and **Humbold,**[34] by applying a solution of *Salt of tartar,* i.e. *Kali tartaricum* (**Translator's note:** the German word used by Hahnemann is *Weinsteinsalz)* was able to produce

---

[32] **Translator's note:** Hahnemann writes this names as only **Kellie** in the first edition (p. XXXVI), but as **G. Kellie** in the fourth edition (p. 84, para)

[33] **Translator's note:** Hahnemann writes this name as **Ferriar** in the first edition (p. XXXVI) but as **J. Ferriar** in the fourth edition (p. 84, para 112).

[34] **Translator's note:** Hahnemann writes **Humbold** here (1st edition, p. XXXVI., or para - 51) but as **Alex. von Humboldt** in 4th edition (para 113 or p. 85. 1st line)

75

Der durch seine ungeheure Kraft, das Befinden des Menschen zu verändern, man weiss nicht, ob in verwegnen Händen mehr fürchterlich, als in der Hand des Weisen eher verehrungswürdig zu nennende Arsenik würde, im *Gesichtskrebse* nach *Gui von Chauliac*, nach *Theodoric*, nach *Valescus von Taranta*, nach *Fallopius*, nach *Pettet*, nach *Rönnov*, (*Cosme*) und mehrern Neuern nicht so grosse Heilungen haben vollbringen können, wenn dieses Metalloxyd nicht die homöopathische Kraft besässe, schon vor sich *sehr schmerzhafte, sehr schwer heilbare Knoten* (nach *Amatus* dem Portugiesen) und tief eindringende, *bösartige Geschwüre* (nach *Heinreich* und *Knape*) zu erzeugen. — Die Alten würden das, Arsenik enthaltende, sogenannte magnetische Pflaster des *Angelus Sala* bei *Pestbeulen* und *Karbunkeln* nicht so einstimmig wohlthätig haben finden können, wenn der Arsenik nicht vor sich (wie *Degner* und *Knape* bezeugen) die Neigung besässe, *schnell in Brand übergehende Entzündungsgeschwülste* hervorzubringen. — Der Arsenik bringt, nach den

the *sensitiveness of the muscles* to such a degree that it excited *tetanic convulsions.* Can the curative properties manifested by *(Caustic) Alkaline salt,* i.e. *Kali tartaricum* [**Translator's note:** the German word used by Hahnemann is *(ätzenden) Laugensalzes*] in that kind of *tetanus,* in which **Stütz** and others have found it to be so helpful, be explained in a simpler or more rational manner than through its effects?

52. *Arsenic* (**Translator's note:** the German word used by Hahnemann is *Arsenik),* which possesses such strong actions on human body that we are unable to decide whether it is more dangerous in the hands of the reckless than it is useful in the hands of the wise,—could never have caused so many remarkable cures of *cancers in the face,* as observed by many physicians such as **Guy von Chauliac, Theodoric, Valescus von Taranta, Fallopius, Penet, Rönnov, (Cosme),** if this metallic oxide did not possess the homoeopathic property of producing, in healthy persons, *very painful tubercles which are very difficult to cure,* (as observed by **Amatus, the Portuguese**); *deep and infiltrating malignant ulcers,* (as witnessed by **Heimreich**

Wahrnehmungen *Dan. Crüger's* und *J. C. Grimm's* die meisten Zufälle einer *bösartigen rothen Ruhr* hervor; was Wunder, wenn ihm schon *Galenus* in Klystiren und *Zacutus* der Portugiese, *Slevogt* und *Molitor* innerlich als *Heilmittel in einer Art rothen Ruhr* haben heilsam finden können? Und wo käme seine so tausendfach bestätigte (nur noch nicht behutsam genug angewendete) Heilkraft in einigen Arten von *Wechselfeber* her, die seit Jahrhunderten schon von *Myrepsus*, nachgehends von *Slevogt, Molitor, Jacobi, J. C. Bernhardt, Jungken* und *Fowler* nicht unzweideutig gepriesen worden ist, wenn sie nicht in der eigenthümlichen Fieber erregenden Kraft des Arseniks gegründet wäre, welche fast alle Beobachter der Nachtheile dieser metallischen Substanz, und insbesondre *Amatus* der Portugiese, *Degner, Buchholz, Henn,* und *Knape* deutlich bemerkten? — Ganz wohl läßt sich *Alexander'n* glauben, daß der Arsenik ein Hauptmittel in (einigen Arten?) der *Brustbräune* sei, da schon *Otto Tachenius* und *Guilbert Beklemmung des Athemholens, Greiselius* fast *erstickende*

and **Knape)**. The ancient physicians would not have agreed totally in their praise of *Arsenic*, so-called *magnetic plaster* of **Angelus Sala** in *plague buboes* and *carbuncles*, if *Arsenic* did not have the tendency to produce (according to the observations of **Degner** and **Knape)** *inflammatory swellings* which *quickly become gangrenous*. From where can *Arsenic* get power to bring symptoms of a *very severe blood tinged dysentery* (as was observed by **Dan. Crüger** and **J.C. Grimm**) and one wonders how it can be a salutary cure for *bloody dysentery* when given through *enema* by **Galenus** and when given as normal internal medicine by **Zacutus, the Portuguese, Slevogt** and **Molitor?** From where does *Arsenic* bring its curative power, shown so many thousands of times, in certain forms of *intermittent fever* (though it was not used carefully) and highly extolled for centuries, first by **Myrepsus** and subsequently by **Slevogt, Molitor, Jacobi, J.C. Bernhardt, Jungken** and **Fowler,** if it was not within the power of *Arsenic* to cause a *peculiar fever,* as almost every observer of the deleterious effects of this substance have clearly noticed, especially **Amatus, the Portuguese, Degner, Buchholz, Heun** and **Knape?** We may confidently allow **Alexander's** belief that *Arsenic* is a great remedy in some kinds of *angina pectoris* because **Otto Tachenius** and **Guilbert,** have seen it give rise to *oppression*

Schwerathmigkeit, und vorzüglich *Ma*-*jault* ein beim Gehen plötzlich entstehendes *Asthma* mit Sinken der Kräfte vom Arsenik wahrgenommen haben. —

Die *Konvulsionen*, welche nach *Ramsay, Fabas* bei *Unzer*, und *Closmier* der Genuß *kupferner* Dinge, und die wiederholten *epileptischen Anfälle*, welche eine verschluckte Kupfermünze unter *Lazermes* und der Kupfersalmiak unter *Pfündel's* Augen erregt haben, erklären dem nachdenkenden Arzte deutlich genug, woher die Heilung des *Veitstanzes* durch Kupfer, wovon *R. Willan* — und die vielen Heilungen einer Art *Fallsucht* durch die Bereitungen eben dieses Metalls kamen, wovon *Weissmann, Pasquallati, Duncan, Russel, Cullen* und Andre so glückliche Erfahrungen aufzeichneten.

Haben *Poterius, Wepfer, Wedel, Fr. Hoffmann, R. A. Vogel, Thierry* und *Albrecht* mit Zinn eine Art *Schwindsucht*, hektisches *Fieber, langwierige Katarrhe* und *feuchte Engbrüstigkeit* geheilt, so geschah es vermittelst der eigenthümlichen Kraft des Zinnes, eine Art *Schwindsucht* erzeugen zu können, welche schon *J. E. Stahl* beobachtet hatte. — Wie wäre es wohl möglich, daß Zinn, wie *Gutschläger* berich-

of the respiration, **Greiselius** saw a *dyspnoea almost amounting to suffocation;* and **Majault** specially, saw it produce *sudden attacks of asthma increased by walking, associated with sinking of the vital powers.*

53. The *convulsions* caused by *Copper* (**Translator's note:** the German word used by Hahnemann is *Kupferner),* and by the ingestion of substances containing *Copper,* as observed by **Ramsay, Fabas,** according to **Unzer** and **Cosmier,** through the recurrent episodes of *epilepsy* which **Lazerme** saw, occurring after swallowing a copper coin, which **Pfundel** saw produced by copper, sufficiently evident to explain to the thinking physician how *Copper* has been able to cure a kind of *St. Vitus dance,* as reported by **R. Willan,** has cured a case of *epilepsy,* about which **Weifsmann, Pasquallati, Duncan, Russell, Cullen,** and others have recorded their pleasant experience of so many successful cures from *preparations of this metal Copper.*

54. Poterius, Wepfer, Wedel, Fr. Hoffmann, R.A. Vogel, Thierry and **Albrecht** have cured a kind of *phthisis, hectic fever, long-lasting catarrh* and *humid asthma* with *Tin,* i.e. *Stannum metallicum* (**Translator's note:** the German word used by Hahnemann is *Zinn)* because this metal possesses

tet, *Magenschmerzen* heilen könnte, wenn es nicht vor sich schon dergleichen erregen könnte. Und das kann es, wie auch *Geisschläger* selbst sah, und ehedem *Stahl* (mat. med. C. 6. p. 83).

Amelung's Kur einer Art *geschwäriger Lungensucht* durch den innern Gebrauch des Bleies deutet auf die von *Boerhaave* beobachtete Tendenz dieses Metalls, selbst unter seiner äufsern Auflegung eine Art *Schwindsucht* zu erzeugen. — Sollte die schädliche Kraft des Bleies, *Ileus* hervor zu bringen, wie *Thunberg*, *Wilson*, *Luzuriaga* und Andre sahen, nicht diese schreckliche Krankheit, wenn sie Menschen aus andern, unmechanischen Ursachen befällt, zu besiegen geschaffen worden seyn? Und wirklich heilte *Angelus Sala* durch innern (homöopathischen) Gebrauch dieses Metalles den *Ileus* und *Agricola* eine andre *heftige Leibesverstopfung*. — Wenn *Otto Tachenius* und *Ettmüller* ehemals *hartnäckige hypochondrische Beschwerden* mit Blei heilten; so erinnere man sich der diesem Metalle anerschaffnen Neigung, *hypochondrische Uebel* vor sich zu erzeugen, wie in *Luzuriaga's* Beschreibung seiner schädlichen Wirkungen zu sehen ist.

the power of producing a kind *of phthisis,* as **J.E. Stahl**[35] saw. How could it cure *the stomach-ache,* as **Geischläger** says it does, if it did not have the power of causing a similar disease? **Geischläger** and **Stahl** [*Mat. Med.* Cap. 6, p. 83] before him, have proved that it possesses this power.

55. Amelung's cure of a type of *ulcerative lung disease* by the internal administration of *Lead,* i.e. *Plumbum metallicum* (**Translator's note:** the German word used by Hahnemann is *Bleies)* indicates the tendency of this metal to cause *a kind of phthisis* when applied externally, as was observed by **Boerhaave.** The bad effects of *Lead* produces the most *obstinate constipation* and even *ileus*[36] as **Thunberg, Wilson, Luzuriaga** and others have seen; do not these bad effects also give us indications to understand that this metal possesses a corresponding curative power? **Angelus Sala** cured (homoeopathically) a type of *ileus,* and **Agricola,** another *serious constipation* by administering this metal internally. When **Otto Tachenius** and **Ettmüller** previously cured *tenacious hypochondriacal complaints* with the help of *Lead,* we should keep in mind that this metal has a tendency to cause *hypochondriacal sufferings,* as can be seen in the description of its bad effects in the records of **Lazuriaga.**

---

[35] **Translator's note:** Hahnemann (1st edition, p. xxix) writes **J.** E. Stahl, whereas in 2nd edition and 4th edition (p. 88, serial para no. 116) as **G.** E. Stahl.

[36] **Translator's note:** Mechanical, dynamic, or adynamic obstruction of the bowel; may be accompanied by severe colicky pain, abdominal distension, vomiting, absence of passage of stool, and often fever and dehydration.

Man darf sich nicht wundern, daſs *Marcus* (Magaz. II. 2.) eine *Entzündung und Geschwulst der Zunge und des Rachens* schnell und dauerhaft mit einem Mittel geheilt hat, welches nach der täglichen, tausendfachen Erfahrung aller Aerzte ganz specifisch Entzündung der innern Theile des Mundes erzeugt (mit Quecksilber) welches dergleichen schon bei äuſserer Auflegung (der merkurialischen Salbe, Pflaster oder des Sublimats) auf die Haut des übrigen Körpers thut, wie *Degner* nebst Andern erfuhr. — (Die *Gemüthstörung* und die *Herzensangst*, welche, unter Andern, *Hill* vom Quecksilbergebrauche wahrnahm, und die bekannte, fast specifische Tendenz dieses Metalls, *Speichelfluſs* zu erregen, erklärt sehr einleuchtend, wie *W. Perfect* eine mit *Speichelfluſs* abwechselnde *Melancholie* mit Quecksilber dauerhaft heilen konnte. — Woher kömmt des Quecksilbers guter Ruf in der häutigen *Bräune*? Warum war *Seelig* in Heilung der von Frieselfieber begleiteten *fürartigen Bräune* so glücklich mit Kalomel? Macht wohl irgend eine Arznei in der Welt vor sich eine schlimmere *Bräune* als Kalomel? — Heilte *Sauter* jene *geschwürige Mundentzündung* mit

56. We should not be surprised if **Marcus** (*Magaz. II, 2*) cured rapidly and permanently *an inflammation* and *swelling of the tongue* and *of the fauces* with *Mercury* (**Translator's note:** the German word used by Hahnemann is *Qucksilber*) a remedy which, according to the every-day experience of many physicians, has a particular tendency to produce *inflammation of the interior of the mouth,* the manifestation which it causes ever when just applied to the surface of the body (in the form of ointment containing *Mercury* or its plaster or its sublimates as was observed by **Degner** and others. The *disturbance of the intellectual faculties* and *mental anxiety,* from the use of *mercury* (**Hill**) combined to the almost specific power of this metal to excite *salivation,* is the reason of why **W. Perfect** could, by using *mercury,* cure permanently a case of *melancholia.* How could the preparations of *Mercury* bring so much of good fame and success to **Seelig**, in the treatment of *membranous quinsy* accompanying *purpura*[37]? How can any physician in the world not know to treat with a sure enough medicine like *Calomel* (**Translator's note:** the German word used by Hahnemann is *Kalomel)* for *quinsy?* **Sauter** cured homoeopathically an *ulcerous inflammation of the mouth accompanied with aphthae* and *flow of foetid saliva,* by prescribing

---

[37] **Translator's note:** A condition characterized by haemorrhage into the skin. Appearance of the lesions varies with the type of purpura, the duration of the lesions and the acuteness of the onset. The colour is first red, gradually darkens to purple, fades to a brownish yellow, and usually disappears in 2 or 3 weeks; colour of residual permanent pigmentation depends largely on the type of unabsorbed pigment of the extravasated blood; extravasations may occur also into the mucous membranes and internal organs

Schwämmchen und Speichelflussgestan-
ke durch Gurgeln mit Sublimatauflösung
wohl anders als 'homöopathisch, das ist,
durch eine ähnliche arzneiliche Krankheitspotenz? — Mehrerer Gemische von Arzneien bediente sich *Hecker* in der *caries*
von Pocken mit sichtbarem Erfolge; zum
Glücke dafs in allen diesen Mischungen
Quecksilber mit befindlich war, von welchem nur allein diefs Uebel besiegt werden
konnte, homöopathisch, da Quecksilber unter allen je bekannt gewordnen Arzneien,
die einzige Potenz ist, welche *Knochen-*
frass specifisch selbst erzeugen kann, wie
so viele übertriebne Merkurialkuren, auch
unvenerische Kuren (Michaelis) bezeugen.
Eben so wird auch dieses bei seinem langwierigen Gebrauche durch Erzeugung des
Beinfrasses so fürchterliche Metall, homöopathisch höchst wohlthätig in Heilung
der *caries* bei Verwundungen der Kno-
chen, wovon uns *Justus Schlegel*, *Joerdens*
und *J. Matth. Müller* (obs. med. chir. Dec. II.
Cas. X.) sehr merkwürdige Beobachtungen
geliefert haben.

Bei Lesung der Schriften über die medicinische *Elektrisität* mufs man über
die nahe Beziehung erstaunen, mit welcher
die von ihr hie und da erzeugten Körperbe-

a solution of *Calomel* (**Translator's note:** the German word used by Hahnemann is *Kalomel)* as a gargle. **Hecker** used various medicinal compounds successfully in a case of *caries occurring after small-pox*. Fortunately all of these mixtures and combinations contained *Mercury,* to which it can be surmised that such diseases yielded (homoeopathically), because *Mercury* is one of the few medicinal substances which can cause *caries of bones,* as is expressed by the many mercurial courses used in the treatment of *venereal* and other diseases, such as those described by **Michaelis**. This metal (*Mercury*), the long use of which is so harmful due to its tendency to cause *caries of bones,* brings a very beneficial homoeopathic influence in the *caries* which follows severe injuries of the bones, some very remarkable cases of which have been observed by **Justus Schlegel, Joerdens**, and **J. Matth. Müller** (*Obs. med. chir.* Dec. II, Cas. X).

57. On perusal of the published writings on the subject of *medical electricity,* one is surprised to see what similarity exists between the morbid symptoms occasionally produced

schwerden und Krankheitszufälle den ganz ähnlichen Körperbeschwerden und Krankheiten entsprechen, welche sie mit Glück und dauerhaft durch Homöopathie geheilt hat. Ich sage hier nichts von den Heilungen die sie schon als entgegengesetzt wirkendes Arzneimittel,[*] bei neu entstandnen Fällen von Gefühlsverlust, Schlagfluss, Lähmungen und schwarzem Staare bei vollkräftigen Körpern zuweilen vollführte — da sie dergleichen auf diese opponirte Weise in chronischen alten Lähmungen und Amaurosen der Natur der Sache nach, nie auszurichten im Stande ist, so wenig als irgend ein andres Palliativ. Ich erwähne blos ihrer homöopathischen Wirkungen. Unzählig sind die Schriftsteller, welche in der Primärwirkung Beschleunigung des Pulses von der positiven Elektrisität wahrnahmen, vollständig *feberhafte Anfälle* aber, blos durch Elektrisität erzeugt, sahen *Sauvages*, *Delas* und *Barillon* bei *Bertholon*. Diese ihre febrilische Tendenz war Ursache, dass *Gardini*, *Wilkinson*, *Syme*, und *Wesley* eine Art *Tertianfieber* einzig mit

[*] Blos in der Nachwirkung sehr heftiger und ungeheurer elektrischen Schläge sind Anwandlung von Lähmung der Glieder, Gefühlsverlust, und Lähmung der Gehör- und Seh-Nerven enthalten.

by this agent and the natural diseases which it has cured homoeopathically in a permanent manner. I am not speaking here about the cures which *Electricity*, as a medicine[Fn] acting in an opposite manner has performed in acute cases of *loss of sensation – apoplexy, paralysis and blindness* in healthy persons, because like other palliatives, according to nature, it is never able to do this in opposite way in old chronic cases of *paralysis and blindness*. I am talking only about its homoeopathic action of electricity, an oppositely acting medicines, were noticed in *recent* cases of *loss of sensation, fits, paralysis and loss of vision*, in robust persons, because, like other palliatives, according to the nature of things, it is *never* able to do this in this opposite manner in *old chronic cases of paralysis* and *blindness*. I have seen instances of homoeopathic effects in the innumerable writings of various authors. Many authors like **Sauvages, Delas, Barillon** and **Bertholon** have observed and recorded the *primary action* produced by *positive electricity* like *acceleration of pulse* very similar to that occurring during *attacks of fever*. **Gardini, Wilkinson, Syme** and **Wesley** were able to cure

---

Fn (Hahnemann's Footnote): It is only during the secondary action of very violent and dangerous electric shocks that one can observe the traces of *paralysis of the limbs, loss of sensation and paralysis of the nerves of hearing and vision.*

Elektrisität heilen konnten, *Zetzel* aber und *Willermoz* sogar *Quartanfieber*. — Sie erregt, wie bekannt, eine den *Zuckungen* ähnliche Verkürzung der Muskeln, und *de Sans* konnte durch sie, so oft er wollte, sogar anhaltende *Konvulsionen* am Arme eines Mädchens erregen; und eben mittelst dieser konvulsivischen Tendenz konnten *de Sans* und *Francklin* (bei *Sauvages*) krankhafte *Konvulsionen* mit Elektrisität stillen. — *Hamilton* und *de Haen* sahen die Elektrisität *rheumatische Schmerzen* hervorbringen, und eben *rheumatische Schmerzen* sind es, welche unzählige Mahle schon von der Elektrisität homöopathisch und dauerhaft geheilt worden sind, wie eine unnennbare Menge Aerzte und Naturforscher bezeugen. — Auch *Hüftweh* selbst, erregte die Elektrisität (*Jallabert* und Philos. Trans. Vol. 63.) und konnte also auch leicht das *Hüftweh* heilen, wie *Hiortberg*, *Lovet*, *Arrigoni*, *Daboueix*, *Mauduyt*, *Syme* und *Wesley* durch ihre Erfahrungen bewährt haben. — Eine Menge Aerzte haben eine Art *Augenentzündung* durch Elektrisität gehoben, nämlich vermittelst eben der Tendenz derselben, wodurch sie selbst *Augenentzündungen* (nach *Patrick*, *Dickson* und *Bertholon*) erzeugen kann. — *Buisson* sah eine *Verhärtung*

types of *tertian fever* because of its tendency to produce such fever and **Zetzel** and **Willermoz** were able to cure a type of *quartan fever* with it only. It is by virtue of this power which electricity possesses to produce *convulsive shortening of muscles* seen by **de sans** and **Franklin** (recorded by **Sauvages**), that **de Sans** was able to stop *convulsions* in the arm of a young girl. **Hamilton** and **de Haen** saw that *electricity* produces *rheumatic pains*, and such pains have been homoeopathically and permanently cured in innumerable cases, as has been testified by a great number of physicians and naturalists. *Electricity* likewise produces a kind of *sciatica* [**Jallobert** and *Philos. Trans. Vol. 63*] and it has also cured *sciatica* as was confirmed by the experiences of **Hiortberg, Lovet, Arrigoni, Daboueix, Mauduyt, Syme** and **Wesley.** Many physicians have cured a type of *ophthalmia* by electricity, that is, many through the power which it possesses of producing similar *inflammation of eyes* (according to the works of **Patrick, Dickson** and **Bertholon**). **Buisson** observed that an *induration of the mammary glands* disappeared by lightning, and **Manduyt** cured *induration of cervical glands* with *electricity;* he could not have done

der Brustdrüsen vom Blitze verschwinden
und *Mauduyt* heilte *verhärtete Halsdrüsen* mit Elektrisität; er hätte es nicht vermocht, wenn dieses Agens nicht schon vor
sich im Stande wäre, *Geschwülste der
Halsdrüsen* zu erzeugen, wie *de Haen* von
ihr sah. — *Fuschel* heilte *Aderkröpfe* (varices) mit Elektrisität, welche diese Heilkraft blos mittelst ihrer (von *Jallabert* beobachteten) Eigenschaft, *Venengeschwul-
ste* zu erregen, besitzt.

Der *Galvanische Metallreitz*, wel-
cher schon vor sich (wie *Ritter*, *Bischoff* und
Geiger vielfältig beobachteten) die Kraft besitzt, die *Muskeln* (der positive Pol die
Strecke - der negative aber die Beuge - Muskeln) *zu verkürzen*, konnte jene dreizehn-
jährige Stummheit (Hufel. Journ. XXIV.) welche in einer *Steifigkeit der Zunge* bestand, in wenigen Tagen, in kleiner Gabe
angewendet (mit einem einzigen Plattenpaa-
re) leicht und vollständig heilen, da die Heilung durch Homöopathie geschah. — Der *un-
erträglich brennend stechende* Schmerz,
den der *Galvanismus* nach Schliessung der
Kette, wie bekannt, an jeder empfindlichen
Stelle unsers Körpers hervorbringt, erklärt
von selbst, wie vor einiger Zeit eine Art
Gesichtsschmerz (tic douloureux) von ei-

this if this agent were not able to cause *swelling of the cervical glands* as seen by **de Haen**. **Fuschel** cured *varices* with *electricity*, and it was because of this property of *electricity* (as observed by **von Jallabert**) to produce *varicose tumours*.

58. The *galvanic metallic current* has the power (according to **Ritter, Bischoff** and **Geiger** after repeated observations) of shortening the muscles (the positive pole acts on the extensor muscles and, the negative pole on the flexor muscles) was able to cure easily and completely in a few days a case of *loss of voice* of thirteen years' standing (*Hufeland's Journal.,* xxiv) which was caused by a *stiffness of the tongue*. A small dose was employed (a single pair of pellets) because the cure was homoeopathic. As is well known, *the intolerable burning pricking pain* which, *Galvanism* produces, after the circuit is closed, in every sensitive part of our body, explains why a kind of *face-ache (tic douloureux)* could be cured by a physician by the use of the Voltaic dry battery.

nem Arzte durch die Voltaische Säule geheilt werden konnte.

Starke *Hitze* eines akuten Fiebers mit 130 Pulsschlägen ward von einem *heisen* Bade von 100° Fahr. sehr gemildert und der Puls bis zu 110 Schlägen herabgestimmt (Albers).

Und so finden sich noch mehrere Heilungen in allen Zeitaltern durch Arzneien von ähnlicher Krankheitspotenz als die zu heilende Krankheit war, schnell und dauerhaft vollführt, deren Urheber ohne zu wissen, was sie thaten, selbst im Widerspruche mit den Lehren aller bisherigen Systeme, und wider ihren Willen, das wohlthätige Heilgesetz der Homöopathie faktisch bestätigen mussten, das sie scientiv anzuerkennen von ihren symbolischen Büchern gehindert wurden.

So hat auch sogar die Hausmittelpraxis der mit gesundem Beobachtungssinn begabten unärztlichen Klasse von Menschen diese Heilart als die sicherste und gründlichste in der Erfahrung befunden.

Auf frisch erfrorne Glieder legt man Schnee oder gefrornes Sauerkraut. — Eine mit kochender Brühe begossene Hand hält der erfahrne Koch in einiger Entfernung dem Feuer nahe, und achtet den anfänglich

59. As was observed by **Albers** that the potent heat of *an acute fever with a pulse of 130* (per minute) was reduced considerably and the pulse brought down to 110 (per minute) by a *warm bath of 100° Fahr.*

60. The rapid and permanent cures that have been brought about by the medicines having similar disease producing power to that of the disease to be cured is in fact in contradiction to the doctrine of the main and existing system of medicine. The illustrations in the various books have become embarrassing to the existing system because it, against their inclination and will, only confirms and helps to recognise the scientificity of homoeopathy.

61. Even in the practice of domestic medicine the non-medical class of people, with sound sense of observation, on the basis of their experience in *domestic practice* have found this healing art as the safest and most rational (well-founded) one.

62. Frozen *Sauerkraut*[38] is frequently applied or rubbed to recently frost-bitten[39] limb; an experienced cook who scalds his hand, holds his scalded hand at a certain (small) distance

---

[38] **Translator's note:** Pickled cabbage salad-a German dish of shredded cabbage fermented in its own juice with salt.

[39] **Translator's note:** Local tissue destruction resulting from exposure to extreme cold; in mild cases, it results in superficial, reversible freezing followed by erythema and slight pain; in severe cases, it can be painless or paresthetic and result in blistering, persistent edema, and gangrene.

dadurch vermehrten Schmerz nicht, da er weifs, dafs er hiemit in kurzer Zeit die verbrannte Stelle zur gesunden, schmerzlosen Haut wieder herstellen kann; — andre verständige Nichtärzte legen auf die verbrannte Stelle ein ähnliches, Brennen erzeugendes Mittel, starken Weingeist oder Terbenthinöl, und stellen sich binnen ein Paar Stunden damit wieder her, während die kühlenden Salben, wie sie wissen, diefs in eben so viel Monaten oft nicht ausrichten. — Der alte kluge Schnitter wird, wenn er auch sonst keinen Brantwein trinkt, doch in dem Falle, wenn er in der Sommergluth sich bis zum hitzigen Fieber angestrengt hat, nicht kaltes Wasser (contraria contrariis) trinken (er kennt das Nachtheilige dieses palliativen Verfahrens), sondern einen mäfsigen Schluck Branntwein; die Lehrerin der Wahrheit, Erfahrung, überzeugte ihn von dem Vorzuge dieses homöopathischen Verfahrens.

Ia es gab sogar von Zeit zu Zeit Aerzte, welche ahneten, dafs die Arzneien durch ihre Kraft, analoge Symptomen zu erregen, analoge Krankheitszustande heilen. So sagt *Hippokrates*, oder der Verfasser des Buchs περὶ τόπων τῶν κατ' ἄνθρωπον (Basil. Frob. 1556. S. 72.) die merkwürdigen Worte: διὰ τὰ ὅμοια

from the fire and does not pay attention to the increase in pain which occurs first, because he knows from his experience that by doing so he can change the burnt (scalded) part into healthy painless skin in a very short time. Other intelligent non-medical persons, for example, the manufacturers of lacquered substance apply to a scalded part with a substance that causes a similar *burning* sensation, such as strong *spirits of wine,* or *oil of turpentine* and by it they cure themselves in the course of a few hours, whereas cooling ointment, as they know well, would not bring a cure in as many months. Experience, the teacher of truth, has convinced an old prudent harvester of the advantage of the homoeopathic procedure and taught him that if the heat of sun causes a violent feverish condition in him, he will not drink cold water *(contraria contrariis)* — as he knows the danger of this palliative procedure rather he takes a small quantity of a *heating* liquor, a mouthful of brandy.

63. There have been physicians who had presentiments that medicines cure analogous symptoms due to its power of producing analogous disease conditions. Thus the author of the book: περι τπων κατ' ανθρωπον[40], (Basil Frob. 1538, S.72) which is among the writings credited to **Hippocrates**, has the following notable words: δια σα δμοια νουσοσ γιυεται και δια σα ομοια προσΦερομενα εκ νοσευντων υγιαινονται, —— δια το

---

[40] **Translator's note:** *On the Localities of Human Beings or On Places and Individuals:* a book by *Hippocrates.*

νῶσος γίνεται, καὶ διὰ τὰ ὅμοια προσΦερόμενα ἐκ νοσεύντων ὑγιαίνονται — διὰ τὸ ἐμέσιν ἔμετος παύεται. — So haben auch nachgängige Aerzte (aufser dem, was *Thomas Erastus* in seinen Disputationen nur so als scholastische Thesis hinwirft) die Wahrheit der homöopathischen Heilart gefühlt. So sieht z. B. *Boulduc* ein (Mem. de l'ac. roy. 1710.), dafs die purgirende Eigenschaft der Rhabarber die Ursache ihrer Durchfall stillenden Kraft sei; — *Detharding* erräth (Eph. N. C. Cent. 10. obs. 76), dafs der Sensblätteraufgufs Kolik bei Erwachsenen stille, vermöge seiner analogen, Kolik erregenden Wirkung bei Gesunden —; und wenn *Bertholon* (Med. Elektr. II. S. 15, vergl. mit S. 282.) gesteht, dafs die Elektrisität denselben (höchst ähnlichen) Schmerz, den sie selbst errege, in Krankheiten abstumpfe und vernichte — und *Thoury* (memoire lu à l'Acad. de Caen), dafs die positive Elektrisität an sich zwar den Puls beschleunige, aber wenn er krankhaft schon zu schnell. sei, denselben langsamer mache — so scheinen beide die homöopathische Kausalverbindung dieser Erscheinungen mit Ueberzeugung anzuerkennen.

So nahe war man zuweilen der Wahrheit!

εμεειν ευετεσ πανεται[41]. The physicians of later times have also felt and expressed the truth of the homoeopathic method of cure (as is seen in the scholarly thesis *Disputations* of **Thomas Erastus**). Thus, for example, **B. Boulduc** observed (*Mem. de l'ac. Roy., 1710*) that the *purgative property* of *Rhubarb*, i.e. *Rheum officinale* **(Translator's note: the German word used by Hahnemann is *Rhabarber*)** was the cause of its power to cure *diarrhoea*. **Detharding** (*Eph. N. C. Cent. 10. obs. 76*), guessed that the infusion of *Senna*, i.e. *Senna acutifolia* **(Translator's note: the German word used by Hahnemann is *Sensblätter*)** leaves relieved *colic* in adults because of its power to produce a similar *colic* in healthy persons. **Bertholon** (*Med. Elektr. II, S. 15, Vergl. mit. S. 282*) admits that in sick persons *electricity* diminishes and removes *pain* very similar to that which it itself produces, **Thoury** (*Memoire la á Pacad. de Caen*) observed that *positive electricity* possesses the power of *increasing the pulse*, but when that is already increased in a disease it reduces its frequency – thus, it appears that both the observations have homoeopathic association but these phenomena were to be recognised and comprehended.

64. Sometimes, so close, was the man to the truth.

---

[41] **Translator's note:** Translation of these Greek lines are: *Diseases are produced by causes of similar character as itself and by the use of things of similar nature the sick (persons) can be cured; vomitings are stopped by things which cause vomiting.*

Organon

der

rationellen Heilkunde

nach

homöopathischen Gesetzen.

ORGANON OF RATIONAL
ART OF HEALING
by
HOMOEOPATHIC PRINCIPLES

1.

Der Arzt hat kein höheres Ziel, als kranke Menschen gesund zu machen, was man Heilen nennt.

2.

Das höchste Ideal der Heilung ist schnelle, sanfte, dauerhafte Wiederherstellung der Gesundheit, oder Hebung und Vernichtung der Krankheit in ihrem ganzen Umfange auf dem kürzesten, zuverlässigsten, unnachtheiligsten Wege, nach deutlich einzusehenden Gründen. (rationelle Heilkunde).

3.

Sieht der Arzt deutlich ein, was an Krankheiten überhaupt und an jedem einzelnen Krankheitsfalle insbesondre zu hei-

A 2

§ 1

The physician has no higher goal than to make sick men healthy, which is called *cure*.

§ 2

The highest ideal of the healing is the rapid, gentle and lasting restoration of health, or the removal and annihilation of disease entirely, in the shortest, most reliable, and least harmful means[1], on easily understandable *principles* (*The Rational Art of Healing*).

§ 3

If the physician can clearly understand what is in each disease in general and particularly in each single case of sickness which is to be cured (*knowledge of disease, knowledge about the essentials of disease - indication*); if he clearly understands

---

[1] **Translator's note:** Hahnemann in all the editions of the Organon wrote 'WEGE' which is the plural of WEG. In German *Weg* means '*road, trail, path, way, means, methods*'. *Unnachtheiligsten* means *least harmful* or *safest*. Thus these two words **Wege Unnachtheiligsten** means **safest means**.

len ist (Krankheitskenntnifs, Kenntnifs
des Krankheitsbedürfnisses — Indikation—); sieht er deutlich ein, was an
Arzneien überhaupt und an jeder Arznei
insbesondre das Heilende ist (Kenntnifs der
Arzneikräfte) und weifs er nach deutlichen Gründen das Heilende der Arzneien
auf das an der jedesmahligen Krankheit zu
Heilende so, dafs Genesung erfolgen
mufs, anzupassen sowohl in Hinsicht der
Angemessenheit der für den Fall nach ihrer Wirkungsart geeignetsten Arznei (Wahl
des Heilmittels — Indikat —) als in
Hinsicht der genau erforderlichen Menge
derselben (rechte Gabe) und der gehörigen
Wiederholungszeit der Gabe — kennt er
die Hindernisse der Genesung in jedem
Falle und weifs sie hinwegzuräumen, damit die Herstellung von Dauer sei: so versteht er durchaus nach zureichen-
den Gründen zu handeln und er
ist ein rationeller Heilkünstler.

4.

Er ist zugleich ein Gesundheit-Er-
halter, wenn er die, Gesundheit störenden

what is the curative principle in drugs in general and in each drug in particular (*knowledge of the powers of medicines*); if according to the distinct reasons he can adapt the healing powers of the drug to the disease that is to be cured so that recovery must follow, and if he has the ability to select the particular remedy whose mode of action is most suitable to the case (choice of the remedy - *the indicated one*), and also the ability to decide the exact quantity of the remedy required (*the required dose*) and the proper period for its repetition, if, I say that he knows all these things and in addition to it, identifies in each case the obstacles to lasting recovery and knows how to remove them, *then he understands thoroughly how to treat according to proper principles, and he is a rational practitioner of the Healing Art.*

§ 4

He is also a preserver of health, if he knows the causes that may disturb health and excite disease and knows how to keep them away from healthy persons.

und Krankheit erzeugenden Dinge kennt,
und sie von den gesunden Menschen abzu-
halten weiſs.

5.

Es läſst sich denken, daſs jede Krankheit auf einer Veränderung im Innern des menschlichen Organismus gegründet seyn müsse: diese wird jedoch blos nach dem, was die äuſsern Zeichen davon verrathen, vom Verstande ge-
ahnet; an sich erkennbar aber auf
irgend eine Weise ist sie nicht.

6.

Das unsichtbare, krankhaft Veränderte im Innern und die merkbare Veränderung des Befindens im Aeuſsern (Symptomen Inbegriff) machen zusammen aus,
was man Krankheit nennt; beide sind die
Krankheit selbst.

Anm. Ich weiſs daher nicht, wie man jenes
bei Krankheiten im Innern des Körpers
krankhaft Veränderte, für etwas der
Krankheit Auſserwesentliches und vor
sich Bestehendes, für eine Bedingung

§ 5

It must be remembered that every disease does depend upon changes in the interior of the human organism. Thus disease can only be understood in mind by its outward indications and all that these symptoms reveal; *in no other way, whatever, can the disease itself be understood.*

§ 6

The invisible changes that produce disease in the interior of man together with the perceivable alterations in health (the totality of its symptoms) make up that what is called disease - both together actually constitute the disease.

Footnote: Therefore I do not know how the morbid changes which occur in disease in the interior of the body could have been considered as a thing existing by itself and *separate from the disease, a cause, as it's inner, immediate, first cause (prima causa).* A thing or a condition requires a first or proximate cause only in order to be produced but once it is produced; it no longer requires a first or a proximate cause for its continued existence.

Thus a disease, once produced continues to exist independent of its initial cause; exists without further need of its cause for its maintenance, persists even if its cause no

der Krankheit, für ihre innere,
nächste, erste Ursache (prima
causa) hat ausgeben können. Eine Sache oder ein Zustand bedürfen doch nur
zum Werden einer ersten nächsten
Ursache; wenn sie aber schon sind, so
bedürfen sie zum Seyn nun keiner Ent-
stehungs-, keiner ersten und nächsten Ursache mehr.

Eben so dauert die nun einmahl entstandne Krankheit fort, unabhängig von
ihrer nächsten Entstehungs - Ursache und
ohne dafs diese noch dazuseyn braucht:
ohne dafs sie noch da ist. Wie hat man
nun wohl ihre Wegnahme zur Hauptbe-
dingung der Krankheitsheilung machen
können? Unmöglich klebt einer fliegen-
den Kugel eine prima causa ihres Flugs an,
und was wir an ihr Verändertes bemerken können, ist blos eine abgeänderte Art
ihrer Existenz, ein abgeänderter Zustand,
und es würde mehr als lächerlich seyn,
zu behaupten, man könne diesen Zustand
nicht anders gründlich aufheben, man
könne die Kugel nicht besser wieder in Ruhe
bringen, als erst durch Ausforschung der
prima causa ihres Flugs, und dann durch
Hinwegnahme dieser metaphysisch erkann-
ten prima causa — oder durch Hinwegnahme der diesem Fluge zum Grunde lie-

longer exists. How then can its removal be held to be essential to the cure of the disease? It is impossible that a *prima causa* of its flight should adhere to the flying bullet, and the alteration we can observe in it is only an altered kind of existence – an altered state, and it would be more than ridiculous to assert that we cannot radically remove this state, that we cannot bring the bullet to rest unless we first investigate the *prima causa* of its flight, and then remove this metaphysically ascertained *prima causa* (as others would explain this), or remove the alterations produced in the inner essence of the bullet on which its flight depends.

Nothing like this! A single force of equal power opposed to the exact direction of the bullet's flight immediately stops, without any metaphysical search, which is impossible, into the inner essence of the state of the bullet in its flight.

For us it is only required to know the symptoms of the flight of the bullet – in other words, the force and the direction of its motion – so that an opposing counter force of equal power can be set against this state and thus bring it to an immediate halt.

genden, (wie sich Andre ausdrücken) im
innern Wesen der Kugel entstandnen Veränderungen.

Mit nichten! Ein einziger dem Fluge der
Kugel in gerader Richtung opponirter Stoſs
von gleicher Gegenkraft bringt sie augenblicklich zur Ruhe, ohne alle metaphysische, unmögliche Erforschungen der innern Wesenheit des Zustandes der Kugel
beim Fluge.

Man braucht blos die Symptomen des
Fluges dieser Kugel, das ist, die Kraft der
Fortbewegung und ihre Richtung genau
zu kennen, um diesem Zustande ein gerade opponirtes Gegenmittel von gleicher
Kraft entgegen setzen und so augenblickliche Ruhe herstellen zu können.

Dieses ist zugleich (sei's im Vorbeigehn
gesagt) ein Beispiel von den übrigen naturgemäſsen Abänderungen der abnormen Zustände physischer Dinge — nämlich
durch das gerade Entgegengesetzte. So wird
das kochende Wasser schnell durch Zusatz
einer gewissen Portion Schnee zur gemäsigten Temperatur herabgestimmt — so verliert die Säure durch das ihr opponirte Laugensalz ihre Schärfe und wird zum Neutralsalze — das allzu Gedehnte sucht sich
zusammen zu ziehen, das Gepreſste sich
auszudehnen — das allzu Trockne zieht

110

This (may it be said as a passing remark) is at the same time an example of the manner in which other alterations can naturally be produced in abnormal conditions of *physical* things, i.e. through their exact opposite. Thus boiling water can be quickly brought to a lower temperature by adding a certain quantity of ice thus an acid becomes a neutral salt by losing its acidity when opposed it with an alkali, and; the overstretched material tries to contract itself whereas the compressed one tries to expand itself, the too dry absorbs moisture from the air, and so on; and thus most of the

genden, (wie sich Andre ausdrücken) im innern Wesen der Kugel entstandnen Veränderungen.

Mit nichten! Ein einziger dem Fluge der Kugel in gerader Richtung opponirter Stoſs von gleicher Gegenkraft bringt sie augenblicklich zur Ruhe, ohne alle metaphysische, unmögliche Erforschungen der innern Wesenheit des Zustandes der Kugel beim Fluge.

Man braucht blos die Symptomen des Fluges dieser Kugel, das ist, die Kraft der Fortbewegung und ihre Richtung genau zu kennen, um diesem Zustande ein gerade opponirtes Gegenmittel von gleicher Kraft entgegen setzen und so augenblickliche Ruhe herstellen zu können.

Dieses ist zugleich (sei's im Vorbeigehn gesagt) ein Beispiel von den übrigen naturgemäſsen Abänderungen der abnormen Zustände physischer Dinge — nämlich durch das gerade Entgegengesetzte. So wird das kochende Wasser schnell durch Zusatz einer gewissen Portion Schnee zur gemäsigten Temperatur herabgestimmt — so verliert die Säure durch das ihr opponirte Laugensalz ihre Schärfe und wird zum Neutralsalze — das allzu Gedehnte sucht sich zusammen zu ziehen, das Gepreſste sich auszudehnen — das allzu Trockne zieht

alterations of the abnormal states of physical things are affected by Nature by means of their opposites.

But, *the vital* organism of animals is governed by very different laws for the removal of its morbidly altered state; in this case the law of opposites, suitable for the alteration of *non-vital* physical nature, is of no use.

Feuchtigkeit aus der Luft an sich; u. s. w. und so werden wohl die meisten Abänderungen der abnormen Zustände physischer Dinge durch Gegensätze von aussen durch die Natur bewerkstelligt.

Der vitale Organismus der Thiere hingegen bedurfte ganz hievon abweichender Gesetze zurEntfernung seines krankhaft abgeänderten Zustandes; da gilt nicht das Gesetz des opponirten Gegensatzes, was zur Abänderung der Zustände der unvitalen physischen Natur das angemessene war.

7.

In den Arzneien muſs ein heilendes Princip vorhanden seyn; der Verstand ahnet es. Aber sein Wesen ist uns auf keine Weise erkennbar—; blos seine Aeuſserungen und Wirkungen lassen sich in der Erfahrung abnehmen.

8.

Der vorurtheillose Beobachter —, er kennt den Unwerth übersinnlicher Spekulationen, die sich in der Erfahrung nicht nachweisen lassen — nimmt, auch wenn er der scharfsinnigste ist, an jeder einzel-

§ 7

The rationality says that there must be a *curative principle* existing in medicine. *But in no way its inner nature* (**Translator's note:** Hahnemann's German word is **Wesen**) *can be ascertained by us* - its manifestations and its outward effects *only* can be judged by experience.

§ 8

The unprejudiced observer, who knows the uselessness of hyper physical speculation, which cannot be confirmed by experience and, however sharp his observation is unable be may takes note of nothing in any single case of disease, except the alterations in the condition of the body and mind which are perceptible by the senses, the *disease phenomena, symptoms* in fact; in other words, he can note only such deviations from a former state of health as are observed by the patient himself, by those around him and the physician. All these perceptible signs together form the disease.

nen Krankheit nichts, als äußerlich durch
die Sinne erkennbare Veränderungen des
Befindens Leibes und der Seele, Krankheitszufälle, Symptomen wahr, das
ist, in die Beobachtung des Kranken über
sich selbst, und des Arztes und der Umstehenden über ihn fallende Abweichungen
vom gesunden, ehemahligen Zustande desselben. Alle diese wahrnehmbaren Zeichen
bilden zusammen die Gestalt der Krankheit.

9

Da an Krankheiten sonst nichts wahr-
nehmbar ist, als diese; so müssen es
auch einzig diese Symptomen seyn, durch
welche die Krankheit Beziehung zur erforderlichen Arznei hat, wodurch sie Anfode-
rung auf Hülfe macht und auf dieselbe hinweisen kann —, so muß dieser Symptomenkomplex, dieses nach außen re-
flektirte Bild des innern Wesens
der Krankheit das einzige seyn, wodurch es — von Seiten der Krankheit —
möglich ward, ein Heilmittel für sie aufzu-
finden, das einzige, was die Wahl des

§ 9

As, then in disease we can depend on nothing except these perceptible symptoms, the disease can make the required remedy known through the symptoms, in fact, through these only, it makes known, both the things, the need of the patient for help and the kind of help that is required. And thus this symptom-complex, *this outward reflection, which represents the inner nature of the disease,* is the only means by which it is possible to find a curative remedy for it, the only means which can point out the most appropriate instrument of cure.

angemessensten **Heilmittels** bestimmen
kann.

10.

Blos der Komplex aller Symptomen
einer Krankheit repräsentirt diese Krankheit in ihrem ganzen Umfange.

Anm. 1. Alle genauere Erfahrungen lehren,
dafs eine beschwerliche, Hülfe erheischen-
de Krankheit fast nie aus einem einzigen
Symptome bestehe, und ein einziges hefti-
ges Symptom fast nie allein da sei. Fast
immer sind mehrere merkbare Krankheitszeichen und Abweichungen vom natürlichen Zustande zugleich, am Kranken wahr-
zunehmen, welche die Einheit des kranken
Gesamtzustandes bilden, so wenig auch einige derselben auf den ersten Anblick Beziehung auf einander zu' haben scheinen.
Ein einziger, leichter Zufall ist keine,
Hülfe fodernde Krankheit.

Anm. 2. Von jeher suchte man, wenn man
sich nicht anders zu helfen wufste, in
Krankheiten hie und da ein einzelnes
der mehrern Symptomen durch Arzneien
zu bestreiten und wo möglich zu unterdrü-
cken — eine Einseitigkeit, welche un-

§ 10

A disease is represented in its whole extent by this complex of its totality of symptoms.

Footnote No. 1: All accurate experience teaches that a difficult and troublesome disease treatment, never consists of one single symptom, and that a single intense symptom seldom, almost never, occurs alone. Almost always there are several observable signs of disease and deviations from the normal health simultaneously present in the patient, which form the unity of the whole disease condition, although at first sight some of them may seem to be not related to one another. A single mild symptom does not constitute a disease requiring treatment.

Footnote No. 2: In every era human beings, not knowing how otherwise to help in cases of disease, tried to combat, by remedies, *one single symptom* out of many symptoms in an individual and, if possible, to suppress it—an *one-sided method* which under the name of *symptomatic treatment* has rightly brought universal criticism, because in that procedure not only there was no benefit gained, but much damage was caused. One single symptom is not the actual disease as one foot is not the whole man.

ter dem Namen, symptomatische Kurart mit Recht allgemeine Verachtung erregt hat, weil durch sie nicht nur nichts gewonnen, sondern auch viel verdorben wird. Ein einzelnes der Symptomen ist so wenig die Krankheit selbst, als ein einzelner Fufs der Mensch selbst ist.

11.

Es läfst sich nicht denken, auch durch keine Erfahrungen in der Welt nachweisen, dafs nach Hebung aller Krankheitssymptomen (des ganzen Konvoluts der wahrnehmbaren Zufälle), etwas andres als Gesundheit übrig bliebe, übrig bleiben könne, so dafs die krankhafte Veränderung im Innern des Organismus ungetilgt geblieben wäre.

12.

Die unsichtbare krankhafte Veränderung im Innern und der Komplex der von aufsen wahrnehmbaren Symptomen sind hienach beide wechselseitig und nothwendig durch einander bedingt, beide bilden zusammen die Krankheit in ihrem Umfange, das ist, eine solche Einheit, dafs leztere

§ 11

It is not understandable, nor can it be established by any experience in the world, that when all the symptoms of disease (the entire totality of perceptible phenomena) are removed, there should, or could remain, anything but a state of health or that the disease causing alteration in the interior of the organism should remain unremoved.

§ 12

The invisible disease-producing alteration in the interior of man and the complex of outwardly observable symptoms are consequently determined by one another reciprocally and compulsorily; both together constitute the whole of the disease, that is, they constitute such a unity that the latter, complex of symptoms, must exist or disappear together with the former, invisible disease-producing alterations in the interior of man, that they must exist together and disappear

mit ersterer zugleich stehen und fallen, dafs
sie zugleich mit einander daseyn und zugleich mit einander verschwinden müssen,
so dafs, wer (was) im Stande ist, die Gruppe der wahrnehmbaren Symptome hervorzubringen, zugleich die dazu gehörige (von
der äufsern Krankheitserscheinung unzer-
trennliche) innere krankhafte Veränderung
im Körper erzeugt haben niufs — sonst
wäre die Erscheinung der Symptomen unmöglich —, und, folglich, wer (was) den
Umfang der wahrnehmbaren Krankheitszeichen hebt, auch zugleich die krankhafte
Aenderung im Innern des Organismus gehoben haben mufs — weil sich die Hebung
der erstern ohne die Verschwindung der
leztern nicht denken läfst.

Anm. Ein ahnungsvoller Traum, eine abergläubige Einbildung, eine feierliche Schicksal-
Prophezeyung des an einem gewissen Tage
und zu einer gewissen Stunde unfehlbar zu
erwartenden Todes brachte nicht selten alle
Zeichen entstehender und zunehmender
Krankheit, des herannahenden Todes und
den Tod selbst zu der angedeuteten Stunde
zuwege, welches ohne gleichzeitige Bewirkung der (dem von aufsen wahrnehmbaren

together, so that whatsoever is able to produce a group of perceptible symptoms, must have caused in the body that corresponding inner morbid change (which is inseparable from the outward manifestation of disease) – otherwise the manifestation of the symptoms would be impossible – and similarly whatever removes the totality of the outward signs of disease must simultaneously have removed the inner morbid change, because the disappearance of the former, the totality of outward signs, without the disappearance of the latter, the inner morbid change, is not unthinkable.

Footnote: A warning dream, a superstitious fantasy, a sincere prediction that death certainly would occur on a particular day and at a particular time, have sometimes produced all the signs of the beginning of and increasing illness and of approaching death and have even caused death itself at the hour predicted, which would not be possible without the simultaneous creation of an inward change (corresponding to the outwardly observable conditions); hence

Zustande entsprechenden) innern Veränderung nicht möglich war — ; und eben
so wurden in solchen Fällen durch eine
künstliche Täuschung oder Gegenüberre-
dung wiederum alle den nahen Tod ankün-
digenden Krankheitsmerkmale nicht selten
verscheucht und plötzlich Gesundheit wieder hergestellt, welches ohne Wegnahme
der Tod bereitenden, innern krankhaften
Veränderungen ebenfalls nicht möglich war.

13.

Da nun in der Heilung durch Hinwegnahme des ganzen Inbegriffs der wahrnehmbaren Zeichen und Zufälle der Krankheit zugleich die ihr zum Grunde liegende
innere Veränderung — also jedesmahl das
Total der Krankheit — gehoben wird, so
folgt, daß der Heilkünstler blos den Inbegriff der Symptomen hinwegzunehmen hat,
um mit ihm zugleich die Veränderung im
Innern — also das Total der Krankheit,
die Krankheit selbst, zu heben, als worauf
einzig das erhabne Ziel des rationellen Heilkünstlers beruhen kann; man müßte denn
das Wesen der Heilkunde nicht in Herstellung der Gesundheit, sondern in Er-

in such cases all the signs of approaching death have been frequently removed, and a state of health suddenly restored, by a similar cause by some skilful deception or persuasion to believe in an opposite conviction, and this again could not have happened without the removal, through a moral (psychical) remedy, of the external and inward alterations which threatened life.

§ 13

In cure effected by the removal of the whole totality of the perceptible symptoms and manifestations of the disease, the internal alteration which caused the symptoms is also removed - the totality of the disease - it means that the physician has only to remove the whole complex of the symptoms in order also to annihilate the internal change - in other words, to remove the whole disease, the disease itself, an achievement which must always be the only aim of the rational healer; because the spirit of the Art of Healing consists in helping the restoration of health, not in searching for the change in the internal and hidden things, a search which can lead to nothing but fruitless speculation.

grübelung der Veränderung im verborgnen
Innern, d. i. in fruchtleeren Spekulationen
suchen wollen.

Anm. Blos vom Misbrauche des zu edlern Ab-
sichten dem menschlichen Geiste verliehe-
nen Triebes, das Unendliche zu erreichen,
entstanden jene kecken Eingriffe in das Ge-
biet des Unmöglichen, jene spekulativen
Grübeleien über das innere Wesen des arzneilich wirkenden Stoffs in den Medika-
menten, über Vitalität an sich, über die
innere, unsichtbare Einrichtung des Organismus im gesunden Zustande und über die,
Krankheit bedingende Abänderung dieses
verborgnen Innern, das ist, über die innere Natur und Wesenheit der Krankheit,
fälschlich „innere nächste Ursache" genannt.

Es blieben aber Spiele der Phantasie und
des Witzes (physiogenische und pathogeni-
sche Poesie), weil uns die zur metaphysi-
schen Kenntniß der innern Vorgänge im innern, lebenden Organismus nöthigen festen
Punkte fehlen und in Ewigkeit fehlen werden, von deren nächstem man stufenweise
zu den übrigen bis an den innersten Ur-
punkt übergehen könne, woran der Men-
schenschöpfer die Bedingung der Krank-

Footnote: It is only due to the wrong direction of the desire implanted in the mind of man to reach the infinite for nobler purposes that these arrogant attempts have been made in the realm of the impossible, those speculative thoughts over the essential nature of the medicinal powers of drugs, over the vitality, over the inner invisible workings of the organism in health and over the changes of this hidden interior working which cause disease—in other words, over the inner nature and essence of disease wrongly called the 'internal proximate cause'.

But this remained a mere play of fantasy and in fact (physiogenic and pathogenic poetry) because the concrete data necessary for obtaining a metaphysical knowledge of the processes that go on in the interior of the living organism are, and will forever be lacking. Next we can pass gradually to the remaining data, until we come to the innermost point, upon which the Creator of man implanted the conditioning of the disease in the holy place of that hidden workshop. All that mankind has learnt about Animal Magnetism, Galvanism, Electricity, attraction and repulsion, Earth Magnetism, Thermal, Phenomena of gases and other objects of chemical and physical enquiry, is of no use in the comprehensive, clear, and useful explanation of even the smallest function in the healthy or diseased states of living organism. What innumerable unknown powers and their laws may be involved in operation in the functions of the living organs of which we can form no conception, and for ascertaining which we should require many more senses than we have, and these senses endowed with infinite delicacy! All these requisites for abstract

heit im Heiligthume jener verborgnen Werkstätte knüpfte. Alles was die Menschenkinder vom thierischen Magnetism, Galvanism, Elektricität, Anziehungs - und Abstoßungskraft, Erdmagnetism, Wärmestoff, Gaslehre und von der übrigen Chemie und Physik etwa aufgefaßt haben, reicht bei weitem nicht hin zur aufschließenden, deutlichen und fruchtbringenden Erklärung auch nur der mindesten Funktion im lebenden, gesunden oder kranken Organism. Welche unzähligen, unbekannten Kräfte und ihre Gesetze mögen bei den Verrichtungen der lebenden Organe noch in Wirkung seyn, die wir nicht einmahl ahnen und zu deren Erkennung uns unendlich mehr Sinne, als wir haben, und von unendlicher Feinheit verliehen seyn müßten! Alle diese zu einer solchen abstrakten Erforschung nothwendigen Erfordernisse, alle jene festen Punkte und Mittelglieder fehlen dem Sterblichen gänzlich — und es ist Mißkenntniß der menschlichen Fähigkeiten und Verkennung der Erfordernisse zum Heilgeschäfte, wenn der Arzt die Ergrübelung solcher Dinge für nöthig ausgiebt, deren Kenntniß ihm so unnöthig ist, als unfähig er zu ihrer Erforschung geschaffen ward.

investigations, all these fixed data and media are withheld from mortal man, and it shows a misconception of human capabilities and of what is required in the business of curing, when the physician insists that the investigation of such things is necessary, then he shows a misconception of the capacities of men and a misunderstanding of the requisites for the process of healing.

Many great thinkers who devoted themselves to this attempt to penetrate into the secrets of nature and so many baseless hypotheses full of contradictions arose. History teaches this, and so does the sound judgement of the most learned brains. If only they had been of the slightest use to practical medicine; if these speculations had only been able to reveal the true remedy for the slightest disease, we might tolerate them! So thought the honest and wise **Sydenham**, who said -

"Quantulacumque in hoc scientiae genere acces sio etsi nil magnificentius quam odontalgias aut clavorum pedibus innascentium curationem, edoceat, longe maximi facienda est, prae inani subtilium speculationum pompa,—quas fortasse medico ad abigendos morbos non magis ex usu futura est, quam architecto ad construendas aedes musicae artis peritia."

Original Page Missing

(**Translator's note:** translation of the above paragraph is:

It is of insignificant importance to have the knowledge about how odontalgia is produced or know the origin of callus of foot which are opinions of totally empty speculation. It is of far-fetched significance, rather, to cure the sickness based on the skills and experience as the skill of a musician become more skilled by experience.)

But what have we seen! all conceivable hypothesis concerning the functions, the inner nature, and composition of different parts of the living brain in health and in disease, all those uncountable conjectures regarding the nature of inflammation, all theories about the nature of water and caloric, were never able, in the world's history, to give a hint or an indication of the specific remedy for the phrenitis caused by sunstroke! **Löffler** discovered it accidentally to consist in sprinkling the skin with hot water, and the rational (Homoeopathic) system of medicine can easily and quickly find by its simple laws this and other specific remedies, without metaphysical elaboration and without having to wait for its coincidental occurrence for another thousand years.

131

Original Page Missing

§ 14

So far, then, as in diseases nothing that indicates the need for help can be discovered by observation except the complex of symptoms, it follows that it is exactly the totality of the perceptible symptoms, and that alone must give the significant indication in disease for the choice of a remedy.

15

Hinwiederum, da das heilende Wesen in Arzneien nicht an sich erkennbar ist, und in reinen Versuchen selbst vom scharfsinnigsten Beobachter an Arzneien sonst nichts, was sie zu Arzneien machte, wahrgenommen werden kann, als jene Kraft, im menschlichen Körper deutliche Veränderungen seines Befindens hervor zu bringen, besonders aber den gesunden Menschen umzustimmen, und mehrere, bestimmte Krankheitssymptomen in und an demselben zu erregen; so folgt, dafs, wenn die Arzneien als Heilmittel wirken, sie ebenfalls nur durch diese Symptomenerregung ihr inneres Heilprincip an den Tag legen und ihr Heilvermögen in Ausübung bringen können, und wir uns also einzig an die krankhaften Zufälle, die die Arzneien im gesunden Körper erzeugen (als die einzige Offenbarung ihrer inwohnenden Heiltendenz) zu halten haben, um zu bestimmen, welche unter den einzelnen Arzneien dem jedesmahligen Krankheitsfalle am angemessensten sei (sobald gefunden ist, worauf diese Angemessenheit beruht).

§ 15

On the other hand, because the curative principle of medicine itself cannot be correctly perceived, and because in pure experiments even by the most acute observers nothing can be observed in drugs which makes them medicines except their power to produce perceptible changes in the health of the human body and to excite, especially in the healthy, distinct symptoms of disease; it becomes clear that, drugs act as remedies because they only make known their inner healing principle and bring their healing power into play through this ability to produce symptoms. And it is more clear further that, if we wish to ascertain which among the several remedies is the most appropriate for any individual case of illness, we can depend on only those disease-phenomena which medicines produce in healthy bodies (for these are the only proof of their inherent healing power).

16.

Da nun Krankheiten nichts aufzuweisen haben, was an ihnen hinwegzunehmen sei, um sie in Gesundheit zu verwandeln, als den Komplex ihrer Symptomen, und auch die Arzneien nichts Heilkräftiges aufweisen können, als ihre Neigung, Krankheits-Symptome zu erzeugen, so folgt, dafs wenn Arzneien wirklich Heilmittel zu werden, das ist, Krankheiten vernichten zu können im Stande sind, dieses nur dadurch erfolgen kann, dafs von gewissen Symptomen, die das Heilmittel erzeugen kann, gewisse Symptomen der Krankheit aufgehoben und vertilgt werden.

17.

Fände man nun in der Erfahrung (wie man auch findet!), dafs ein gegebnes Symptom einer Krankheit blos von demjenigen Arzneistoffe gehoben würde, welcher ein ähnliches unter seinen (im gesunden Körper von ihm erzeugten) Symptomen aufzuweisen hat, so würde es schon wahrscheinlich, dafs diese Arznei durch ihre Tendenz, gleichartige Symptomen zu

§ 16

Now, if diseases have nothing to manifest by removal of which it can be changed into health, excepting the complex of its symptoms, and further, if medicines can show nothing of their curative power except their tendency to produce disease-symptoms, it follows that medicines, to be true remedies, must annihilate and remove the symptoms of disease by the power of the symptoms which they themselves can produce.

§ 17

Now only if, we find in experience (and we do find!) that a particular disease-symptom is only removed by the same medicine (which has produced a similar symptom in a healthy body), then it would be possible that this remedy is capable to annihilate that disease-symptom by virtue of its tendency to bring out similar kind of symptoms.

erregen, fähig werde, an dieser Krankheit
Symptomen gleicher Art zu tilgen.

18.

Fände sichs dann ferner (wie sichs
auch in-der That findet!), dafs diejenige
Arznei, welche in ihrer Einwirkung auf
den gesunden menschlichen Körper alle die
Symptomen zu erkennen gegeben hat, die
die zu heilende Krankheit in sich fafst, bei
ihrem arzneilichen Gebrauche in derselben
auch den ganzen Komplex der Krankheitssymptomen, die ganze gegenwärtige
Krankheit aufhebe und in Gesundheit ver-
wandle, so liefse sich nicht zweifeln, dafs
das Gesetz gefunden sei, nach welchem
diese Arznei auf diese Krankheit heilbrin-
gend gewirkt habe, das Gesetz: gleichartige Symptomen dieser Arznei heben Symptomen gleicher Art in dieser gegebnen
Krankheit auf.

19.

Da sichs nun aber ohne Widerrede,
und ohne den mindesten Zweifel übrig
zu lassen, in Rücksicht j e d e r Arznei und

§ 18

Then if, by experience it is should be found (and, indeed, it is found!) that the same medicine which has caused, in a healthy body, all the symptoms manifested by the disease which it is desired to cure, can remove when used as medicine the entire complex of disease-symptoms that is, the whole existing disease, and change the condition into a state of health, then it cannot be doubted that the law has been discovered whereby this medicine has brought recovery to this disease, namely, the law: *Similar symptoms in the medicine remove similar kind of symptoms in the disease.*

§ 19

Now, as experience proves unquestionably in regard to *every* medicine and *every* disease, that all medicines without exception cure quickly, rationally and permanently, the disease whose symptoms are similar to its own symptoms, we are justified in asserting that *"the curative power of medicines depends on the similarity of their symptoms to the symptoms of disease: or in other words, every medicine which, among the symptoms which it can cause in a healthy body, reproduces most of those present in a particular disease, is capable of curing that disease in the quickest, most rationally and in a most permanent manner."*

jeder Krankheit in der Erfahrung findet, daſs alle Arzneien die ihnen an Symptomen konformen Krankheiten ohne Ausnahme schnell, gründlich und dauerhaft heilen, so hindert uns nichts, festzusetzen; „das Heilvermögen der Arzneien beruht auf ihren, mit den der Krankheit übereinkommenden Symptomen,“ oder mit andern Worten: „jede Arznei, welche unter ihren, im gesunden menschlichen Körper von ihr erzeugten Krankheitszufällen die meisten der in einer gegebnen Krankheit bemerkbaren Symptome aufweisen kann, vermag diese Krankheit am schnellsten, gründlichsten und dauerhaftesten zu heilen.“

20.

Dieses ewige allgemeine Naturgesetz, daſs jede Krankheit durch die ihr ähnliche künstliche Krankheit, die das passende Heilmittel zu erzeugen Tendenz hat, vernichtet und geheilet wird, beruht auf dem

§ 20

This eternal, universal law of Nature, that every disease is annihilated and cured by the similar artificial disease which the proper remedy has the tendency to produce, depends on the following maxim: *that only one single disease can exist in the body at any one time, and therefore one disease must completely yield to another.*

Footnote: The few illustrations which have been brought forward against it are very much under suspicion of being possible misinterpretation and difficult to be taken as clear and indubitable observations.

Satze: daſs immer nur eine einzige Krankheit im Körper bestehen kann, daher durchaus eine Krankheit der andern weichen muſs.

Anm. Die wenigen Beispiele, welche man vom Gegentheile hat anführen wollen, waren der Täuschung allzu sehr unterworfen, als daſs man sie reine, über alle Zweifel erhabne Beobachtungen nennen könnte.

21.

Der Organism erhält nämlich von jeder Krankheit eine besondre Stimmung; eine zweite andre Stimmung von einer neuen Krankheit kann er, seiner an unwandelbare Einheits - Gesetze gebundnen Natur wegen, entweder überhaupt nicht annehmen, oder doch nicht, ohne die erstere krankhafte Stimmung fahren zu lassen; die neue krankhafte Stimmung müſste denn bei ihrer Unfähigkeit die ältere aufzuheben, dem Organism allzu lange aufgedrungen werden, da dann beide verschmelzen zu einer ebenfalls einzigen (dritten) Krankheit, die man mit dem Namen, kom-

§ 21

From every disease the organism receives a particular impression; it either cannot accept another impression from a new disease because of its nature being bound down to unchangeable uniform laws of unity or at least, not without letting the first morbid impression disappear; if the new morbid impression is unable to remove the older one, and is forced upon the organism too long, the two join together to form a single (third) disease, which is termed a complicated disease. This maxim is based on the following facts.

plicirte Krankheit belegt. Diese Satze
gründen sich auf folgende Thatsachen.

§ 2.

Eine chronische, im Körper schon
vorhandne, natürliche Krankheit hält die
Entstehung einer neuen chronischen
Krankheit ab, aufser wenn wenigstens die
neue eine miasmatische oder endemische
ist, deren Ansteckung der Körper fortwäh-
rend geraume Zeit über ausgesetzt blieb.
In diesem Falle, da beide gewöhnlich un-
gleichartig sind, die neue folglich die
alte nicht homöopathisch vernichten kann,
wird entweder die ältere, wenn sie schwa-
cher ist, von der neuen, so lange diese dauert, suspendirt (so verschwand, wie
Schoepf sah, die Krätze, als der Scharbock
eintrat, kam aber nach Heilung des Schar-
bocks wieder hervor), oder es verschmelzen beide zusammen in eine sogenannte komplicirte Krankheit; welche denn aber immer nur eine einzige bildet (einen Mittelzustand von beiden) und
blos wie eine einfache zu behandeln und
homöopathisch zu heilen ist nach dem To-

§ 22

A natural chronic disease already existing in the body opposes the appearance of a new chronic disease, unless at least the latter be a *miasmatic*[2] or *endemic* disorder and the body has been unduly exposed to it over a long period of time. In such a case, as mostly the two diseases are dissimilar, the new disease cannot senove the earlier homoeopathically, and either the former, if it is a weaker disease, is suspended as long as the latter lasts (as **Schoepf** saw an itching skin eruption disappear when the patient was affected by Scurvy, only to return, however, after the Scurvy was cured), or the two diseases combine into one so-called complicated disease; which, though complicated, always present a single disease-picture, (intermediate between the two disease-pictures), and can be treated and cured homoeopathically by the totality of the newly united symptom-complexes just like a simple disease. From the time of the second contagion up to the time of the combination of both into a (third) single (complicated) disease, the first affection remains latent.

---

[2] **Translator's note:** The word *miasm* has been used here not in the sense that we understand after reading the later editions of Organon and Chronic Diseases. It does not mean the fundamental cause here. Here the *miasm* is used to mean the miasma or the pollutant which as was understood during the time to be responsible for most of the severe diseases.

tal des neu vereinigten Symptomenkomplexes. — Von der Zeit der zweiten Ansteckung an bis zur Verschmelzung beider in eine (dritte) einzige (komplicirte), schweigt die ältere.

> Anm. So kann eine ganz frisch entstandne Krätze an einem noch ungeheilten venerischen Kranken zwar noch, während die venerischen Symptomen indefs schweigen, mit der ihr eigenthümlichen Arznei geheilt werden; kommen aber die (durch die Krätze abgeänderten) venerischen Symptomen wieder hervor, so ist die Vereinigung beider zu einer dritten (komplicirten) Krankheit geschehen, und der Ausschlag kann nun nicht mehr mit Schwefel geheilet werden.
> Die Vereinigungen (Komplikationen) des Scharbocks, der venerischen Krankheit, des Wichtelzopfs u. s. w. sind nicht selten.

23.

Ungleich häufiger aber als die von selbst verschmelzenden (und sich so komplicirenden) natürlichen Krankheiten sind die künstlichen, wenn auf einen mit einem chronischen Uebel behafteten Körper

Footnote: So, a quite newly developed scabies on a still unhealed venereal patient can regress by its specific medicine; but the venereal symptoms again recurs (with the altered scabies) and its combination forms a third (complicated) disease, and the eruption now can not be cured by Sulphur.

The combination of scurvy, venereal diseases, matted hairs, etc. are not rare.

§ 23

But incomparably more common than the combination (and, therefore, the complication,) of natural diseases, are the artificial diseases, caused by unsuitable treatment applied for a prolonged time to the bodies suffering from chronic disease. Such a treatment, which does not have power similar to that of the disease for which it is given, is unable to remove it and cure it homoeopathically; but on the contrary they attack the organism over a long period of time in a dissimilar way, and thus gradually produce an inner condition of a dissimilar type. In short, an artificial chronic disease combines with

langwierige, unpassende Kuren wirken, das ist, künstliche Krankheitspotenzen, welche durch keinen analogen Gegenreiz die alte Krankheit aufzuheben vermögen und sie nicht homöopathisch heilen können, sondern den Körper in einer disparaten Richtung geraume Zeit lang angreifen, und ihm so nach und nach eine andersartige innere Umstimmung, eine künstliche andersartige chronische Krankheit beibringen, die mit dem alten chronischen Uebel sich vereinigt und so ein neues monströses Uebel, eine komplicirte Krankheit bildet, oft von sehr empörender Art.

Anm. Mehrere in ärztlichen Iournalen zur Konsultation aufgestellte Krankheitsfälle sind von dieser Art, so wie andre in medicinischen Schriften erzählte chronische Krankengeschichten. Von gleicher Art sind die häufigen Fälle, wo die venerische Krankheit unter langwieriger Behandlung mit unpassenden Quecksilberpräparaten nicht heilt, sondern sich mit dem indels allmählig erzeugten chronischen Quecksilbersiechthume zu einem grausamen Mitteldinge von komplicirter Krankheit (verlarvte venerische Krankheit) verbindet, die nun

the original chronic disease and so forms a new monstrous malady, *a complicated disease,* which is often of a very difficult kind.

Footnote: Numerous cases of diseases which are published in medical journals seeking advice for the treatment are of this type, and are similar to many case-histories of chronic diseases described in medical writings. To the same type belong those numerous cases in which venereal disease is not cured by prolonged treatment with unsuitable preparations of Mercury, rather it joins together with *chronic Mercury poisoning* to make a terrible combination of complex disease (Masked Venereal Disease), which now can not be cured with Mercury (the remedy for venereal disease), but must be treated with Potassium sulphide (the remedy for Mercury poisoning).

nicht mehr weder mit (dem Heilmittel
der venerischen Krankheit) Quecksilber,
noch mit (dem Heilmittel der Quecksilberkrankheit) Schwefelleber zu heilen ist.

24.

Wird hingegen einem mit einer chronischen Krankheit behafteten Körper eine
neue, mehr lokale und deshalb weniger
mit jener verschmelzbare Krankheit künstlich aufgedrungen, welche keine
Aehnlichkeit mit ersterer hat, folglich die ältere nicht homöopathisch heilen
kann, so wird gewöhnlich die chronische
natürliche Krankheit so lange suspendirt, als die künstliche unterhalten wird.

Anm. Zwei mit Fallsucht behaftete Kinder
wurden durch Ansteckung mit Grindköp-
fe von den epileptischen Anfällen, an denen sie gelitten hatten, indefs frei; sobald aber die Köpfe wieder heilten, war
auch die alte Fallsucht bei beiden wieder
da, wie *Tulpius* sah. — Schon mehrere
Epileptische blieben von ihren Anfällen
frei, so lange die ihnen gelegten Fontanel-
len im Gange erhalten wurden; verfielen
aber sogleich wieder in die bisher nur aus-

§ 24

On the other hand, if a chronic disease is present in an organism, and if the patient is attacked with a new, more local, and hence less severe artificial disease, which has no similarity to the first and therefore cannot cure it homoeopathically, then usually the chronic natural disease is suspended as long as the artificial disorder lasts.

Footnote: Tulpius observed that two children affected with epilepsy remained free from epileptic fits after they were infected with ringworm of the scalp. But as soon as their scalp had become free from ringworm the old epilepsy appeared again. Even severe epilepsy remained suppressed by a cautery[3] – wound or issue[4] created but the suspended epilepsy, reappeared with greater violence when the artificial ulcers were allowed to heal as was seen by **Pechlin** and many others.

---

[3] **Translator's note:** *Cautery:* An agent used for scaring or burning the Skin or tissues by means of heat or of caustic chemicals. It was formerly a method of checking or controlling humours.

[4] **Translator's note:** *Issue:* A suppurating sore, acting as a counter – irritant maintained by the presence of foreign body in the tissues; it was formerly regarded as means of escape for peccant humors.

pendirte Fallsucht, wenn man die künstlichen Geschwüre (und wenn es erst nach
vielen Iahren geschah) wieder zuheilen
liefs. *Pechlin* und mehrere Andre führen hiervon Beispiele an.

25.

Ist schon eine alte chronische, entweder künstliche oder natürliche Krankheit
im Körper, so wird von dieser, als der stärkern, eine neue akute andersartige
natürliche Krankheit, auch oft eine künstlich aufgedrungene akute Krankheit vom
Organism abgehalten.

Anm. Leute, die an Flechten leiden, sind
nach *Larrey* frei von der Pestansteckung,
und durch unterhaltene Fontanelle und
beständige Blasenpflaster (d. i. künstliche
(lokale) chronische Krankheiten) bleiben die
Europäer in Syrien frei von der Ansteckung
der levantischen Pest, wie in neuern Zeiten *Larrey*, in ältern aber *van Hilden* und
F. Plater beobachtet haben. Mehrere chronische Krankheiten, (flechtenartige Aus-
schläge und andre Hautkrankheiten, *Ien-
ner*) vorzüglich aber die Rachitis lassen die
Schutzpockenimpfung nicht haften, so wie
das durch tägliches Koffertrinken bei Kin-

§25

When a chronic disease, either artificial or natural, is already present in an organism, and because it is stronger, it will repel from the organism a new acute *dissimilar* natural disease, and will often *restrain* an artificial acute disease from manifesting on the organism.

Footnote: According to **Larrey** people who suffer from Herpes are free from infection of Plague and by maintaining continuous Issues or blistering-plaster on fontanelles [i.e. artificial (local) chronic wound), the Europeans in Syria had remained free from being infected by Plague of Levant as it had been observed by **Larry** in the recent times and **van Hilden & F. Plater** in the olden times. Several chronic diseases (herpetic eruptions and other skin diseases as per **Jenner**), the Rachitis prevents cow-pox vaccine from taking effect, just as drinking of coffee everyday by children creates chronic ill health as this vaccine produces defence by generating false vaccine-pustules.

dern erzeugte Siechthum diese Impfung mächtig abwehrt, oder doch öfters unächte Vaccinepusteln erzeugt.

26.

Wird aber einem mit einem chronischen Uebel behafteten Körper eine neue akute Krankheit dennoch a u f g e d r u n g e n, und leztere ist stärker, aber u n g l e i c h a r t i g, so schweigt die chronische Krankheit nur so lange (wird s u s p e n d i r t), als die akute ihren Verlauf hält und kömmt dann ungeändert wieder hervor.

A n m. Wie die geschwürige Lungensucht stillsteht, wenn die Menschenpocken ausbrechen, und sich wieder erneuert, sobald sie abgetrocknet sind.

27.

Wird ein schon mit einer akuten Krankheit behafteter Körper mit einer neuen akuten, aber andersartigen Krankheit angesteckt, so weicht die eine, welche die schwächere ist, wird aber nicht vernichtet, sondern blos so lange s u s p e n d i r t, bis die stärkere ihren Lauf vollendet hat.

§ 26

When the organism suffering from a chronic illness, is affected by a new and acute disease and the new acute disease proves to be stronger than the first disease, but is not similar to it, then the chronic disease does not produce symptoms (is *suspended*) while the acute disease runs its course, and then reappears in an unchanged form afterwards.

Footnote: Just as ulcerous phthisis remains latent, when small-pox erupts, and would again reappear as soon as it dries up.

§ 27

When the organism suffering from an acute disease is affected with another new acute disease of a *dissimilar* type, the disease which is the weaker of the two disappears, but is not annihilated, and remains *suspended* until the stronger disease has run its course.

Anm. Die zuerst ausgebrochenen Masern verschwinden sogleich, sobald die Kindblattern ausbrechen, und erst wenn diese ab-
geheilt sind, kommen die bis dahin suspen-
dirten Masern wieder zum Vorscheine, und
vollenden ihren Lauf. — Einen Bauerwä-
zel (Mumps) sah ich sogleich verschwinden, als die Schutzpockenimpfung gehaf-
tet hatte, und erst nach Beendigung der
Vaccine, als die peripherische Entzündung
vergangen war, kam die fieberhafte Ohr-
und Unterkiefer-Drüsengeschwulst (Bau-
erwäzel) wieder hervor, und verlief wie
gewöhnlich. — Wie die Vaccinepusteln am
achten Tage zur Vollkommenheit waren,
brachen die (den Körper schon vorher angesteckt habenden) Masern aus und die Kuhpocke stand still; erst nachdem die Masern
sich abschuppten, gieng die Vaccine ihren
Weg wieder fort bis zu Ende (*Kortum*) —.
Schon entwickeltes Scharlachfieber mit
Bräune ward vier Tage unterbrochen und
suspendirt, während die Kuhpocke und
ihre Areola entstanden (*Jenner*).

23.

Wird dagegen dem schon mit einer
akuten Krankheit behafteten Organism die

Footnote: The earlier eruption of Measles disappears as soon as Small-pox eruptions appear, and not until these are healed, the eruption of Measles, which remain suspended till then, appear again and complete its regular course. I have seen that of Parotitis (Mumps) disappeared when cow-pox vaccine took effect, the febrile tumefaction of the parotid and sub-maxillary glands (Parotitis) appeared and ran its usual course only after the effect of vaccination disappeared. Even after the measles had broken out (the body already infected earlier) the cow-pox vaccine took effect, but did not run its course until these vaccine-pustules had disappeared (**Kortum**). Furthermore, a case of Scarlet Fever with Tonsillitis was halted for four days and suspended while the Cow-pox and its areola developed (**Jenner**).

§ 28

On the contrary, if an acute disease attacks an organism which is already suffering from a *similar* acute disease, then the *stronger of the two diseases annihilates the weaker completely and removes it homoeopathically.*

Footnote: So, the small-pox abrogates an already manifesting cow-pox completely; the cow-pox does not complete, its full course but is destroyed, whereas sometimes it has an appearance as if the cow-pox had been transformed into small-pox which then continues to run its course till the end.

gleichartigen Krankheit aufgedrungen, so hebt die stärkere die schwächere gänzlich auf und vertilgt sie homöopathisch.

Anm. So hebt die zu Schutzpocken kommende Kindblatterkrankheit erstere gänzlich auf; die Schutzpocken kommen nicht zur Vollendung, sondern werden vernichtet, wo es dann zuweilen den Anschein hat, als ob die Schutzpocken sich in Kindblattern verwandelten, welche leztern dann einzig ihren Lauf fortsetzen bis zu Ende.

29.

Zwei akute zu einander in denselben Körper kommende Krankheiten verschmelzen nicht mit einander; die etwa hievon angeführten Fälle sind nur scheinbar.

Anm. Durch die ihrer Reise schon nahe gekommene Vaccinepustel werden die nun ausbrechenden Kindblattern oft zwar sehr in ihrem Anschn geändert, gutartig, einzeln stehend, von einem breitern, rothen Hofe umgeben, sind mehr warzenartig, und enthalten wenig Eiter; aber dieser Eiter bringt bei der Fortimpfung dennoch nichts

§ 29

When two acute diseases meet together in the same organism, they never complicate each other; as is only apparent from the cases cited.

Footnote: When the cow-pox vaccine-pustule, approaches to its time of maturity, it more than often changes the appearance of the small-pox that has already broken out – benign, single and separately, surrounded by broad red areolae, root-like in shape and contain little pus. But this pus produces nothing different from real small-pox with further vaccination (**Muhry**). Two acute diseases mingle so little with one another that one has examples where few moments before the fever of pox had appeared with vaccination and still many children were vaccinated successfully with the lymph from the vaccine-pustules were affected with artificial cowpox (**Hardege D.J.**). *Two similar acute diseases never strengthen one another and they destroy one another homoeopathically (the stronger- the weaker)*

anders als wahre Kindblattern hervor (*Muhry*). Zwei akute Krankheiten verschmelzen so wenig mit einander, dafs man Beispiele hat, wo wenige Augenblicke vorher, ehe bei der Vaccination das Fieber des Menschenblatterausbruchs erschien, mit der Lymphe aus den Vaccinepusteln noch andre Kinder geimpft wurden, mit dem reinen Erfolge, dafs blos ächte Kuhpocken davon erschienen (*Hardege d. j.*). Z w e i
a k u t e g l e i c h a r t i g e K r a n k h e i t e n
h e b e n e i n a n d e r b l o s a u f, u n d
v e r n i c h t e n e i n a n d e r h o m ö o p a-
t h i s c h (die stärkere die schwächere).

30.

Eben so, wenn schon eine chronische
Krankheit im Körper liegt, und es wird ihm
eine s e h r ä h n l i c h e akute Krankheit aufgedrungen, s o w i r d d i e c h r o n i s c h e
v o n d e r a k u t e n g ä n z l i c h v e r n i c h-
t e t u n d h o m ö o p a t h i s c h g e h e i l t.

A n m. So heilt die Schutzpockenimpfung, deren Miasm nächst der Kraft, Kuhpocke hervorzubringen, zugleich einen Ansteckungszünder zu einem Hautausschlage von kleinen, in ihrem Umkreise rothen Pusteln (pimples) enthält (und bei einigen Körpern

§ 30

Further more, if a chronic disease is already present in body, and a very similar acute disease attacks the patient, *the chronic disease is completely annhilated by the acute and is homoeopathically cured.*

Footnote: Inoculated small pox, whose miasm possesses besides the power to produce cow-pox, to excite a contagion of a small, skin rash containing (as produced by actually coalescing the bodies), which it can cure, completely and permanently, some of the similar, often very old skin-rash, as many of the factual observation proves.

Thus, an old humid herpes was completely cured by breaking out of the measles (Hufeland's Journal, XXIII).

Leroy [Heilkunde für Mütter, p. 384, **(Translator's note: The Therapy for the Mother, p. 384)]** saw one lingering, very obstinate ophthalmia in a boy disappear after appearance of small pox, whose nature is to produce ophthalmia in its acute stage.

wirklich hervorbringt) einige diesem ähnliche, oft sehr alte Hautausschläge vollkommen und dauerhaft, wie eine Menge
Thatsachen erweisen. —

Eben so ward ein älter feuchtender Herpes durch die hinzugetretenen Masern vollkommen geheilt (*Huf.* Iourn. XXIII).

Leroy (Heilk. f. Mütter S. 584) sah eine
langwierige, sehr hartnäckige Augenentzündung bei einem Knaben durch die Men-
schenblatterkrankheit auf immer verschwinden, in deren Natur es liegt, Augenentzündung selbst zu erzeugen in ihrem akuten Stadium.

Durch Einimpfung der Menschenblattern
ward eine hartnäckige Augenentzündung
gehoben von *Dezoteux* (traité de l'inoculation S. 189). Und so sind mehrere dergleichen Fälle bei den Krankheitsbeobach-
tern anzutreffen.

51.

Auf diesem uns von der Erfahrung aufgestellten Gesetze der Menschennatur, daſs
Krankheiten b l o s von gleichartigen Krankheiten vernichtet und geheilet werden, beruht das groſse homoopathische Heilgesetz:
daſs eine Krankheit blos von einer
Arznei vernichtet und geheilet

According to Dezoteux [*Traité* de *L'inoculation*, p. 189 **(Translator's note:** A Treatise on Inculcation, p.189)], an obstinate ophthalmia was cured by the inoculation of small pox. In additions it, several similar cases of the disease were observed.

§ 31

The great Homoeopathic Law of Cure, taught by experience, is based on a Law of nature that diseases are annihilated and cured by a similar disease. The Homoeopathic Law of Cure is : *A disease can only be annihilated and cured by a remedy which has the tendency to produce a similar and homogenous disease, because the effects of such medicines are nothing but (artificial) diseases.*

werden kann, welche eine gleichartige und ähnliche Krankheit zu
erzeugen geneigt ist — denn die
Effekte der Arzneien vor sich sind
nichts anders, als künstliche
Krankheiten.

32.

Die Tinktur von einer Unze Chinarinde mit ein Paar Pfund Wasser gemischt
und in Tag und Nacht allmählig ausgetrun-
ken, bringt nicht weniger gewifs ein mehr-
tägiges Chinafieber, und ein laues Fufs-
bad von Arsenikauflösung oder eine auf den
Haarkopf gestrichene Arseniksalbe nicht
weniger gewifs ein wenigstens vierzehnt.-
giges Arsenikfieber zuwege, als der
Aufenthalt in herbstlicher Sumpfluft ein
gewöhnliches Wechselfieber zuwege
bringt. Ein Gürtel von Merkurialpflaster
um die Hüften gelegt *) bringt wohl noch
schneller und gewisser die Quecksilberkrankheit hervor, als das angelegte Hem-
de von einem Krätzigen die Wollarbei-

---

*) Eine der ältesten Gebrauchsarten des Quecksilbers zu
Anfange des sechszehnten Iahrhunderts.

C

§ 32

The tincture of an ounce of Cinchona-bark **(Translator's note:** *Cinchona officinalis)* mixed with two pounds of water and taken in the course of a day and night (twenty-four hours) will definitely cause a *China fever* of many days duration; and warm foot-bath of a solution of Arsenic or the application of an arsenical ointment on the scalp will as certainly produce *Arsenic fever* lasting at least a fortnight, as living in a marshy area in autumn will cause *Intermittent fever.* A girdle made of mercurial plaster around the hips[Fn] will cause *Mercurial disease* (poisoning) as quickly and certainly as wearing the shirt of a person affected with the itch will produce an attack of the itch. A strong infusion of *Hollunderblüthen* **(Translator's note:** the German common name of Elder flower, i.e. *Sambucus nigra.* However it is interesting to note that in paragraph no. 29 of Introduction, Hahnemann has used a different German common name of elder, i.e. *Schwarzholder)* or a few berries of Belladonna **(Translator's note:** Atropa belladonna) are just as surely disease-producing or pathogenetic forces as inoculated vaccine matter or a viper bite, or a great fright, and each of these influences being disease-forces can as soon as face to face with a similar disease already present in the body, becomes a remedy and a force for the purpose of expelling it, become for the same

ter-Krätze hervorbringt. Ein kräftiger Hollunderblüthen - Aufguſs, oder einige verschluckte Belladonnebeeren sind eben so gewiſs krankmachende Potenzen, als eingeimpfter Kindblatterstoff, oder ein Viperbiſs, oder ein Schreck, und jeder dieser Einflüsse kann aus gleichem Grunde, als er Krankheits-Potenz ist, sobald er einer schon im Körper vorhandnen ähnlichen Krankheit zu ihrer Vertreibung entgegen gesetzt wird, aus gleichem Grunde zur Gegenkrankheitspotenz, zum Heilmittel werden, so daſs alles was wir Arznei nennen, nichts anders als Krankheit erregende Potenz, und alle wahre Heilmittel nichts anders als Potenzen sind, welche eine ähnliche Gegenkrankheit im Organism kunstlich zu erzeugen fähig und dadurch die ähnliche natürliche Krankheit aufzuheben und zu vernichten im Stande sind.

33.

Freilich wird, wenn wir nach den Regeln der rationellen Heilkunde eine der zu

reason a counter-disease-force, a remedy; *so that all that we call medicine is nothing but a pathogenetic force, and all true remedies are only forces which are able to produce, artificially, a similar counter-disease in the organism, and thereby to remove and annihilate the similar natural disease.*

Footnote: One of the oldest similar uses of mercury at the beginning of the 16th Century.

§ 33

When, according to the rules of the Rational Therapy we have found the medicine which is most suitable for curing a disease under treatment and have used it as a remedy, it is clear that the sick organism is, as it were, affected with a new disease (counter-disease) by virtue of the disease-producing power inherent in the drug; but it must be accepted that this artificial counter-disease possesses greater advantages over all natural counter-diseases.

kurirenden Krankheit möglichst angemessene Arznei gefunden haben und sie nun als Heilmittel anwenden, durch eine solche künstliche Krankheitspotenz dem schon kranken Organism eine neue Krankheit (Gegenkrankheit) gewissermasen eingeimpft und, so zu sagen, aufgedrungen; aber, man muſs gestehen, eine Gegenkrankheit von ungemeinen Vorzügen vor allen natürlichen Gegenkrankheiten.

34.

Die unsichtbaren Einflüsse, von welchen die gewöhnlichen Krankheiten des Menschenlebens erregt zu werden pflegen, sind uns allzu wenig bekannt, stehen auch allzu wenig in unsrer Gewalt, als daſs wir durch sie Krankheiten bequem und nach Willkühr hervorbringen, sie mehrern ältern Krankheiten als Heilmittel entgegen setzen, und so Gesundheit, wo es nöthig, damit wiederbringen könnten.

35.

Selbst der zur Entfernung einiger Krankheiten einzuimpfenden Miasmen sind zu wenig, als daſs man von ihnen auch nur

C 2

§ 34

The invisible influences by which the common diseases of human beings are usually produced are very little known, and are all very little under our control, to help us to use them for producing (artificial) diseases at our will, and thus use them as remedies against many diseases of longer standing so that we can restore health whenever necessary.

§ 35

Even those miasms[5], which might conceivably be inoculated for the removal of some diseases, are very few in number to enable us to make even a limited use of them as remedies.

---

[5] **Translator's note:** Miasms meant pollutants. Here the *miasm* is used not in the sense of dynamic fundamental cause of disease rather to mean the material factors which supposedly cause the disease.

einen mäfsig ausgedehnten Gebrauch als Heilmittel machen könnte.

36.

Könnten wir auch wirklich mehrere natürliche Krankheiten durch Kunst und nach Willkühr veranstalten, so sind sie entweder der damit zu heilenden Krankheit nicht analog genug, folglich nicht hülfreich, oder sie sind auch selbst von längerer Dauer, und wenn sie ja das ältere Uebel bezwungen hätten, so behaupten sie sich dagegen selbst oft noch geraume Zeit im Körper, verschwinden selten vor sich, und müssen gewöhnlich durch künstliche Hülfe wiederum gezwungen werden, zu entweichen.

Anm. Beispiele giebt die eingeimpfte Wollarbeiter-Krätze, womit man hie und da einige chronische Krankheiten heilte.

37.

Unendlich leichter hingegen, weit gewisser und mit ungemessener Auswahl können wir uns zum Heilzwecke jener Krankheitspotenzen bedienen, die man gewöhn-

§ 36

Even if we were able to produce artificially many kinds of natural diseases and whenever we desired, they are either not sufficiently similar to the disease under treatment, and therefore not useful, or they are themselves of longer duration than the original disease, and hence, even when they have actually over-come the older evil (disease), they frequently remain for a long time in the organism, seldom go away of themselves, and usually require the help of Healing Art to force to be removed them.

Footnote: There are examples where one cured a few chronic diseases now and then with the inoculated wool-sorter's itch.

§ 37

On the other hand, we can use, more easily, with greater certainty and with an almost unlimited varieties; the disease-producing forces generally called *drugs* or *medicines* for the purposes of cure, we can give to the counter-disease thereby caused (which is to remove the natural disease that we are asked to treat) a regulated strength and duration, because we can regulate the size and weight of their doses; and as every medicine differs from all others and possesses a wide sphere of action, we have in the large number of medicinal substances an unlimited number of artificial diseases in our hand, which with a correct selection can oppose the natural course of the diseases and infirmities of human beings, and so, we are able to remove and destroy natural diseases quickly and certainly, by means of artificially produced very similar diseases.

lich Arzneien zu nennen pflegt; der durch
sie zu erregenden Gegenkrankheit (welche
die natürliche Krankheit, zu der wir ge-
rufen werden, aufheben soll) können wir
gemessene Stärke und Dauer geben, weil
Maas und Gewicht ihrer Gaben in unsrer
Gewalt steht, und da jede Arznei abweichend von jeder andern, und vor sich
schon vielfach wirkt, so haben wir in der
grofsen Menge der Anzneistoffe eine uner-
mefsliche Zahl künstlicher Krankheiten in
unsrer Hand, die wir den im Laufe der Natur entstehenden Krankheiten und Gebrechen der Menschenkinder mit treffender
Wahl entgegen setzen und so Naturkrank-
heit mit höchst ähnlicher, künstlich erreg-
ter Gegenkrankheit schnell und sicher aufheben und auslöschen können.

58.

Da es nun weiter keinem Zweifel unterworfen ist, dafs die Krankheiten des
Menschen blos in Gruppen gewisser beson-
drer Symptomen bestehen, durch einen Arzneistoff aber blos dadurch, dafs dieser ähn-

172

§ 38

Now, it is no more a matter of doubt that the diseases of mankind consist only of certain groups of specific symptoms, and may be annihilated and restored into health (such is the process in all genuine cures) truly by a medicine, but only by such a medicine which can artificially produce similar disease-symptoms. Hence the art of cure comprises of finding a solution to the following three points—

I. How can the physician ascertain what he needs to know of the disease in order to cure it?

II. How can he know the individual disease-producing powers of medicines which are to act as opposite-diseases for the cure of natural diseases?

III. How can he employ the most suitable method of using these artificial disease-producing powers (medicines) for the cure of natural diseases?

liche krankhafte Symptomen künstlich zu
erzeugen vermag, vernichtet und in Gesundheit verwandelt werden (worauf der
Vorgang aller achten Heilung beruht), so
wird sich das Heilgeschaft auf Beantwor-
tung folgender Punkte beschranken:

I. Wie erforscht der Arzt was er von der
   Krankheit zu Heilabsichten zu wissen
   nöthig hat?

II. Wie erforscht er die als Gegenkrank-
    heit, zur Heilung der natürlichen
    Krankheiten bestimmte, krankmachen-
    de Potenz der Arzneien?

III. Wie wendet er diese künstlichen
     Krankheitspotenzen (Arzneien) zur
     Heilung der naturlichen Krankheiten
     am zweckmasigsten an?

39.

Was den ersten Punkt betrifft, so
kann die ungeheure Verschiedenheit und
Menge der Krankheiten leicht verleiten,
zu glauben, man könne ihre übergrofse

§ 39

In regard to the first point, the huge number and number of diseases might easily mislead us into a believing that due to their enormous variety it is impossible to retain them in the memory and keep in mind their great diversity; and that they cannot be cured if one is notable to have a comprehensive view of the whole and if we can not arrange them into small compartments so as to be able to treat each subject in reference to common characteristics and similarities from numerous and varied individual cases of disease, as if they were a single disease, by which their treatment and alleviation would be possible.

Mannigfaltigkeit unmöglich ins Gedächt-
nifs fassen und überschauen und sie daher nicht heilen, wenn man keinen fafs-
lichen Ueberblick über das Total gewin-
nen, und sie nicht in wenige Fächer von
kleinem Umfange vertheilte, um die da in
jedes einzelne Fach nach einigen gemeinsamen Beziehungen und Aehnlichkeiten
aufgestellten vielen und mancherlei Krankheitsindividuen sämtlich überein, gleichsam als eine einzige Krankheit, nach allgemeinen Formen arzneilich behandeln,
und sich so ihre Kur erleichtern zu können.

40.

Die Krankheiten, Gebrechen und
Siechthume sind aber so unendlich mannig-
faltige Erscheinungen, dafs eine brauch-
bare Klassification derselben nicht einmahl
möglich wäre, wenn auch eine solche ge-
zwungene Zusammenfassung derselben in
getrennte Fächer zur Heilabsicht erforderlich zu seyn scheinen sollte.

Anm. Die bisherigen systematischen Einthei-
lungen der Krankheiten (fast jede Patho-

§ 40

The diseases, infirmities and chronic ill-healths are such infinitely diverse phenomena that their useful classification is not possible, even if such a forced compilation of them into separate classes seem to be necessary requisite for cure.

Footnote: I shall not go over the prevailing systematic classification of diseases though (almost every work on pathology has a different classification, which suits him). Had there been only one classification from the numerous one, which makes sense and is of real use, it undoubtedly would have achieved and retained universal approval, because truth is omnipotent.

logie hat eine andre, ihr eigne) übergebe
ich. Wäre nur eine einzige von den unzähligen von einleuchtendem, wahren
Nutzen, so würde sie unstreitig den allgemeinen Beifall — durch die Allmacht,
die der Wahrheit eigen ist — errungen
und behalten haben.

41.

Am meisten schien die Eintheilung in
allgemeine und in Lokal-Krankheiten ge-
feiert zu werden.

42.

Der menschliche Organism ist aber im
lebenden Zustande ein völlig geschlosse-
nes Ganze, eine Einheit. Iede Empfindung, jede Kraftauferung, jedes Mi-
schungsverhältnifs der Stoffe des einen
Theils hangt mit der Empfindung, der
Funktionen und dem Mischungsverhält-
nisse der Stoffe aller übrigen Theile innig
zusammen. Kein Theil kann leiden, ohne
dafs alle übrige zugleich — mehr oder
weniger — mit leiden, mit verandert werden.

§ 41

The most common classifications of diseases observed are into *general* and *local diseases*.

§ 42

But the human organism in its living condition, is a complete whole, a unity. Each sensation, each manifestation of power, every affinity of the component part of one part is intimately associated with the sensation, the functions and inter-relationship of all other parts. No part can suffer without all other parts more or less sympathising and undergoing, at the same time, greater or lesser alterations.

43.

Diese lebendige Einheit verstattet nicht, daſs an unserm Körper eine Krankheit je blos örtlich, vollkommen und absolut örtlich bleibe, so lange das für lokal gehaltene Uebel noch an einem, vom übrigen Körper nicht völlig getrennten Theile sich befindet. Immer leidet der übrige Körper mehr oder weniger mit, und legt dieſs Uebelbefinden durch dieses oder jenes Symptom an den Tag. Immer macht jede, selbst an ganz entfernten Orten angebrachte oder innerlich eingenommene kräftige Arznei auch auf diesen örtlich scheinenden Fehler einen ändernden Eindruck und das für die Gesamtkrankheit (wovon das Lokalübel immer nur ein Theil, immer nur ein Symptom ist) specifisch passende Heilmittel pflegt zugleich das, obschon ganz entfernt und isolirt scheinende Lokalübel selbst mit zu heilen.

44.

Eine zweite hoch aufgenommene Eintheilung der Krankheiten in fieberhafte

§ 43

This living unity does not allow any disease on the body to remain only local, completely and absolutely local as long as the suffering, wrongly named local, is not confined to a part entirely separate from the rest of the body. The rest of the body always sympathises more or less and expresses this sympathy by suffering some symptom or other. Every powerful medicine even when applied to a quite distant part or given internally, causes a change-making effect on this apparently local affection also, and the remedy specifically suitable for the general disease (of which the local suffering is always only a part, only a symptom) generally cures the local suffering, although it may be in a very distant part and apparently separated.

§ 44

A second highly respected division of diseases into *febrile* and *afebrile*, is equally unsatisfactory. There is no agreement as to what characteristic signs and symptoms should and can be included in the definition of fever, and what should be rejected; and among the greater number of theories and definitions of fever there is not single one which does not include symptoms which are also found, more or less, in diseases which are universally considered among the most afebrile in character. The most febrile pass over into the most afebrile by imperceptible degrees, a fact which shows that a sharp division between the two is only done in pathology and is not in conformity with nature.

und fieberlose leidet gleiches Schicksal.
Es fehlt sogar noch die Uebereinkunft,
welche Charakterzüge und Symptomen in
die Fieberdefinition aufgenommen werden
sollen und können, und welche auszu-
schliefsen sind, und es ist keine unter der
grofsen Zahl der Fieber-Theorien und Defi-
nitionen, welche nicht Zufälle in sich begriffe, die auch in den fieberlosest geachteten Krankheiten mehr oder weniger statt
finden. In unmerklichen Abstufungen gehen die fieberhaftesten in die fieberlosesten
über und zeigen, dafs eine scharfe Tren-
nung beider nur pathologisch, aber nicht
naturgemäfs ist.

45.

An sich würde die Benahmung
oder Klassifikation der unzählig verschiednen Krankheiten, wenn sie nur ei-
nigermafsen richtig und vollständig möglich wäre, für den Arzt, als Naturhi-
storiker, eben den Nutzen haben, den
die Klassification andrer Naturerscheinun-
gen und Naturkörper in der allgemeinen

§ 45

The *nomenclature* or *classification* of the innumerable varieties of diseases, even if it were possible to achieve tolerably accurate and complete, would serve the physician only as a *natural historian,* in the same way as the classification of other natural phenomena and natural objects is of value in general natural history, in other words, it would facilitate his historical perception by furnishing him with a tabular arrangement; but for the *physician as a practitioner of the art of medicine* it is of no use at all, for the true healing art cannot be satisfied with such simple one-sided similarity of several individual diseases with one another which is sufficient for the classification of diseases into *genera* and *species,* but must have the most complete view of every single case of disease before it can select an accurately suitable remedy, that is, before it can deserve to be called a *well-founded and rational art of healing.*

Naturgeschichte leistet, nämlich seine historische Ansicht durch einen tabellarischen Ueberblick zu erleichtern; aber für den Arzt als Heilkünstler hat sie gar keinen Nutzen, da die wahre Heilkunde sich mit der flachen, einseitigen Aehnlichkeit mehrerer Krankheitsindividuen unter einander, die zur Zusammenkoppelung in Gattungen und Arten zureicht, nicht begnügen darf, sondern die vollständigste Ansicht jedes zu heilenden, individuellen Krankheitsfalles auffassen muſs, ehe sie ein genau passendes Heilmittel wählen, das ist, den Namen der gründlichen und rationellen Heilkunde verdienen kann.

46.

Die Natur hat keine Benahmung oder Klassifikation der Krankheiten. Sie schafft einzelne Krankheiten, und will, daſs der wahre Heilkünstler an seinem Menschenbruder nicht die systematisch vereinte Krankheitsgattung (eine Art von Verwechselung verschiedner Krankheiten mit-

§ 46

Nature does not have nomenclature or classification of diseases. It produces *single* diseases, and demands that the true healer shall treat his fellow-beings not as the systematic combination which constitute a *genus* of disease (a kind of confusing different diseases together), but shall always treat the individuality of each individual case of disease; but she forbids the therapeutic treatment of groups of diseases constructed only by the imaginative men, because such treatment is deforming of the divine work of healing; on the contrary she enjoins the treatment of individual disease, (*which it has wisely created as separate entities*).

Footnote: Huxham, who deserves high honour for his acute insight and equally for his tender conscience says (*Op. Phys. Med., tom.1*): *Nihil sane artem medicam pestiferum magis unquam irrepsit malum, quam generalia quaedam nomina morbis imponere, iisque aptare velle generalem quandam medicinam.*[6]

---

[6] **Translator's note:** Huxham's words can be translated as: *In reality no other dangerous evil has ever creeped into the art of medicine than the imposition of some general names to the diseases as well as the desire to apply (or adapt) a certain general medicine to them.*

einander), sondern jedesmahl nur das In
dividuum seiner Krankheit individuell behandeln soll; den therapevtischen Leisten
aber, für die von Menschen blos in der
Idee zusammengefügten Krankheitszünfte
geschnitzt, verbietet sie, an die (weis-
lich von ihr eigenartig geschaffe-
nen) Krankheitsindividuen anzulegen, und
so das göttliche Heilwerk zu verkrüppeln.

Anm. Der eben so sehr seiner Einsicht, als
seines zarten Gewissens wegen verehrungs-
werthe *Huxham* sagt (Op. phys med.
Tom. I.): „Nihil sane in artem medicam
„pestiferum magis unquam irrepsit malum,
„quam generalia quaedam nomina morbis
„imponere, iisque aptare velle generalem
„quamdam medicinam.‟

47.

Wenn nun die Rationalität der Heilkunde, wenn wo irgend, vorzüglich darinn besteht, daſs sie alle systematische und
andre Vorurtheile unterdrücke, wo möglich nie ohne Grunde handle, wo möglich
nie einige sich darbietenden Grunde zum

§ 47

If the rationality of the art of medicine manifests itself at all it is prominently in this that it rejects all systematic and other prejudices, in its refusal to act without good reasons, in the adoption of every possible measure that may make the treatment appropriate and in concentrating as much as possible to that which can be definitely ascertained. *Thus the characteristic of the rational and thorough physician is, chiefly, attention to the varieties and differences of diseases, (as also of drugs) or, that is to say, the careful investigation of the individual phenomena of every single disease and of the peculiar mode of action of every single medicine.*

zweckmäsig Handeln vernachlässige, und
sich möglichst an das Erkennbare der Dinge halte; so wird vorzüglich die Berücksichtigung der Abweichung
und Verschiedenheit der Krankheiten (so wie der Arzneimittel),
das ist, die sorgfältige Aufsuchung der individuellen Zeichen
der jedesmahligen Krankheit und
die der individuellen Wirkungsart jeder einzelnen Arznei den rationellen, den gründlichen Arzt
charakterisiren.

48.

Blos der rationelle Heilkünstler wird,
da jede Krankheits-Epidemie in der Welt
(mit Ausnahme jener wenigen mit einem
festständigen, unabänderlichen Miasma)
von der andern, und selbst jeder einzelne
Krankheitsfall epidemischer und sporadi-
scher Art, am meisten aber jeder nicht zu
einer solchen Kollektivkrankheit gehörige Krankheitsfall von jedem andern ab-
weicht —, auch jedes ihm zur Heilung

§ 48

Every epidemic of disease in the world (excepting those few which have a fixed, unchangeable miasm[7]) differs from all other, and even every single case of *epidemic* and *sporadic* disease, and specially in every case of disease not belonging to such collective diseases, described elsewhere, differs from every other, so the rational physician will judge every disease coming under his care just as it is according to its individual differentiating features. When he has investigated its individual peculiarities and noted all its signs and symptoms (because that is why they are there, so that they should be taken care) he will treat it according to its individuality, *i.e.* according to the particular group of symptoms it manifests, with a suitable individual remedy corresponding to it. By proceeding in this honest, unprejudiced and rational manner, he will prove the difference between himself and every other physician

---

7 **Translator's note:** Though the homoeopathic concept of chronic disease and that of fundamental cause has not yet been formulated when this book was published and hence the word *miasm* was used here totally in a different context. However, it will be an interesting exercise for any serious student of homoeopathy to read the first sentence of this aphorism (§48 of 1st edition) and 1st paragraph of aphorism 46 of 5th edition and the last few lines of aphorism 73 of 5th edition, in addition to aphorism 49 of 1st edition and aphorism 73 of 5th and 6th editions. This will give an insight into the evolution of the concept of *fixed miasm* and that of *epidemic disease*. In 1st edition (aphorism-48) he calls it *feststständigen [definite, fixed, established] miasma* while in 5th and 6th edition (aphorism-46) he calls it *feststchenden miasm.*

angetragene Siechthum nach seiner indi
viduellen Verschiedenheit nehmen, wie es
ist, und wenn er dessen Eigenheiten und
alle seine Zeichen und Symptomen erforscht hat (denn dazu sind sie, dafs auf
sie soll geachtet werden), auch nach seiner Individualität, d. i. nach der sich an
ihm zeigenden Gruppe von Symptomen
mit einem individuell passenden Heilmittel behandeln und sich durch ein so recht-
liches und vorurtheilfreios, als rationelles
Verfahren vor jeden andern Arzte auszeich-
nen, der den Krankheitsfall gründlich auszuspähen nicht würdigt, sondern ihn, der
Bequemlichkeit zu Gefallen, nach Gutdun-
ken generalisirt, ihm seine systematische
Vermuthung anheftet, und blos nach dieser, seine Behandlung modelt.

49.

Einige Krankheiten, welche einen
eignen Ansteckungsstoff (ein eignes, sich
ziemlich gleichbleibendes Miasm) zum
Grunde haben, z. B. die levantische Pest,
die Menschenpocken, die Masern, das äch-

who does not take trouble to investigate the case of disease thoroughly, but generalizes it in a careless way to suit his own convenience, gives a label from one of his systematic names, and plans a treatment to suit his conjecture.

§ 49

Some of the diseases are caused by a peculiar agent of contagion (a particular miasm of a sufficiently fixed character), for example, *the Plague of the Levant, Small-pox, Measles, true smooth Scarlet Fever, Venereal disease, the Itch of wool-sorters,* as well as *Rabies, Whooping cough, Plica polonica,* etc. These diseases appear to be so definitely fixed in their *course* and *character* that, whenever they appear, they can always be recognized by their already well known symptoms. Therefore, it is possible to give each of them a definite name and to work to lay down for each of them a regular and fixed method of treatment suitable, as a rule, for each of them.

te glatte Scharlachfieber, die venerische
Krankheit, die Wollarbeiterkrätze—, auch
wohl die Hundswuth, der Keuchhusten,
der Wichtelzopf u. s. w. erscheinen in ihrem Charakter und Verlaufe so selbstständ-
dig, dafs sie, wo sie sich zeigen, wie
schon bekannte Individuen an ihren sich
gleichbleibenden Zeichen immer kennbar
bleiben. Man konnte ihnen daher, jeder
einen eignen, Namen geben, und sich be-
mühen für jede derselben eine feststän-
dige Heilart, als Regel, einzuführen.

50.

So mögen wohl noch einige andre
Krankheiten, denen wir ein Miasm noch
nicht nachweisen können, so wie jene an
gewisse Gegenden und klimatische Verhältnisse gebundene, nebst den hie und da
endemischen: das herbstliche Sumpfwech-
selfieber, das gelbe Fieber, der See-Schar-
bock, der Pian, die Yaws, die Sibbens,
die Pellagra u. s. w. auch sonst noch einige wenige Krankheiten entweder aus einer einzigen, sich gleichbleibenden Ursa-

§ 50

It may be that there are still some other diseases which till now we can not prove to be due to a "miasm" as also those diseases that belong to certain localities and appearing under particular climatic conditions and those that are *endemic* in certain scattered areas, *e. g. Autumnal Marsh-Fever, Yellow Fever, Sea-scurvy, Pian, Yaws*[8] *the Sibbens, Pellagra*[9], etc. Similarly, there are a few diseases produced either by a single uniformly acting cause or from a combination of several definite causes acting simultaneously, which can readily be classed together to some extent, (as, for example, *Gout,* and possibly also *Membranous croup* and *Millar's asthma*). These diseases equally deserve to get their particular names because the group of symptom remains, on the whole, tolerably the same, in each of them, and so each is eligible to a definite and almost fixed method of treatment.

---

[8] **Translator's note:** An infectious tropical disease caused by *Treponema pertenue* and characterized by the development of crusted granulomatous ulcers on the extremities; may involve bone, but, unlike syphilis, does not produce central nervous system or cardiovascular pathology.

[9] **Translator's note:** An affection characterized by gastrointestinal disturbances, erythema (particularly of exposed areas) followed by desquamation, and nervous and mental disorders; may occur because of a poor diet, alcoholism, or some other disease causing impairment of nutrition; commonly seen when corn (maize) is a main nutrient in the diet, resulting in a deficiency of niacin.

che, oder aus einem, öfterer sich vereini-
genden Zusammenflusse mehrerer, bestimmter Ursachen, die sich leicht auf eine
bestimmte Art zusammen gesellen (wie z.
B. bei der Knotengicht; auch wohl der
häutigen Bräune und dem Millarischen
Asthma der Fall seyn mag), entspringen,
und wohl nicht viel weniger verdienen,
jede ihren eignen Namen zu führen, da
die Gruppe der Symptomen bei jeder derselben, im Ganzen, sich doch ziemlich
gleich bleibt, und daher einer eigenarti-
gen, fast feststehenden Behandlung fähig
ist.

51.

Aber schon anders ist es mit einer
Menge der übrigen Krankheiten, welche
vermuthlich aus dem Zusammenflusse einiger sich nicht auf gleiche Art zur Erzeugung des Uebels verbindenden, krankmachenden Ursachen entspringen, daher oft
in mehrern wichtigen Symptomen von einander abweichen, und deshalb nie überein
ein mit denselben Mitteln ärztlich behan-

§ 51

But it is very different matter with many other diseases which probably are caused by the concurrent effect of several pathogenic causes which do not combining in the same way for the production of the malady, hence these diseases often differ from one another in regard to many important symptoms, and so all of them cannot ever be treated with the same remedies. To this class of disease belong the widely different kinds of *Epilepsy, Catalepsy, Tetanus, Chorea, Pleurisy, Phthisis, Diabetes, Angina pectoris, Prosopalgia, Dysentery,* and other conditions represented by names which the schools have given to disease-states that often differ fundamentally and only resemble one another in a few symptoms they have in common, because by regarding them as identical it was easy to lay down an identical treatment for them. But the very different results obtained by following this method were alone enough to discard the supposed identity of diseases upon which the method is founded. As collective names they may have some use, but not at all as the special names of supposed identical morbid states because then they lead the physician astray into a uniform empirical medical treatment, which is detrimental for the patients.

delt werden können. Hieher gehören die
sehr verschiednen Arten von Fallsucht,
Katalepsie, Tetanus, Veitsdanz, Pleuritis,
Lungensucht, Diabetes, Brustbräune, Gesichtsschmerz, Ruhr und andre Namen,
welche die Schule oft wesentlich abweichenden, und nur durch ein Paar gemein-
schaftliche Symptome einander ähnlichen
Krankheitszuständen gab, um unter Vor-
aussetzung ihrer Identität für sie eine
gleichartige Kurbehandlung festsetzen zu
können, deren sehr ungleicher Erfolg in
der Erfahrung schon allein die supponirte
Identität derselben widerlegt. Als Kollek-
tivnamen mögen sie gelten, nur nicht als
Eigennamen angeblich identischer Krankheitszustände; denn dann verführen sie zu
einer gleichförmigen, empirisch arzneilichen Behandlung zum Verderben der Kranken.

Anm. So giebt es z. B. im Diabetes mehrere Verschiedenheiten, d. i. mehrere wesentlich von einander abweichende Krankheiten, unter diesen einzigen Namen zusammen gedrängt, welche blos dem ersten
flüchtigen Anblicke nach, in einem oder

D

Footnote: Thus, for instance, there are many varieties of diabetes, i.e., several diseases basically different classed together under this single name, which at the first casual glance seem to resemble one another in one or more symptoms, but are erroneously believed to be, separate that they are, one and the same disease. If the individual cases are more carefully examined it will be found in almost every one of them that there are symptoms differing widely from those present in other cases, and symptoms present in some and absent in others, and that even the urine often varies much in its character, although the inventors of the name *diabetes* attached a very great importance to their discovery as if it were a great discovery of a special character therein; sometimes it passes rapidly into vinous and acetous fermentation, at other times it only becomes mouldy, and so forth. If one kind of diabetes was curable with Ammonium sulphate, many other kinds will not be benefited by this remedy. Alum would seem to be beneficial in a few cases, and again in others neither Alum nor Ammonium sulphate would be of any use. Can these

dem andern Symptome einander scheinbar
ähneln, aber sehr mit Unrecht für eine
und dieselbe Krankheit sind gehalten
worden. Wurden die einzelnen Fälle
genauer untersucht, so fanden sich fast in
jedem sehr abweichende, in den andern
Fällen nicht vorhandne Zufälle, und selbst
der Harn, auf welchen sich die Erfinder
dieses Namens, als auf einen wichtigen
Fund viel zu Gute thaten, wich oft in
seiner angegebnen Beschaffenheit ab; der
eine ging schnell in geistige und saure
Gährung über, der andre schimmelte blos,
u. s. w. Wenn die eine Art Diabetes mit
geschwefeltem Ammonium geheilt werden
konnte, so vermochte man doch viele andre Arten nicht mit diesem Mittel zu heilen. Da schien hingegen Alaun die hülfreiche Arznei in einem Paar Fällen zu
seyn, und wieder in andern weder Alaun,
noch geschwefeltes Ammonium. Soll das
einerlei Krankheit seyn, was im Inbegriffe
seiner Symptomen so verschieden ist, und
eine so abweichende Heilart verlangt?
Arten von Diabetes könnte man diese
mancherlei Krankheitszustände allenfalls
wohl nennen, aber nur nicht schlechthin
Diabetes, um nicht eine sich gleichblei-
bende, einfache Krankheit unter diesem
Namen fälschlich vermuthen zu lassen.

be the same disease which differ so much in their collective symptoms and require such different modes of treatment? These manifold disease-conditions may indeed be called *kinds of Diabetes,* but not simply *Diabetes*, so as to convey the false impression that they are all of one simple identical disease. Any one who has cured one case of *facial neuralgia* with mercurial ointment will soon find three or four cases for which this ointment will not be of least use, although he will call them all by the same name. If each of these names only indicated diseases which were always identical in character, then it would be impossible that the remedy which succeeded once should ever fail, because if the diseases were identical they must yield to same treatment. But as they do not do so, which clearly demonstrates that in spite of bearing the same name they are essentially different disease, wherein no trouble is taken

Wer einmahl einen Gesichtsschmerz mit Quecksilbersalbe heilte, wird wohl noch drei, vier Fälle erleben, die er alle unter demselben Namen begreift, und in deren keinem doch je wieder diese Salbe hilft. Wenn jeder dieser Namen nur Krankheiten bezeichnete, die sich immer gleich wären, so wäre dieses Fehlschlagen der Kur mit demselben, schon einmahl sich hülfreich erwiesenen Mittel ganz unmöglich; sie müßten sämtlich gleicher Kurart weichen, wenn sie selbst gleich wären. So wie sie dieß aber nicht thun, so zeigen sie klärlich an, daß sie, trotz des gleichen Namens, wesentlich verschiedne Krankheiten sind, nach deren unterscheidenden Symptomen zu forschen, man sich nur nicht die Mühe nahm. Arten von Gesichtsschmerz könnte man diese mancherley Krankheitszustände allenfalls wohl nennen, nur nicht schlechthin Gesichtsschmerz, da es durchaus nicht immer eine und dieselbe Krankheit ist. So ist es mit den übrigen genannten, und andern Krankheitsnamen solcher Art.

52.

Und so werden vollends in den übrigen Krankheiten die Namen immer unei-

D 2

to investigate the differentiating symptoms. Certainly these various disease-states might be called *kinds of facial neuralgia*, for it is not always one and the same disease. And so it is with the other diseases mentioned, and with other disease-names of this kind.

§ 52

And so ultimately, with regard to other diseases, the names are even more inappropriate, and the empirical treatment they lead to is still more dangerous, when they comprise a still greater diversity of morbid states which bear a distant resemblance to one another by hardly *one or two* similar symptoms, whilst the greater number of their other phenomena and characteristics

gentlicher, und ihre Verführung zur em-
pirischen Behandlung immer gefährlicher,
wenn sie eine noch gröfsere Verschiedenheit von Krankheitszuständen unter sich
begreifen, welche kaum mit ein Paar
ähnlichen Symptomen sich einander, blo:
in der Entfernung, nähern, während die
grofse Zahl ihrer übrigen Zufälle und Ei
genheiten sehr weit von einander abwei
chen. Die vieldeutigen Namen von kal
ten Fiebern, Gelbsucht, Wassersucht,
Schwindsucht, Leukorrhöe, Hämorrhoiden, Rheumatism, Schlagflufs, Krämpfe,
Lähmung, Melancholie, Manie, u. s. w.
mogen zu Beispielen dienen.

Anm. Welche unzählige, höchst von einander
    abweichende Arten von sogenannten Wech-
    selfiebern giebt es nicht, die höchstens
    das Phänomen von Frost und Hitze, und
    etwas typusähnliches, und oft auch wohl
    dieses nicht einmahl, mit einander gemein
    haben! Bei näherer Erforschung ihrer
    übrigen Zeichen findet man, dafs fast je-
    de dieser abweichenden Arten eine Krank-
    heit sui generis ist. — Mit welchem Rech-
    te könnte man die vielen höchst verschied-
    nen Krankheiten, die in ihren übrigen

differ widely from one another. The vague names of ague, jaundice, dropsy, consumption, leucorrhoea, haemorrhoids, rheumatism, apoplexy, cramps, palsy, melancholia, mania, etc., may be cited as examples.

Footnote: What countless number of so-called *Malarias* there are not, differing widely from one another, having in common at most the phenomena of chills and heat and something of an intermittent nature, and not always even that! On closer investigation of their other symptoms we find that almost every one of these differing types of disease is a disease *of its own kind*. With what right we can call the many very different diseases by the one name of *jaundice*, which presupposes identity, when all their symptoms except one are different, and that one, *yellowness of the skin*, depends on a disturbance of bile-excretion which may arise from very different causes? So also among the symptoms of various very different illnesses there is found *oedema*; but who would on account of this single symptom, which is certainly very conspicuous but not on that account always the most important—often,

Symptomen keine Verwandschaft, und nur in dem einzigen Zufalle, der Haut-Gilbe, einige Aehnlichkeit mit einander haben, welche sich auf eine Störung der Gallabsonderung gründet, die wiederum höchst verschieden ist — mit dem, Identität voraussetzenden Namen, Gelbsucht belegen? — Eben so ist bei unzähligen höchst verschiednen Siechthumen unter den vielen andern Symptomen, auch Haut-Oedem zugegen; wer wollte nun dieses einzelnen, zwar sehr in die Augen fallenden, aber deshalb nicht immer wichtigsten, oft nicht einmahl wichtigen Symptoms wegen, alle jene höchst verschiednen Krankheiten für eine einzige, unter dem gemeinsamen Namen Wassersucht, ausgeben, und so alle die übrigen höchst bedeutsamen Symptomen unbeachtet lassen, die diese Krankheiten weit von einander entfernen? Und so in den übrigen Beispielen. —

55.

Wie könnte man auch nur mit einem Scheine von Rationalität jene höchst verschiednen Krankheitszustände, welche oft nur ein einziges Symptom mit einander

indeed, not at all important—assert that all these very various diseases were one single disease called *dropsy,* thereby leaving unnoticed the other highly important symptoms which differentiate these diseases from each other? And so it is with other examples.

§ 53

How could any one with any semblance of reason, include under general names those very dissimilar diseases when they have often only single symptom in common, and how can such a classification justify their identical medicinal treatment? And if the medicinal treatment is not to be same in all the cases—as it cannot be without causing harm to the patients—what is the use of identical names which imply an identical treatment? These names, therefore, are so misleading, useless, and harmful that they ought to exercise little influence upon the treatment of a rational physician. He, at least, knows that he has to form a judgment on diseases and to cure them not on the basis of a vague nominal similarity of the a single symptom, but by the indication of the entire totality of all signs and symptoms presented by each individual patient,

gemein haben, unter generelle Namen zu-
sammenziehen, und so fur jeden eine gleichartige arzneiliche Behandlung rechtfertigen
wollen? Und soll die arzneiliche Behandlung nicht gleichartig seyn, — wie sie es
auch ohne Verderben des Kranken nicht seyn
darf —; wozu der, gleiche Heilart voraus-
setzende identische Namen? So misbräuch-
lich, nutzlos und schädlich diese Namen also sind, so wenig dürfen sie je Einfluss auf
die Kurart eines rationellen Heilkünstlers
haben, welcher weifs, dafs er die Krankheiten nicht nach der vagen Namensähnlich-
keit eines einzelnen Symptoms, sondern
nach dem ganzen Inbegriffe aller Zeichen
des individuellen Zustandes jedes einzelnen Kranken zu beurtheilen und zu heilen
habe, dessen Leiden er genau auszuspähen
die Pflicht hat, nie aber hypothetisch vermuthen darf.

54.

Selbst jene Volkskrankheiten, welche
sich wohl auch bei jeder einzelnen
Epidemie durch einen Ansteckungsstoff
fortpflanzen mögen — die Menge jener soge-

whose sufferings it is his duty to investigate accurately and to the exclude mere hypothetical guesses.

§ 54

Even those mass-affecting-diseases which *during every epidemic* may spread by a contagion - the large number of so-called putrid, bilious, nervous fevers (hospital, jail or camp fevers), or other spreading fevers, vary very much in their manifestation and their course at every time of their occurrence. Every fresh epidemic, for instance, of the so-called putrid fever appears in many of its most striking symptoms unlike all previous epidemics of the same name, because there is a different miasm at the root of each epidemic. It is counter to the principles of logical exactitude

nannten (Spital-Kerker-Lager-) Faul-Gal-
len- Nerven- und andrer herumgehenden
Fieber sind sehr abweichend in ihrem jedesmahligen Verhalten und Verlaufe. Iede
neue Epidemie derselben, z. B. des sogenannten Faulfiebers, zeigt sich, weil jeder Epidemie ein abgeändertes Miasm zum
Grunde lag, selbst in mehrern der auffallendsten Symptomen allen vorher-gegan-
genen Epidemien seines Namens so un-
ähnlich, dafs man alle logische Genauig-
keit in Begriffen verleugnen müfste, wenn
man diesen, von sich selbst so sehr abweichenden Seuchen den alten, oder überhaupt einen sehr eingeführten Namen geben und sie mit den ehemaligen Epidemien
gleicher Benennung überein, arzneilich behandeln wollte, verführt durch den mis-
bräuchlichen Namen.

55.

Nur die einzelnen Fälle jeder solchen
epidemischen oder sporadischen Seuche
insbesondre, die man in dieser Rücksicht
eine Kollektivkrankheit nennen möch-

to give to this very different disorder the old name and thus to be misled by the misuse of a name into employing the same medicinal treatment for this epidemic as for former epidemics of the same name.

§ 55

We can only consider as similar for curative purposes the cases of each of such epidemic or sporadic affections, which in this regard may be appropriately called a *collective disease,* and treat them similarly, (with due regard to the greater or lesser variations from the type which appear in each individual case).

te, kann man bei der Heilung für ähnlich
ansehen, und (mit Berücksichtigung der
gröfsern óder kleinern Verschiedenheiten
jedes einzelnen Falles insbesondre) ähnlich
behandeln.

56.

Iede Epidemie begreift nämlich eine
Menge einander sehr ähnlicher Krankheitsindividuen in sich; die Epidemien selbst
aber weichen sehr von einander ab, und
können nicht mit einem ähnlichen oder
gleichen Namen belegt, nicht unbesehens
mit gleicher Arznei behandelt werden.

57.

Diese, keines festständigen, speciel-
len Namens fähigen Epidemien, welche bei
jeder neuen Erscheinung im Volke in abgeänderter Form und mit einer veränderten
Gruppe von Zeichen und Symptomen hervortreten, werden als Kollektiv-
krankheiten, am füglichsten zu der un-
geheuer grofsen Klasse aller übrigen Krankheiten; Gebrechen, und

§ 56

Each epidemic includes a number of very similar individual cases of disease; but different epidemics differ very markedly from one another and can not be appropriately called by the similar or a same name, nor can it be treated without examination or inspection with the same remedy.

§ 57

These epidemics, to which no fixed and special name can be given, which at every new occurrence in the different nations they present a changed form and different groups of signs and symptoms, are most appropriately classed as *collective diseases* and *under this vast class should be grouped all other diseases, infirmities and chronic ill-healths* which arise from the concurrence of causes and forces differing widely in their number, strength and kind, these influences are of an extremely complex nature, and hence arises the infinite varieties of the diseases from which the great race of mankind on the globe is suffering and has always suffered.

Siechthume des menschlichen Körpers gerechnet, welche aus einem sehr verschiednen Zusammenflusse ungleichartiger Ursachen und Potenzen, die an Zahl, Stärke und Art sich aufserst ungleich sind, entspringen; — Einflüssen von unendlich gemischter Natur, aus welchen jene so unendlich verschiedenen Krankheiten hervorsprießen woran das grofse Geschlecht der Menschen auf dem Erdenrunde leidet und je gelitten hat.

58.

Alle Dinge, die nur einigermasen wirksam sind, (ihre Zahl ist unübersehlig) vermögen auf unsern, mit allen Theilen des Universums in Verbindung und Konflikt stehenden Organismus einzuwirken und Veränderungen hervorzubringen, jedes eine verschiedenartige, so wie es selbst verschiedenartig ist.

59.

Wie abweichend, ich möchte sagen, unendlich abweichend von einander müs-

§ 58

Thing which (its number is beyond imagination) can influence and cause changes in our organism, because stands in association and conflict with all parts of the universe, and everything causes a different change, because it differs from all other things.

§ 59

Then, what a difference, I should say, what infinite difference, must there be in those diseases, which are caused by the effect of these innumerable, usually highly inimical forces when they affect our bodies more or less together, or one after the other in different qualities and different strengths; in addition to this *our bodies differ so much from one another in so many external and internal properties and peculiarities and the conditions of life are so diverse that no human being exactly resembles another in any imaginable respect.*

sen nun nicht die Krankheiten, das ist,
die Erfolge der Einwirkung dieser unzähligen, oft sehr feindseeligen Potenzen seyn,
wenn ihrer wenigere oder mehrere zugleich
und in verschiedner Succession, Qualität
und Starke auf unsere Körper influiren, da
leztrre zugleich so sehr in einer
Menge ausserer und innerer Eigenheiten und Verschiedenheiten unter einander abweichen, und in den
mancherlei Zuständen des Lebens
sich dergestalt abändern, dafs kein
menschliches Individuum dem andern gleich ist in irgend einer erdenklichen Rücksicht!

Anm. Einige dieser, Krankheit vorbereiten-
den oder erzeugenden Einflüsse sind z. B.
die unzählige Menge mehr oder weniger
schädlicher Ausdünstungen aus leblosen
und organischen Substanzen —, die so
verschiedentlich reitzenden mancherlei
Gasarten, die in der Atmosphäre, in
unsern Werkstätten und Wohnungen auf
unsre Nerven ändernd oder zerstörend
wirken, oder uns aus Wasser, Erde, Thie-
ren, Pflanzen entgegen strömen —; Mangel an dem unentbehrlichen Nahrungsmit-

Footnote: Some of these influences, which predispose to disease or produce it, are, for example, the countless numbers of more or less harmful emanations, from organic and inorganic substances; the many different irritating types of gas which cause changes and injuries to our nerves, in our atmosphere, dwelling and working places, or which stream out against us from water, earth, animals and plants; the deficiency of indispensable food for the maintenance of our vitality, of pure, fresh air; excess or deficiency of sunlight or of electricity; varying atmospheric pressure and varying humidity or dryness of the air; the properties and possible bad effects, as yet unknown, of high mountainous regions and of low-lying lands and deep valleys; the peculiarities of climate and location in extensive plains, in deserts without

tel für unsere Vitalität, der reinen, freien Luft —; Uebermaas oder Mangel des Sonnenlichts —; Uebermaas oder Mangel der elektrischen Stoffe —; abweichende Druckkraft der Atmosphäre, ihre Feuchtigkeit oder Trockenheit —; die noch unbekannten Eigenheiten und Nachtheile hoher Gebirgsgegenden und dagegen die der niedrigen Orte und tiefen Thäler —; die Eigenheiten der Klimate und andrer Ortslagen auf grofsen Ebenen, auf gewächs - oder wasserlosen Einöden, gegen das Meer hin, gegen Sümpfe, Berge, Wälder oder gegen die verschiednen Winde —; Einflufs sehr veränderlicher oder allzu gleichförmig lange anhaltender Witterung; Einflufs der Stürme und mehrerer Meteore —; allzu grofse Wärme oder Kälte der Luft, Blöfse, oder übertriebne künstliche Wärme unsrer Körperbedeckung oder der Stuben; Beengung einzelner Glieder durch verschiedne Anzüge —; der allzu hohe Grad der Kälte und Wärme unsrer Nahrungsmittel und Getränke; Hunger oder Durst oder Ueberfüllung mit Speifsen und Getränken und ihre schädliche arzneiliche, den Körper umändernde Kraft, die sie theils vor sich besitzen (Wein, Branntwein, mit mehr oder weniger schädlichen Kräutern gewürzte Biere, mit fremdartigen Stoffen

216

water or plant life, on the sea coast or in marshy areas, on hills, in forests or in places exposed to different winds; the influence of very changeable weather or of long-continuance of the same weather; the influence of storms and other meteorological conditions; exposure to air that is too hot or too cold; the effect of excessive or deficient artificial heat, either from clothing or heated rooms; the constriction of limbs by certain forms of dress; the habitual taking of food or drink which is too hot or too cold; hunger, or thirst; or excessive eating, or excessive drinking; or some articles of diet which possess the power to harm the body medicinally, (wine, brandy, beer adulterated with more or less harmful herbs, impure drinking water polluted with foreign substances; coffee, tea, indigenous or exotic spices and food, sauces, liqueurs, chocolate, or cake, seasoned with them; the unknown but possibly injurious character of certain plants and animals used as food) or injurious properties that articles of diet

geschwangertes Trinkwasser, Kaffee, Thee,
ausländische und inländische Gewürzkräuter und die damit reitzend gemischten Speisen, Saucen, Liqueure, Schokolade, Kuchen; die unerkannte Schädlichkeit einiger Gemüse und Thiere im Gemüse) —
theils sie durch nachlässige Zubereitung,
Verderbniß, Verwechselung oder Verfälschung bekommen (z. B. schlecht gegohrnes und nur halb ausgebackenes Brod,
halbgekochte Fleisch- und Gewächsspeisen, oder andre vielfach verdorbne, gefaulte, verschimmelte Nahrungsmittel, in
metallenen Geschirren zubereitete oder aufbewahrte Speisen und Getränke, gekunstelte, vergiftete Weine, mit ätzenden
Substanzen verschärfter Essig, Fleisch
kranker Thiere, mit Gyps oder Sand verfälschtes Mehl, mit schädlichen Samen
vermischtes Getreide, mit gefährlichen Gewächsen aus Bosheit, Unwissenheit oder
Durftigkeit vermischte oder vertauschte
Gemüse) —; Unreinlichkeit des Körpers,
der Körperbedeckungen der Wohnungen —; nachtheilige Substanzen, die durch
Unreinlichkeit oder Nachlässigkeit bei der
Zubereitung und Aufbewahrung in die
Nahrungsmittel gerathen —; Einhauchung
schädlicher Dünste in Krankenstuben, in
Bergwerken, Pochwerken, Rösten und

may acquire through careless preparation, spoiling, substitution or adulteration (e.g., ill-fermented or only half-baked bread, under-done meat and vegetables, or putrid or mouldy food, food and drinks prepared or kept in metal vessels, made-up, poisoned wines, vinegar adulterated with corrosive substances, the meat of diseased animals, flour mixed with gypsum or sand, grain mixed, with harmful seeds; dangerous plants given out of malice, ignorance or poverty); uncleanliness of body or clothes or dwelling places; injurious substances that get into food through uncleanliness or carelessness in preparation or storage; inhaling injurious vapours in sick rooms in mines, stamping-mills, the roasting and smelting houses; the dust laden with many harmful substances that come from stuffs made in factories and workshops; neglect of various police arrangements for the safety of the common welfare; inordinate active or passive exercise; excessive exertion of bodily powers; overworking of one

Schmelzhütten —; der auf uns eindringende Staub mancherlei schädlichen Gehalts von den Stoffen unsrer Fabrikationen und Gewerbe —; Vernachlässigungen mehrerer Anstalten der Policei zur Sicherheit des allgemeinen Wohls —; allzu heftige Anspannung unsrer Körperkräfte, allzu schnelle aktive oder passive Bewegung, übermäsige Exertionen einzelner Körpertheile oder Sinnorgane; mancherlei unnatürliche Lagen und Stellungen, welche die verschiednen Arbeiten der Menschen mit sich bringen —, Mangel des Gebrauchs einzelner Theile oder allgemeine unthätige Körperruhe —; ungeregelte Zeiten der Ruhe (langer Mittagsschlaf), der Mahlzeiten, der Arbeit —; Uebermaas oder Mangel des Nacht - Schlafs —; Anstrengung in Geistesarbeiten überhaupt, oder in solchen, welche widrig und gezwungen sind, oder einzelne Seelenkräfte besonders erregen oder ermüden —; empörende, gewaltsame Leidenschaften, Zorn, Schreck, Aergernifs, oder entnervende Leidenschaften durch wollüstige Leserei, Erziehung, Angewöhnung und Umgang erregt —, Misbrauch des Geschlechtstriebes —; Gewissensvorwürfe, Furcht, Gram, u. s. w.

or other organs of body or mind, or of the organs of sense; various unnatural postures acquired in various occupations and trades; lack of use of certain parts of the body or general laziness; irregularity in the times of rest (long mid day sleep), of meals, of work; excess or deficiency of sleep at night; excessive mental exertion, or mental work of a compulsory but unpleasant nature, or such as excites or tires certain faculties of the mind; violent uncontrollable emotions, such as, anger, fear, and vexation, or debilitating passions excited by reading lascivious books, by injudicious education, by indulgence, by conversation; abuse of sexual functions; reproaches of conscience, fear, grief, &c.

6o.

Daher die unaussprechliche Zahl ungleichartiger Leibes - und Seelengebrechen,
welche unter sich so verschieden sind, daſs
genau genommen, jedes derselben
vielleicht nur ein einziges Mahl
in der Welt existirt, und daſs (jene
wenigen Uebel mit unabänderlichem Miasm
[§. 49.] und etwa sonst noch einige [§. 5o.]
abgerechnet) jede epidemische oder spora-
dische Kollektivkrankheit, und, auſser
ihnen, jeder vorkommende andre Krankheitsfall als eine namenlose, individuelle
Krankheit angesehen und behandelt werden
muſs, die sich noch nie so ereignete als in
diesem Falle, in dieser Person und unter
diesen Umständen, und genau eben so,
nie wieder in der Welt vorkommen kann.

61.

Da die Natur selbst die Krankheiten
so individuell verschieden hervorbringt, so
kann keine rationelle Heilkunde statt finden ohne strenge Individualisation jeden
Krankheitsfalles beim Heilgeschäfte, ohne

§ 60

Thus arises the unaccountable number of dissimilar diseases of body and mind; diseases so different that, strictly speaking, *each has only existed once in the world* and [except for those few evils (diseases) caused by an unchangeable miasm, (§49) and perhaps excluding a few others (§50)]; every epidemic or sporadic type of collective disease and besides these every other case of disease we see is to be regarded and treated as a nameless, individual disorder, which has never occurred before exactly as in this case, in this person and these conditions, and can never occur in the same form in the world again.

§ 61

As Nature herself produces so much various individual types of diseases, therefore there can be no rational healing art without strict individualisation of each case of disease for the purpose of treatment, and without the physician considering each case of disease coming under his care as individual and unique, which is what it precisely is. Then will there be an end to all those empirical generalisation which is so closely related to the impudent conjectures and the arbitrary errors.

daſs der Arzt jede ihm dargebotene Krankheit einzeln und vor sich allein so nehme,
wie sie genau ist. Dann hört all jenes em-
pirische Generalisiren auf, was mit dem
kecken Vermuthen und dem eigenmächti-
gen Verwechseln so nahe verwandt ist!

62.

Diese individualisirende Untersuchung jeden vorkommenden Krankheitsfalles, so wie er an sich selbst ist, verlangt von dem Heilkunstler nichts als Unbefangenheit und gesunde Sinne, Aufmerksamkeit im Beobachten und Treue im
Kopiren des Bildes der Krankheit.

63.

Der Kranke klagt den Vorgang seiner
Beschwerden; die Angehorigen erzählen
seine Klagen, sein Benehmen; der Arzt
sieht, hört und bemerkt durch die übrigen Sinnen was verändert und unge-
wöhnlich in ihm ist. Er schreibt alles
mit den genauen Ausdrücken auf, deren
der Kranke und die Angehorigen sich be-

§ 62

An individualizing examination of every case of disease as is apparent demands from the physician nothing but freedom from prejudice, sound sense, attention in observation and fidelity in tracing the portrait of the disease.

§ 63

The patient describes the course of his sufferings; his attendants tell of his complaints, his general condition; the physician sees, hears and observes by his other senses, what is altered and unusual in the patient. He writes down all the exact expressions the patient and his relatives have said. He keeps himself silent, allows them to say all they want, when possible without interruption; at the outset, the physician requests them to speak slowly so that he can write down as much as he wants.

Footnote: Each interruption disturbs the sequence of thought, and all they would have said in the beginning does not occur to them again exactly as before.

dienen. Stillschweigend laſst er ſie aus-
reden, wo moglich ohne Unterbrechung.
Blos langsam zu sprechen, ermahne sie
der Arzt gleich anfangs, damit er den
Sprechenden im Nachschreiben folgen
konne. ·

Anm. Iede Unterbrechung stört ihre Gedan-
kenreihe, und es fällt ihnen hinterdrein
nicht alles genau wieder so ein, wie sie
Anfangs sagen wollten.

64.

Mit jeder Angabe des Kranken oder
der Angehörigen bricht er die Zeile ab, damit die Symptomen alle einzelnen unter
einander zu stehen kommen. So kann er
bei jedem nachtragen, was ihm anfänglich allzu undeutlich und unbestimmt an-
gegeben worden war.

65.

Sind beide fertig mit dem, was sie
von selbst sagen wollten, so tragt er bei
jedem einzelnen Symptome die nähere Bestimmung nach, auf folgende Weise er-

§ 64

Every statement of the patient or his relatives is written in a separate paragraph, so that each single symptom is arranged one below the other. Thus the physician can make additions to any record which was too inarticulate or vague in the beginning.

§ 65

After both (**Translator's note:** the patient and his friends) have finished what they wanted to say, he (**Translator's note:** the physician) scrutinizes each single symptom more closely and enquires in the following manner. He reads over the symptoms one by one as they were related to him and particularly asks for further details about each one; e.g., at what time did this complaint occur? before taking the medicine? whilst taking the medicine? or only some days after discontinuing the medicine? what kind of pain was it described exactly? Where was its exact location? did the pain come in paroxysms at different times, unaccompanied by any other symptom? how long did it last? at what time of day or night was it worst, and at what hour did it stop? what was the exact character, in simple words, of this or that symptom or circumstance?

kundigt. Er liest die einzelnen ihm ge-
sagten Symptomen vor, und fragt bei jedem insbesondre: z. B. zu welcher Zeit
ereignete sich dieser Zufall? In der Zeit
vor dem Arzneigebrauche? während dem
Arzneinehmen? oder erst einige Tage hernach, als er schon mit aller Arznei aufge-
hört hatte? Was für ein Schmerz, genau
beschrieben, war es, der sich an dieser
Stelle ereignete? Welche genaue Stelle war
es? Erfolgte der Schmerz abgesetzt, nur
einzeln, in verschiednen Zeiten? Wie lange setzte er jedesmahl aus? Zu welcher
Zeit des Tages oder der Nacht war er am
schlimmsten, oder setzte ganz aus? Wie
war dieser, wie war jener angegebne Zufall, oder Umstand, mit deutlichen Worten beschrieben, genau beschaffen?

66.

Und so läfst der Arzt sich die nähere
Bestimmung von jeder einzelnen Angabe
noch dazu sagen, ohne doch jemahls dem
Kranken die Frage so in den Mund zu legen, dafs er blos mit Ia, oder Nein drauf

E

§ 66

In this manner the physician obtains more exact information of each symptom, but he does never frame his questions in such a way that the patient can simple answer with a *Yes* or *No*; because if care is not taken in this matter, the patient will be misled into giving an affirmative or negative answer which is untrue or half-true or incorrect, in order to save himself trouble or to please his questioner, and from it a false disease portrait and an unsuitable treatment will certainly be the result.

Footnote: In other words, the physician should never ask the patient or his attendants in his inquiry, in the first place, "Was not this or perhaps that circumstance present?" "Is it not a fact that it was so and so?" He should never be guilty of making such suggestions, which persuade the patient into giving a false information.

antworten könnte, sonst wird derselbe verleitet, etwas Unwahres, Halbwahres oder anders Vorhandnes aus Bequemlichkeit oder dem Fragenden zu Gefallen, zu bejahen oder zu verneinen, wodurch ein falsche Bild der Krankheit und eine unpassende Heilart entstehen mufs.

> Anm. Er darf, mit einem Worte, weder den Kranken, noch den Krankenwarter bei der ersten Erkundigung fragen: „war nicht etwa auch dieser oder jener Umstand da?" „Nicht wahr, es war so und so?" Dergleichen zu einer falschen Angabe verführende Suggestionen darf sich der Arzt nie zu Schulden kommen lassen.

67.

Ist nun bei diesen freiwilligen Angaben von mehrern Theilen oder Funktionen des Körpers nichts erwähnt worden, so fragt der Arzt, was in Rucksicht dieser Theile und dieser Funktionen noch zu erinnern sei, aber in allgemeinen Ausdrucken, damit der Berichtgeber genothigt sei, sich speciell daruber zu äufsern.

§ 67

If during the course of these voluntary informations if nothing has been said about some parts or some functions of the body, the physician ask respectively about those parts and function, but he always uses general expressions, so that his informants are forced to explain in special detail.

Anm. Z. B. Wie ist es mit dem Stuhlgange?
Wie geht der Urin ab? Wie ist es mit
dem Schlafe bei Tage, bei der Nacht?
Wie ist sein Gemüth, seine Laune beschaffen? Wie ist es mit dem Durste?
Wie mit dem Geschmacke so vor sich im
Munde? Welche Speisen und Getränke
schmecken ihm am besten, welche sind
ihm am meisten zuwider? Hat jedes seinen natürlichen, vollen oder andern Geschmack? Ist etwas wegen des Kopfs, der
Glieder oder des Unterleibes zu erinnern?

68.

Hat nun der Kranke (— denn nur diesem ist in Absicht seiner Empfindungen,
außer in Verstellungskrankheiten, der
meiste Glaube beizumessen —) auch durch
diese freiwilligen oder fast unveranlaßten
Aeußerungen dem Arzte gehörige Auskunft gegeben und das Bild der Krankheit
ziemlich vervollständigt, so ist es diesem
erlaubt, speciellere Fragen zu thun.

Anm. Z. B. Wie oft hatte er Stuhlgang,
von welcher genauen Beschaffenheit? War
der weißlichte Stuhlgang Schleim oder

E 2

Footnote: *For example :-* What is the character of the stools ? How does he pass urine? How does he sleep by day, and in night? What is his disposition and mood? How about the thirst? What is taste he has in his mouth? What kinds of food and drink are most liked, what does he dislike most? Has each kind of food its full natural taste or a changed one? Is there that he remembers about the head, the limbs, or the abdomen?

§ 68

It is on the patient (because greatest faith must be attributed only to his sensations, except in cases of feigned diseases); if the patient has given the physician the necessary

Koth? Waren Schmerzen beim Abgange oder nicht? Welche genaue und wo? Was brach er aus? Ist der garstige Geschmack im Munde faul oder bitter oder sauer, oder wie sonst? Ist dieser Geschmack, auch wenn er nichts geniefst, im Munde? zu welcher Tageszeit am meisten? oder entsteht er nur während dem Essen oder Trinken, oder gar erst nachher? Läfst er den Urin gleich trübe, oder wird er erst beim Stehen trübe? Von welcher Farbe ist er, wenn er eben gelassen ist? Von welcher Farbe ist der Satz? Wie gebehrdet und äufsert er sich im Schlafe? Wimmert, stöhnt, redet, oder schreiet er im Schlafe? Erschrickt er im Schlafe? wirft er sich öfters herum? schnarcht er beim Ein-oder Ausathmen? Liegt er blos auf dem Rucken oder auf welcher Seite? Deckt er sich selbst fest zu, oder leidet er das Zudecken nicht? Wacht er leicht auf, oder schläft er allzu fest? Wie oft kömmt diese, wie oft jene Beschwerde, auf welche jedesmahlige Veranlassung, im Sitzen, im Liegen, im Stehn oder bei der Bewegung, blos nuchtern und fruh, oder blos Abends, oder blos nach der Mahlzeit?. Wann kam der Frost? War es blos Frostempfindung, oder war er zugleich kalt, (an welchen

information either voluntarily or at least without prompting, so that the portrait of the disease is workably complete, then the physician may ask more detailed questions.

Footnote: For example, How often do the bowels act, and what is the exact character of the stools? Is passing of stool painful? Of what did the vomitus consisted? Is the bad taste in the mouth bitter, or sour, or putrid, or of what character? What is his behaviour during sleep? Does he moan or cry out or talk during sleep? Does he lie only on his back? If not, on which side? When did the rigor come? How long did the cold stage last? And how long the hot stage stayed? How great was the thirst? When did he perspire? etc.

Theilen?), oder wohl gar bei der Frostempfindung heiß anzufühlen? War es
blose Empfindung von Kälte ohne Schau-
der? War er heiß ohne Gesichtsröthe?
An welchen Theilen war er heiß anzufühlen? Oder klagte er Hitze ohne heiß
zu seyn beim Anfühlen? Wie lange dauerte der Frost, wie lange die Hitze?
Wann kam der Durst; beim Froste? bei
der Hitze? wie stark war er, worauf?
Wann kommt der Schweiß? beim Anfange, oder zu Ende der Hitze? oder wie
viel Stunden nach der Hitze? Wie stark
ist der Schweiß? heiß oder kalt? an welchen Theilen? von welchem Geruche?
Was klagt er an Beschwerden vor oder
bei dem Froste, was bei der Hitze, was
nach derselben? u. s. w.

69.

Ist er mit Niederschreibung dieser
Aussagen fertig, so notirt er sich, was er
selbst an dem Kranken wahrnimmt, und
erkundigt sich, was dem Kranken hievon
in gesunden Tagen eigen gewesen.

Anm. z. B. wie sich der Kranke bei dem
Besuche geberdet hat; ob er verdrußlich,

236

§ 69

When complete recording of the have been done of all these statements, he **(Translator's note:** the physician) notes what he himself has observed in the patient and enquires if these peculiarities were present in the patient before his sickness.

Footnote: For example: how the patient behaved during the visit; whether he was morose, quarrelsome, hasty, lachrymose, anxious, despairing or sad, or hopeful, calm. whether he was drowsy or in any way slow in understanding; whether his voice was hoarse or feeble, or incoherent, or how else he talk? what was the colour of his face? of his eyes? and of his skin generally? whether liveliness and power was there in his expression and eyes? the state of his tongue? of his breath? the smell from his mouth, and his hearing? whether his pupils were dilated or contracted? and how quickly and to what extent they reacted to dark and to light? what was the character of the pulse? what the condition of the abdomen? how moist or hot, how cold or dry to the touch, was

zänkisch, hastig, ängstlich, verzweifelt, oder getrost, ob er schlaftrunken, oder überhaupt unbesinnlich war, ob er heisch, sehr leise, oder ob er unpassend, oder wie anders er redete; wie die Farbe des Gesichts und der Augen, und die Farbe der Haut überhaupt, wie die Lebhaftigkeit und Kraft der Mienen und Augen, wie die Zunge, der Odem, der Geruch aus dem Munde, oder das Gehör beschaffen ist; wie sehr die Pupillen erweitert sind, wie schnell, wie weit sie sich im Dunkeln und Hellen verändern; wie der Puls, wie der Unterleib: wie feucht, oder heiss die Haut an diesen oder jenen Theilen anzufühlen ist; ob er mit zurückgebognem Kopfe, mit halb oder ganz offnem Munde, mit über den Kopf gelegten Armen, ob er auf dem Rucken, oder in welcher andern Stellung er liegt; mit welcher Anstrengung er sich aufrichtet, und was vom Arzte sonst auffallend bemerkbares an ihm wahrgenommen werden konnte.

70.

Die Zufälle und das Befinden des Kranken während des Arzneigebrauchs ge-

the skin of any particular part, or generally? whether he lay with head thrown back, with mouth half-open or wholly open, with the arms placed above the head, on his back, or in what other position? what efforts he made to raise himself? and anything else which the physician perceives as noteworthy ?

§70

The accidents and the condition of disease of the patient *during* a course of administration of treatment do not furnish a real portrait of the disease. On the contrary, those symptoms and complaints from which he suffered, *before* the use of the medicine or *some time after* he has stopped taking the medicine, give the real basis of conception of the original form of the disease, and the physician must take special note of these. Indeed, if the disease is chronic and the patient has been taking medicine up to the time of his case-taking, he should be left completely without medicine for few days,

ben nicht das reine Bild der Krankheit;
die Symptomen und Beschwerden hingegen, welche er vor dem Gebrauche
der Arzneien, oder nach ihrer mehr-
tagigen Zurücksetzung litt, geben
den achten Grundbegriff von der ursprünglichen Gestalt der Krankheit,
und vorzüglich diese muſs sich der Arzt
aufzeichnen; er kann auch wohl, wenn
die Krankheit chronisch ist, den Kranken,
wenn er bis zu der Zeit noch Arznei genommen hatte, einige Tage ganz ohne
Arznei lassen und bis dahin die genauere
Prüfung der Krankheitszeichen verschie-
ben, um die dauerhaften, unvermischten
Symptomen des alten Uebels in ihrer Reinheit aufzufassen, und ein untrügliches Bild
von der ursprünglichen Krankheit entwerfen zu können.

71.

Leidet aber der dringende Zustand der
akuten Krankheit keinen Verzug, so muſs
sich der Arzt mit dem, selbst von Arzneien geänderten Krankheitszustande be-

and the physician should defer the more exact examination of the disease-symptoms until the permanent features of the old disease in their purity appear and a clear portrait of the original diseases can be constructed.

§ 71

But if the dangerous character of an acute disease does not permit to give much time, the physician must be satisfied with the observation of the diseased condition, though it may be modified by the use of medicines (if he can not find out the symptoms experienced before the employment of the medicine), so that he may at least handle the existing disorder with a suitable remedy.

gnugen (wenn er die vor dem Arzneigebrauche bemerkten Symptomen nicht erfahren kann), um wenigstens die gegenwärtige Gestalt des Uebels mit einem passenden Heilmittel bestreiten zu können.

72.

Ist die Krankheit durch ein auffallendes Ereigniſs verursacht worden, so wird
der Kranke (oder wenigstens die in Ge-
heim befragten Angehörigen) sie schon angeben entweder von selbst und aus eignem
Triebe, oder auf eine behutsame Erkundigung.

> Anm. Den entehrenden, etwanigen Veran-
> lassungen, welche die Kranken oder die
> Angehörigen nicht gern, wenigstens nicht
> von freien Stücken gestehen, muſs der Arzt
> durch klügliche Wendungen der Fragen,
> oder durch andre Privaterkundigungen auf
> die Spur zu kommen suchen; dahin ge-
> hören: Vergiftung oder intendirter Selbst-
> mord, Onanie, Ausschweifungen in ge-
> wöhnlicher oder unnatürlicher Wollust,
> Schwelgen in Wein, Liqueuren, Punsch,
> Kaffee — Schwelgen in Essen überhaupt,

§ 72

If the disease has any striking and apparent cause, the patient (or, at least, his friends when questioned privately) will mention it, either voluntarily or in answer to careful questioning.

Footnote: Any cause of a disgraceful character, which the patient or his friends may not confess, at least not voluntarily, requires tactfully framing of questions on the part of the physician or by private information. Such causes, for instance, can be poisoning, attempted suicide, onanism, indulgence in ordinary or unnatural debauchery, over indulgence in wine, cordials, punch and other ardent beverages, or coffee — over-indulgence in eating generally, or in some particular food of a hurtful character, venereal disease, unfortunate love, jealousy, domestic unhappiness, worry, grief on account of some family misfortune, ill-usage, balked revenge, injured pride, embarrassment of monetary nature, superstitious fear, hunger — or an imperfection in the private parts, a rupture, a prolapsus, etc.

oder in besonders schädlichen Speisen, venerische Krankheit, unglückliche Liebe, Eifersucht, Hausunfrieden, und Gram über ein Familienunglück, erlittene Mishandlung, verbissene Rache, gekränkter Stolz, Zerrüttung des Vermögenszustandes, abergläubige Furcht, Hunger — oder ein Körpergebrechen an den Schamtheilen, ein Bruch, ein Vorfall, u. s. w.

73.

Bei Erforschung des Zustandes chronischer Krankheiten müssen die Verhältnisse des Kranken in Absicht seiner gewöhnlichen Beschäftigungen, seiner gewöhnlichen Lebensordnung und Diät, seiner häuslichen Lage u. s. w. wohl erwogen und geprüft werden, was sich in ihnen Krankheit Erregendes oder Unterhaltendes befindet, um durch seine Entfernung die Genesung befördern zu können.

Anm. Vorzüglich muss bei den chronischen Krankheiten des weiblichen Geschlechts Rücksicht auf Schwangerschaft, Unfruchtbarkeit, Neigung zur Begattung, Niederkünften, Fehlgeburten, Kindersäugen, und den Zustand des monatlichen Blut-

§ 73

In enquiry of the condition of a patient suffering from a chronic disease, the physician must investigate and weigh carefully the circumstances of the patient, i.e., his ordinary occupation, his usual mode of living, his diet, the surroundings of dwelling place and so forth, so that the factor exciting or maintaining the disease may be discovered and removed.

Footnote: In chronic diseases of the female gender pregnancy, sterility, tendency towards copulation, child berth, miscarriages, breast-feeding and the state of menstruation must be specially taken into consideration. We should not neglect to ascertain if it recurs as too short intervals, or is delayed beyond the proper time, how many days it lasts, whether its flow The inquires as to whether menstruation recurs within a too short intervals or occurs long after the due date, how many days it lasts, whether its flow is continuous or interrupted, the amount of flow/discharge, its colour and whether it is preceded or followed by leucorrhoea before its appearance or after its termination. Also enquiries regarding the complaints of the body and the mind, the kind of sensation and pain, it is preceded, accompanied or followed the menstrual flow - should also be taken note of.

flusses genommen werden. Insbesondre ist in Rücksicht des leztern die Erkundigung nicht zu versäumen, ob er in zu kurzen Perioden wiederkehrt oder über die gehörige Zeit aufsen bleibt, wie viel Tage er anhält, ununterbrochen oder abgesetzt? in welcher Menge überhaupt, wie dunkel von Farbe, ob mit Leukorrhöe vor dem Eintritt oder nach der Beendigung? — vorzüglich aber mit welchen Beschwerden Leibes und der Seele, mit welchen Empfindungen und Schmerzen vor dem Eintritte, bei dem Flusse, oder nachher?

74.

Die Erforschung der obgedachten und aller übrigen Krankheitszeichen muſs deshalb bei chronischen Krankheiten so sorgfältig und umständlich als möglich geschehen und an die kleinsten Einzelheiten gehen, theils weil sie bei diesen Krankheiten am sonderlichsten sind, denen in den schnell vorübergehenden Krankheiten am wenigsten gleichend, und bei der Heilung, wenn sie gelingen soll, nicht genau genug genommen werden können; theils weil die Kranken der langen Leiden so gewohnt

§ 74

The investigation in chronic diseases of the manifestations of disease described above and of other things must be as careful and in as detail as possible and must take note of the minutest peculiarities. It is necessary, partly because these minute peculiarities are specially characteristic of chronic diseases and resemble very little with the features of acute diseases, and so for the purpose of cure has to be very correctly noted; and partly because patients become so accustomed to their prolonged sufferings that they pay little or no attention to the lesser accessory symptoms, which are very characteristic (often very decisive in the search of the curative medicine), in fact they consider these symptoms as a necessary part of their condition, almost as a state of health; because after five, ten, or twenty years of suffering they have almost forgotten the feeling of real health and can hardly believe that these lesser or greater deviations from the normal state of health have any relation to their main disease.

worden sind, dafs sie auf die kleinern charakteristischen (bei Aufsuchung des Heilmittels oft viel entscheidenden) Nebenzu-
fälle wenig oder gar nicht mehr achten und
sie fast für einen Theil ihres nothwendigen
Zustandes, fast für Gesundheit ansehen,
deren wahres Gefühl sie bei der funf-,
zehn-, zwanzigjährigen Dauer ihrer Leiden ziemlich vergessen haben, es ihnen
auch kaum einfällt, zu glauben, dafs die
übrigen kleinern oder gröfsern Abweichungen vom gesunden Zustande mit ihrem
Hauptübel im Zusammenhange stehen
konnten.

75.

Zudem sind die Kranken selbst überhaupt von so abweichender Gemüthsart,
dafs einige, vorzüglich die sogenannten
Hypochondristen und andre sehr gefühlige
und unleidliche Personen ihre Klagen in
allzu grellem Lichte aufstellen und um den
Arzt zur Hülfe aufzureitzen, die Beschwerden mit überspannten Ausdrücken bezeichnen.

§ 75

Moreover, the patients differ so much from one another in their temperament that some of them especially so-called hypochondriacs and other hypersensitive persons, tired of suffering, describe their complaints in exaggerated expressions in order to make the physician more anxious to relieve them.

Footnote: A pure imagination of symptoms is never met with in hypochondriacs, even in the most impatients (a comparison of the symptoms they complain of at various times, as when the physician gives them nothing at all, or gives them something only quite unmedicinal, demonstrates this); but something must be deducted on account of the exaggeration and the use of superlatives, or at least the strength of their expressions must be attributed

Anm. Eine reine Erdichtung von Zufällen
wird man wohl nie bei Hypochondristen,
selbst bei den unleidlichsten nicht, wahr-
nehmen (welches die Vergleichung ihrer zu
verschiednen Zeiten geklagten Beschwerden, während der Arzt ihnen nichts oder
etwas ganz unarzneiliches eingiebt, deutlich zeigt); nur muſs man von ihren Hy-
perbeln und Supperlativen etwas abziehen,
wenigstens die Stärke ihrer Ausdrücke
auf Rechnung ihres übermäsigen Gefühls
setzen — in welcher Hinsicht selbst diese
Hochstimmung ihrer Ausdrücke über ihre
Leiden vor sich schon zum bedeutenden
Symptome in der Reihe der übrigen wird,
welche das Bild der Krankheit konstitui-
ren. Bei Wahnsinnigen und böslichen
Krankheitserdichtern ist es ein andrer
Fall.

76.

Andre, entgegen gesetzte Personen
aber halten theils aus Indolenz, theils aus
misverstandner Scham, theils aus einer
Art milder Gesinnung eine Menge Beschwerden zurück, bezeichnen sie mit undeutli-
chen Ausdrücken, oder geben mehrere als
unbeschwerlich an.

to their hypersensitiveness – in which case this very exaggeration that marks the descriptions of their symptoms becomes an important symptom in the list of features of the picture of the disease. It is a different case when we are dealing with the insane or with rascally malingerers.

§ 76

Other persons of an opposite type of character omit to mention a many of symptoms, partly from indolence, partly from false modesty, partly from lack of intelligence, or else they describe them indistinctly or assert that some of them are of no consequence.

77

So gewiſs man nun auch vorzüglich
den Kranken über seine Beschwerden und
Empfindungen zu hören und vorzüglich
seinen eignen Ausdrücken, mit denen er
seine Leiden auszudrücken vermag, Glauben beizumessen hat, weil sie in dem
Munde der Angehörigen und Krankenwärter verändert und verfälscht zu werden
pflegen; so gewiſs erfordert doch auf der
andern Seite bei allen Krankheiten, vorzüglich aber bei den chronischen die Erforschung des wahren vollständigen Bildes
derselben und seiner Einzelheiten besondre
Umsicht, Skepticismus, Menschenkennt-
niſs, Behutsamkeit im Erkundigen und Ge-
dult in hohem Grade.

78.

Im Ganzen wird dem Arzte die Erkundigung akuter, oder sonst seit kurzem ent-
ständener Krankheiten leichter, weil dem
Kranken und Angehörigen alle Zufälle und
Abweichungen von der nur unlängst ver-
lornen Gesundheit noch in frischem Ge-

§ 77

Now certainly, on the one hand, the physician must listen most carefully to the patient's description of his suffering and sensations, and especially he must believe the actual expressions which the patient himself uses to explain his sufferings, because they are frequently changed and incorrectly stated by friends and attendants, and as surely, on the other hand, in all diseases and especially in chronic diseases, the discovery of the true and complete picture of disease and of its peculiarities needs particular insight, scepticism, knowledge of human nature, caution in conducting enquiry, and patience of the strongest kind.

§ 78

On the whole, the physician will find the investigation of acute diseases or diseases of shorter duration easier, because both patients and friends have recent and clear memories of all the symptoms and deviations from the health which has been recently lost. In such cases also, the physician requires to know all that can be known; but he has less reason for enquiry because the things he wants to know is mostly spontaneously given.

dachtnisse, noch neu und auffallend geblieben sind.   Der Arzt muſs zwar auch
hier alles wissen; er braucht aber weit weniger zu erforschen — man sagt ihm alles
gröſstentheils von selbst.

79.

Bei Erforschung des Symptomeninbegriffs der epidemischen Seuchen und sporadischen Krankheiten ist es sehr gleichgul-
tig, ob schon ehedem etwas Aehnliches unter diesem oder jenem Namen in der Welt
vorgekommen sei, oder nicht.   Die Neu-
heit oder Besonderheit einer solchen Seuche macht keinen Unterschied weder in ihrer Erkennung, noch Heilung, da der
Arzt ohnehin das reine Bild jeder gegen-
wärtig herrschenden Krankheit als neu und
unbekannt voraussetzen und es, vom
Grunde aus, vor sich erforschen muſs,
wenn er ein rationeller Heilkünstler seyn
will, der nie Vermuthung an die Stelle
der Wahrnehmung setzen; nie einen ihm
angetragenen Krankheitsfall weder ganz,
noch zum Theile für bekannt annehmen

§ 79

In the investigation of the symptom-totality of epidemic or sporadic diseases, it does not matter whether or not anything similar has ever appeared in the world before under the same or any other name. The novelty or peculiarity of a disease makes no difference either in the method of examination or of treating it; as in any case the physician must look upon the clear picture of any prevailing disease as something new and unknown, and he must give it a thorough individual examination, if he wants to be a rational practitioner of medicine; for him no conjecture can take the place of truth, nor must he consider that he knows, in whole or in part, any case of disease brought to him, unless he has carefully studied all its manifestations; the more so because every prevailing illness, as proper investigation reveals, is in many respects a unique phenomenon, very different from all previous diseases of a similar name (§54-57) - with the exceptions of those Epidemics which are due to a miasm that remains constant, for example, small-pox, measles, etc.

darf, ohne ihn sorgfältig nach allen seinen
Aeuſerungen auszuspahen, und das hier
um so mehr, da jede herrschende Seuche
in vieler Hinsicht eine Erscheinung eig-
ner Art ist, und sehr abweichend von allen
ehemahligen Seuchen ähnlichen Namens
(§. 54 — 57.) bei genauer Untersuchung befunden wird — wenn man die Epidemien
von sich gleich bleibendem Miasm, die
Pocken, Masern u. s. w. ausnimmt.

80.

Es kann wohl seyn, daſs er beim ersten Krankheitsfalle einer epidemischen
Krankheit nicht gleich zum ersten Mahle
das vollkommne Bild davon zu Gesichte
bekömmt, da jede solche Kollektivkrankheit erst bei genauer Beobachtung mehrerer
Fälle den Inbegriff ihrer Symptomen und
Zeichen an den Tag legt. Indessen kann
der sorgfältig forschende Arzt schon beim
ersten und zweiten Kranken dem wahren
Zustande oft schon so nahe kommen, daſs
er ein charakteristisches Bild davon inne
wird (und selbst schon dann eine passende

§ 80

It may very well happen that in the first case of an epidemic the physician will not get a complete picture of the disease at once; for such a collective disease only reveals the totality of its symptoms and signs to the close observation of several cases. Nevertheless, the physician who examines carefully can often arrive so near to the true state, even with the first or second case of an epidemic that he forms a characteristic portrait of it in his mind (and thereby even at that early stage discovers a suitable counter disease-force for it, a remedy adapted to its requirements).

Gegenkrankheitspotenz, ein angemessenes Heilmittel für sie ausfindet).

81.

Bei Aufzeichnung des Zeichenkomplexes mehrerer Fälle dieser Art wird das entworfene Krankheitsbild immer vollständiger, nicht gröfser und wortreicher, sondern gewöhnlich immer kleiner, aber kenntlicher und charakteristischer, die Totalität dieser Kollektivkrankheit umfassender — denn dann weichen die allgewöhnlichen, nichts Besondres und Auszeichnendes andeutenden Zufälle, z. B. Unlust, Mattigkeit, Mangel an Schlaf und Appetit, u. s. w. in den Hintergrund, und dagegen treten die mehr auffallenden, besondern, wenigstens in dieser Verbindung seltnern, wenig Krankheiten eignen Zufälle hervor und bilden das Charakteristische dieser Seuche.

Anm. Da werden dem Arzte, welcher schon in den ersten Fällen des ziemlich allgemein passenden, oder doch dem specifischen am nächsten kommenden Heilmittels gewifs

§ 81

In the course of writing down the symptom-complex of many cases of this kind, the disease-picture, at first only sketched, becomes steadily more complete; not longer and not in too many words, but almost always shorter, more easily recognizable, more characteristic, including more of the totality of this collective disease – the general symptoms of little importance and individuality, e.g. malaise, tiredness, want of sleep, want of appetite, etc., disappear into the background, and the more striking and special symptoms, belonging to few diseases and of rarer occurrence, begin to become prominent and to constitute the characteristic picture of this disease.

Footnote: If the physician has already been able to select for the earlier cases a remedy approximately suitable, and still more if he has found the remedy almost specific, he will either verify in the later cases the suitableness of his first choice (selected upon a true, although incomplete, conception of the disease), or he will find a more appropriate remedy, and finally to the most appropriate, the specific, remedy.

geworden; die neuern Fälle entweder die
Passendheit des zuerst (nach treuen, obgleich unvollständigen Krankheitsumris-
sen) gewählten bestätigen oder ihn näher-
hin auf das noch passendere, passendste,
specifische Heilmittel hinweisen.

82.

Ist nun der Inbegriff der Symptomen,
das Bild der Krankheit irgend einer Art einmahl genau aufgezeichnet, so ist auch die
schwerste Arbeit geschehen. Der Heilkünstler hat es dann auf immer vor sich
liegen; er kann es festhalten in allen seinen
Theilen, um ein treffendes Gegenstück dazu, eine dem gegenwärtigen Uebel treffend
ähnliche, künstliche Gegenkrankheitspotenz aus den Symptomenreihen aller ihm
bekannten Arzneien darnach aussuchen zu
können; und wenn er sich während der
Kur nach dem Erfolge der Arznei erkundigt, braucht er von der ursprünglichen
Gruppe der Krankheitssymptomen blos ab-
zuziehen, was sich gebessert hat, oder an-
zumerken, was etwa an neuen Beschwerden hinzu gekommen ist.

§ 82

If once the totality of symptoms, the portrait of any type of disease, is perfectly drawn, then his most difficult part of the task is finished. The healer, then, always has it (the portrait) before himself; he can study it in all its details, for discovering an effective opposing force, an artificial opposing disease-force, similar to the existing disease, chosen out of the symptom-lists of all the medicines which are known to him; and when in the course of treatment he wants to ascertain the effect of the remedy, he need only to strike out from the original group of disease-symptoms those that have been ameliorated, and to mark any new sufferings that has appeared.

83

Der zweite Punkt des rationellen Heilgeschäftes betrifft demnach die Wahl des homöopathischen Heilmittels, jener künstlichen Krankheitspotenz, durch deren Einnahme dem Kranken ein ähnliches Leiden (ομοιον παθος), eine künstliche Gegenkrankheit, gleichsam eingeimpft wird, welche die Krankheit, woran er leidet, durch Symptomenähnlichkeit zu überstimmen und auszulöschen (gründlich zu heilen) fähig ist.

84.

Zu dieser Absicht müssen die einzelnen Arzneien in ihrer ganzen Wirksamkeit als Krankheit erregende Potenzen bekannt seyn, das ist, möglichst alle die krankhaften Symptomen und Körperveränderungen, die jede derselben insbesondre zu erzeugen fähig ist, müssen erst bekannt seyn, ehe man eine derselben als Gegenkrankheitspotenz einer natürlichen Krankheit, um sie zu heben, entgegen stellen kann.

§ 83

The second point in the business of a rational healing concerns *the selection of the homoeopathic remedy,* that is, that artificial disease-producing power which can conquer a disease with similar suffering, (υμοιον πάςοζ), as if by inoculation of an artificial counter-disease which by its symptom-similarity is capable of overcoming and annihilating (radically cure) the disease from which he (the patient) suffers.

§ 84

For this purpose each remedy must be known in their entire effectiveness as disease-producing powers, that is, as far as possible, all the morbid symptoms and deviations in the body which each remedy have the power to produce must be known before any one opposing disease-force can be selected to combat the natural disease under treatment.

85.

Giebt man, diefs zu erforschen, Arzneien kranken Personen ein, so sieht man von ihren reinen Wirkungen wenig oder nichts, weil die von den Arzneien in Veränderung des Befindens des menschlichen Körpers besonders zu erwartenden Effekte, mit den Symptomen der gegenwärtigen natürlichen Krankheit vermengt, nur undeutlich oder gar nicht wahrgenommen werden können.

86.

Diefs zu vermeiden, war nichts natürlicher *), als dafs man die einzelnen Arzneien versuchsweise gesunden Menschen in

---

*) Schon der grofse *Albrecht von Haller* sah die Nothwendigkeit hiervon ein (in der Vorrede zur Pharm. Helvet. S. 12.): „Nempe primum in corpore sano medela tentanda est, sine peregrina ulla miscela; odoreque et sapore ejus exploratis, exigua illius dosis ingerenda et ad omnes, quae inde contingunt, affectiones, quis pulsus, qui calor, quae respiratio, quaenam excretiones, adtendendum. Inde ad ductum phaenomenorum, in sano obviorum, transeas ad experimenta in corpore aegroto, cct. "

F 2

§ 85

In order to investigate this, if a medicine be given to a sick person, little or nothing of its true effects is seen, because the effects which is especially desired to observe, namely, the deviations in the state of the human organism particularly the awaited effects together with symptoms resulting from the medicine, are so mixed-up with the symptoms of the existing natural disease that they can be recognized vaguely or not at all.

§ 86

To prevent this, nothing can be more natural[Fn] than to experimentally administer medicines singly to healthy persons in moderate doses and to discover what changes, symptoms and signs it produces in the health of the body and of the mind, that is to say, what disease-elements they tended to produce.

Fn: Footnote: The great Albrecht von Haller recognized this necessity long ago (in the Preface to the *Pharmacopoeia Helvet.*, Basil, 1771, p. 12): "Nempe primum in corpore sano medela tentanda est, sine peregrina ulla miscela, odoreque et sapore ejus exploratis, exigua illius dosis ingerenda

masiger Menge eingab, um zu sehen, welche Veranderungen, Symptomen und Zeichen ihrer Einwirkung jede besonders in der Gesundheit Leibes und der Seele rein hervorbringe, das ist, welche Krankheitselemente sie zu erregen, geneigt sei.

87.

Da traten dann, indem ich diefs mit Standhaftigkeit unternahm, nicht wenige Potenzen künstlicher Krankheit vor meine, mit vieler Aufopferung und moglichster Aufmerksamkeit geführte Beobachtung, die nun mit bestimmlicher Gewifsheit zu Erregung von Gegenkrankheiten gebraucht, das ist, als homoopathische Heilmittel naturlichen Krankheiten entgegen gesetzt werden konnen.

88.

Es fielen zugleich mehrere Reihen von Symptomen in meine Augen die schon in alteren Nachrichten verzeichnet standen, welche Beispiele erzählten von der Schadlichkeit stark wirkender Substanzen, die

et ad omnes, quae inde contingunt, affectiones, quis pulsus, qui color, quae respiratio, quaenam affection excretiones, adtendendum. Inde *ad ductum phaenomenorum, in sano obviorum*, transeas ad experimenta in corpore aegroto, etc."[10]

§ 87

Since I undertook to tread steadfastly, before me were revealed not a few powers of artificial disease ascertained through an observation conducted at much sacrifice and with the most possible attention, which can now be used with certainty for causing counter-diseases, that is, as homoeopathic remedies firmly against natural diseases.

§ 88

At the same time, several arrays of symptoms already written in older records also came in my view, which are examples of the harmfulness of strong substances when swallowed by healthy persons in large quantities.

---

[10] **SS note:** The translation of these immortal lines are:

In fact remedy, first of all, must be tried on a healthy body, without any admixture of the foreign elements, after the smell and taste of the medicine have been examined, a small amount of its dose should be taken and every change which occurs after it be observed; to the rate of the pulse, to the temperature, the rate of respiration, and the excretions. After the observation of the clear effects of phenomena in the healthy body, one may proceed to its trials in the body of a sick person.

von gesunden Personen in gröſserer Menge
verschluckt worden waren.

Anm. Man ahnete nicht, daſs diese Geschich-
ten von Arzneikrankheiten dereinst die
ersten Anfangsgründe der Arzneistoff-
lehre abgeben würden, die bis hieher faſt
nur in Vermuthungen bestand, das ist,
fast noch gar nicht existirte.

89.

Die Uebereinkunft meiner mit jenen al-
tern (obgleich umhinsichtlich auf Heilbehuf
beschriebenen) Beobachtungen reiner Arzneieffekte und selbst die Uebereinstimmung
dieser Nachrichten mit andern dieser Art,
uberzeugt uns leicht, daſs die Arzneistoffe
bei der krankhaften Veränderung des gesunden menschlichen Körpers nach bestimmten, unabänderlichen Gesetzen wirken, daſs sie gewisse, zu-
verlassige Krankheitssymptomen
zu erzeugen geeignet sind.

90.

Indeſs nimmt man in jenen älteren
Beschreibungen der oft lebensgefährlichen

Footnote: It was never suspected that the first foundation of knowledge about the medicines were laid by these histories of medicinal-diseases; till now this knowledge had remained almost totally conjectural, that is, had not existed at all.

§ 89

The agreement of my own observations on the pure effects of drug with these older records (although they were not recorded for purposes of therapeutics), and even the conformity of these records of other author must easily convince us easily that medicinal-substance produce pathological alterations in the healthy human body in accordance with *definite, unchangeable laws*, by which each can produce some appropriate *reliable disease-symptoms*.

§ 90

In those older descriptions of the dangerous effects produced after swallowing large-doses of medicines, it is often found that symptoms of a kind completely opposite to those which were observed first appear in the later stages of these unfortunate incidences.

Effekte in so ubermasigen Gaben verschluck-
ter Arzneien, auch Zustände wahr, die
nicht Anfangs, sondern beim Ausgange
solcher traurigen Ereignisse sich zeigten,
und von einer, den anfanglichen ganz entgegen gesetzten Natur waren.

91.

Solche nachgängigen Zufalle
nahm zwar auch ich Anfangs nicht selten
wahr, doch weit seltner als in jenen Nachrichten vorkömmt, weil ich nicht so über-
masige Gaben zu Versuchen anwendete.
Ie kleinere Gaben ich aber nachgehends zu
Versuchen dieser Art nahm, in desto klei-
nerer Zahl erschienen dieselben, indefs die
anfänglichen Symptomen auch bei
den kleinern Gaben in gleich reichlicher
Menge und mit gleicher Bestimmtheit erschienen, wenn ich die Aufmerksamkeit
bei der Beobachtung verdoppelte und alles
vermied, wodurch irgend die Reinheit des
Versuchs hatte vermindert werden können.

92.

Der Umstand, dafs die nachgängigen,
die man negative oder Sekundär-

§ 91

Such *secondary symptoms* I myself observed quite frequently at first, but not so often as in those records, because I did not employ such enormously large doses. The smaller the doses I subsequently used for such experiments, the more rarely did these (secondary) symptoms occur, whereas even with the smaller doses the *primary symptoms* presented themselves in great numbers and with equal certainty when I paid great attention during the observation and avoided everything which might interfere with the exactitude of the experiment.

§ 92

The fact that these subsequent symptoms (which may be named '*negative*' or '*secondary*') appear more frequently when large doses are used, and are infrequent in appearance in exact ratio to the diminution of the dose used in the experiments

symptomen nennen kann, am häufigsten bei sehr grofsen Gaben zum Vorscheine kommen und je kleiner die Gabe ist, auch in den Versuchen desto seltner werden, zeiget, dafs die Sekundarsymptomen nur eine Art von Nachkrankheit sind, welche bei grofsen Gaben nach Verflufs der anfänglichen Symptomen (positiven oder Primarsymptomen), entsteht; eine Art gegenseitiger Zustand — nach dem gewöhnlichen Vorgange im Leben, in welchem alles in Wechselzustanden vorzugehen scheint.

> Anm. So wie auf allzu grofse Lustigkeit Traurigkeit — auf Leibesverstopfung Durchfall, auf Durchfall Verstopfung, auf Schlaf Munterkeit, auf Frost Hitze und umgekehrt zu folgen pflegt.

93.

Von jeder kräftigen Arznei zeigt sich eine ansehnliche Zahl Symptomen mancherlei Art, ganze Reihen von Zufällen und Krankheitszeichen, welche samtlich Primärsymptomen sind, wenn die Versuchsgabe nicht heftig war. Die Haupteffek-

proves that the secondary symptoms are only a kind of *after-disease* due to large doses which appear after the cessation of the early *'positive'* or *'primary'* symptoms; a kind of opposite state or reactive condition, in accordance with the usual process of life wherein everything seems to go on by a series of alternating states.

Footnote: As sadness usually follows excessive joy, constipation to diarrhoea, diarrhoea to constipation, wakefulness to somnolence, heat to chilliness, and *vice versa.*

§ 93

After the administration of every powerful medicine a considerable number of symptoms of different kinds are manifested, a whole series of occurrences and morbid phenomena of disease, which are all primary symptoms if the experimental dose was not too large. The *chief effects* of the medicines, understood as artificial disease-producing forces, are these more frequent Primary Symptoms.

te der Arzneien, als kunstlicher Krankheitspotenzen, sind jene haufigern Primar
symptomen.

94.

Unter diesen giebt es nicht wenige,
welche andern, bald vorher erschienenen,
bald nachher erscheinenden Symptomen
zum Theil, oder in Absicht gewisser Ne-
behumstande entgegen gesetzt sind, deswegen aber nicht zu den Sekundärsymptomen oder zur Nachkrankheit der Arzneiwir-
kung gehören, sondern nur den Wechsel-
zustand der verschiednen Wirkungsparo-
xysmen positiver (primarer) Art bilden.

95.

Einige Symptomen bringen die Arzneien öfterer, andre seltner, und einige
sehr selten bei ihrer Anwendung am gesunden menschlichen Körper zum Vorscheine.
Die sonderlichsten und die am oftersten
von ihnen erzeugten Symptomen sind die
vorzüglichsten.

§ 94

Among these are not a few symptoms which are, in part or in some conditions, completely, opposite to other symptoms which have appeared earlier or may appear later, and which are not, therefore, to be regarded as Secondary Symptoms or the after-disease produced by the medicine, but only as the alternating phase of the paroxysmal effects of the positive (or Primary) action of the medicine.

§ 95

Some symptoms are produced by medicines more oftener, some less frequently and some appear only very rarely when they are applied on healthy human body. The uncommon symptoms and those which appear frequently are most valuable.

Footnote: Idiosyncrasies are often only those rare but real peculiar medicinal-effects on persons who, although healthy, possess a special sensitiveness to the action of there particular substances. Thus some species of Sumach (**Translator's note:** Rhus venenata) when touched causes certain skin-eruptions in some persons, and eating mussels (**Translator's note:**

Anm. Idiosynkrasien sind oft nichts als solche zwar selten vorkommende, aber reine, auffallende Arzneieffekte auf Personen, welche obgleich gesund, doch für die Einwirkung dieser besondern Substanzen vorzügliche Empfänglichkeit besitzen; so wie einige Sumach - Arten bei der Berührung nur einigen wenigen Personen gewisse Hautausschläge, und die Flußkrebse nach dem Genusse nur bei einigen Wenigen eine Art Rothlauf und Blasenfieber zuwege bringen (obgleich beide die bestandige Tendenz zu diesen Aeufserungen unter allen Umständen behalten), und so wie selbst nur einige Individuen von Pferden und Kühen vom Genusse der Taxusblätter plötzlich getödet werden, indefs die übrigen nur wenig davon leiden.

96.

Iede Arznei zeigt besondre Effekte, welche sich von keinem andern Arzneistoffe verschiedner Art genau so ereignen.

97.

So gewiſs jede Pflanzenart in ihrer äuſsern Gestalt, in der eignen Weise ihres

Cray fish) causes erysipelas and urticaria in few. (although both of these substances possess *the constant tendency to produce these manifestations* under all circumstances); and so some horses and cows have been suddenly killed by eating leaves of yew (**Translator's note:** Taxus baccata), while other animals of the species are little affected by them.

§ 96

Every medicine produces particular effects which are not produced by any other medicinal substance in exactly the same way.

§ 97

As each species of plant differs from every other species in its external form, particular mode of life and growth, in taste and in smell, and as each mineral and each salt is certainly different from every other in external appearance as well as in its inner physical and chemical properties

Lebens, und Wuchses, in ihrem Geschmacke und in ihrem Geruche von jeder andern Pflanzen-Art und Gattung, so
gewiſs jedes Mineral, jedes Salz in seinen
auſsern sowohl, als innern physischen und
chemischen Eigenschaften (wodurch allein
oft schon alle Verwechslung unmöglich
gemacht wird) verschieden ist, so gewiſs
sind sie alle unter sich, in ihren kränk-
machenden (also auch heilenden) Wirkungen verschieden. Iede dieser Substanzen
wirkt daher auf eine eigne, verschiedne,
doch bestimmte Weise die alle Verwechselung verbietet Abänderungen des Ge-
sundheitszustandes und des Befindens der
Menschen.

Anm. Wer die so sonderbar abweichenden
Effekte jeder einzelnen Substanz von denen
jeder andern genau kennt und zu würdigen
versteht, der sieht auch leicht ein, daſs es
unter ihnen, in arzneilicher Hinsicht, keine gleichbedeutenden Mittel, keine Sur-
rogate geben kann. Blos wer die verschiednen Arzneien in ihren reinen positiven
Wirkungen nicht kennt, kann sich solche
Verwechselungen zu Schulden kommen
lassen. So wurden die Mineralien, in de-

(whereby frequent confusion between one with any other is impossible), so definitely are they all different in their power to produce disease (and also healing). Each substance causes changes in the state of health and condition of the human body according to its own peculiar and definite character, the character which forbids the substitution of any other substance for any one.

Footnote: Whoever has a thorough knowledge and properly give values to the extraordinary difference between the effects of one substance and those of ever other, can easily perceive that, amongst them, from a medical point of view there can be no equivalent remedies, no surrogates. Only those who do not know the pure and definite effects of different medicines can be guilty of such substitutions. Thus the minerals in which the recent and more careful chemistry has discovered new and particular metals, differing widely from all others, were held by our ignorant ancestors for stones and clay of no value; similarly, children also confuse things essentially most different because they do not know their external appearances, much less their true worth and their inner and most different qualities.

nen die neue, sorgfältigere Chemie ganz
eigne, höchst verschiedne neue Metalle
entdeckt hat, nur für gleichgültige Steine
und Erden von unsern unwissenden Vor-
fahren gehalten; so verwechseln Kinder
die wesentlich verschiedensten Dinge, weil
sie sie kaum dem Aeufsern nach, und nicht
nach ihrem Werthe, nicht nach ihren innern, höchst abweichenden Eigenschaften
kennen.

98.

Die Substanzen des Thier- und Pflan-
zenreiches sind in ihrem rohen Zustande
am arzneilichsten.

Anm: Diejenigen Pflanzen und Thiere, derer
wir uns zu Nahrungsmitteln bedienen,
haben den Vorzug einer größern Menge
Nahrungstheile vor den übrigen, und weichen darinn von den andern ab, daß die
Arzneikräfte ihres rohen Zustandes theils
nicht sehr heftig, theils, wenn sie auch
heftig sind, durchs Trocknen (wie bei der
Aron - und Päonienwurzel), durch Aus-
pressen des schädlichen Saftes (wie bei der
Kassave), durch Gähren (saure Gurken),
durch Räuchern, und durch die Gewalt
der Hitze (beim Rösten, Braten, Backen,

§ 98

Substances belonging to the animal and vegetable kingdoms are very powerful as medicines in their crude state.

Footnote: Those plants and animals which are used for food have the preference over others of possessing a larger number of components of food, and differ from the others in that their medicinal powers in the crude state are either not so strong or, when they are strong, are lessened and destroyed by drying [as in Arum (**Translator's note:** Arum triphyllum) and Peony root (**Translator's note:** Paeonia officinalis)], by expression of the poisonous juices [as of Cassava (**Translator's note:** Jatropha manihot or J. gossipyfolia)], by fermentation [as of sour gherkins (**Translator's note:** Cucumis sativus, a small cucumber used for making pickles)], by smoking and by the force of heat (in roasting, frying, baking, boiling), or are antidoted and rendered harmless by the addition of salt, sugar, and especially vinegar (in sauces and salads). Even most medicinal plants lose their medicinal-power partly or completely by such operations. The juice of the heroic plants is often reduced to a powerless pitch-like substance by the heat commonly applied in the preparation of an extract. The expressed juice of the most poisonous plants in their fresh state, (for by putting on top of each other when green, it

Kochen) zerstört und verflüchtigt, oder durch den Zusatz des Kochsalzes, des Zuckers, vorzuglich aber des Essigs (in Saucen und Salaten) antidotisch unschädlicher gemacht werden. Ja selbst die arzneilichsten Pflanzen verlieren ihre Arzneikraft zum Theil, oder ganz durch solche Operationen. Der Saft der heroischen Pflanzen wird durch die Hitze der gewöhnlichen Extraktbereitung oft zur ganz unkräftigen pechartigen Masse. Der ausgepreßte Saft der todlichsten Pflanzen in ihrem frischen Zustande (denn wenn sie grün übereinander liegend, wie man sagt, geschwitzet haben, so ist durch innere Gährung schon ein grofser Theil der Arzneikraft verloren) darf nur Einen Tag an einem temperirten Orte stehen, so ist er in volle Weingährung übergegangen, und hat schon viele seiner Arzneikräfte eingebüßt; steht er aber noch einen oder zwei Tage, so ist die Essiggährung vollendet und alle specifische Arzneikraft ist verschwunden; das Satzmehl ist dann völlig unschädlich, der Weizenstärke gleich.

99.

Um die Effekte der Arzneien auszuspahen, muß man wissen, daß die star-

is said that they sweat, and the greater part of their medicinal power is lost by fermentation) if allowed to stand for only one day in a moderately warm place passes into complete alcoholic fermentation and looses much of its medicinal power; but if it is left to stand for another one or two days till the acetous fermentation is complete, all its specific medicinal power *disappears*; the sediment is then quite harmless and resembles wheat-starch.

§ 99

To find out the effects of medicines it must be remembered that strong drugs, so-called heroic medicines will show their effects when given in quite small doses, in healthy, even strong persons. In order to observe the complete effect, the medicines of weaker power must be given in more considerable quantities and the weakest medicines can only be tested upon disease-free persons who are tender, excitable and sensitive.

ken, so genannten heroischen Arzneien
schon in geringer Gabe ihre Wirkung bei
gesunden, selbst starken Personen zeigen.
Die von schwächerer Kraft müssen zu diesen Versuchen in ansehnlicherer Gabe gereicht werden, die schwächsten Arzneien
aber können, damit man ihre absolute
Wirkung wahrnehme, blos bei solchen
von Krankheit freien Personen versucht
werden, welche zärtlich, reitzbar und em-
pfindlich sind.

100.

Der hiezu aufgelegte, beobachtende
Arzt darf keine Arzneien zu solchen Versuchen, von denen das Wohl ganzer Men-
schengenerationen abhangt, nehmen, als
solche, die er genau kennt und von deren Aechtheit und Vollkraftigkeit er gänzlich überzeugt ist.

101.

Iede dieser Arzneien muſs in ganz einfacher, ungekunstelter Form, in Pulver,
oder als blos mit Weingeist verfertigte

§ 100

The physician observing these experiments, upon which depends the welfare of the entire generations of human beings, should not but select only those medicines which he knows well and of whose genuineness and power he is fully convinced.

§ 101

Each of these medicines must be administered in a perfectly simpler and unadulterated form, in powder, or alcoholic tincture, or in watery solution if they are salts and gums, so as to procure only individual effects of each substance. But because infusions of plants in water and fresh juices of the herbs are spoilt by fermentation within a few hours, the medicines belonging to these classes must either be administered without delay immediately after preparation, or fermentation must be delayed by the addition of a little spirit of wine, or avoided by the use of a larger quantity of alcohol.

Tinktur, die Salze und Gummen in wäs-
seriger Auflösung eingegeben werden, um
ihre eigenthümlichen Wirkungen zu erforschen. Da aber der wässerige Aufguſs
der Gewächse und die frischen Kräuter-
säfte sich schon binnen wenigen Stunden
durch Gährung zersetzen, so müssen beî-
de gleich nach ihrer Verfertigung ohne
Zeitverlust eingegeben werden, wenn man
die Gährung nicht durch Zusatz von etwas Weingeist verzögern oder durch eine
stärkere Menge desselben ganz beseitigen
will.

102.

Ieden Arzneistoff muſs man zu dieser
Absicht ganz allein, ganz rein anwenden,
ohne irgend eine fremdartige Substanz zu-
zumischen, oder dergleichen zu derselben
Zeit, oder kurz vorher oder nachher zu
brauchen.

103.

Man giebt dem zum Versuche bestimmten, gesunden Menschen, während

§ 102

Each medicinal substance, for this experimental purpose, must be given alone and in pure form, without mixture of any unfamiliar substance and nothing of a medicinal nature may be used at the same time, shortly before or afterwards.

§ 103

Healthy persons, on whom the experiments are to be carried on, must take in empty stomach such a dose as is used in common medical practice when needed to care against diseases, best given in solution, and no food is to be allowed for some hours afterwards. He must with good intention be precisely attentive and be undisturbed by it.

er nüchtern ist, ungefähr eine solche Gabe
ein, als man in der gewöhnlichen Praxis
gegen Krankheiten zu brauchen pfleget,
am besten in Auflosung, und läfst die Person noch mehrere Stunden nüchtern. Sie
muſs mit gutem Willen auf sich genau
Acht haben und dabei ungestört seyn.

104.

Will man die Effekte dieser einzelnen
Gabe (wie am besten) mehrere Tage lang
beobachten, so muſs die Diät recht mä-
ſsig eingerichtet werden, möglichst ohne
Gewürze, von blos nahrender, einfacher
Art, so daſs die grünen Zugemüſse und
frischen Wurzeln (welche immer einige
störende Arzneikraft auch bei aller Zubereitung behalten) vermieden werden. Die
Getränke sollen die alltäglichen seyn, so
wenig als möglich reitzend.

105.

Die Person muſs sich vor Excessen
aller Art, auch in Leidenschaften huten.

§ 104

When the effects of this single dose are to be observed (as is best) over a period of several days, the diet must be strictly regulated. It should be of a simple nutritious character without spices as far as possible; and green vegetables and fresh roots (which always possess some interfering medicinal power in their every preparation), should be avoided. The drinks should be those usually taken, as little stimulating as possible.

§ 105

The person **(Translator's note:** the prover) must avoid all kinds of excesses, also passions of mind.

106.

Wäre auf die erste Gabe gar nichts erfolgt, wenigstens nichts Deutliches, Bestimmbares, so wird eine zweite, doppelt stärkere den zweiten Tag, und wenn auch diese der Absicht noch nicht entsprache, allenfalls eine noch stärkere am dritten Tage, ihre Wirkung schon zu erkennen geben.

107.

Diese Wiederholung wird jedoch selten nöthig seyn, wenn die Versuchsperson und der Arzt gleich aufmerksam sind; so wie es auch weit sichrer ist, um einen reinen Erfolg, wenigstens in Hinsicht der Succession der Symptome auf einander, zu sehen, wenn bei einer Person nur mit einer einzigen Gabe der Versuch angestellt wird, und erst nach Wochen vielleicht mit einer zweiten Gabe derselben, oder besser, nach geraumer Zeit, mit einer einzelnen Gabe einer andern Arzneisubstanz.

108.

So erfahrt man die Aufeinanderfolge der Arzneisymptomen genauer, als wann

§ 106

If nothing results after the first dose, or at least nothing clear and definite, a second dose of double the quantity should be given on the second day, and if this also does not produces any effect, then a still stronger dose should be administered on the third day.

§107

But, this repetition, will, however, seldom be necessary if both experimenting person [**Ss: the prover**] and the physician are equally observant. We are more certain of obtaining a pure result, especially in regard to the succession of the symptoms upon each other, if the experiment is made on the person by the administration of a single dose and it is only after some weeks, perhaps, that a second dose of the same medicine may be given. A single dose of a different medicinal substance may be administered only after the lapse of a considerable time.

§ 108

The order of appearance of the medicinal symptoms can be observed better in this way rather than when a second dose of the same medicine is given soon after the first; the duration of the action of a medicine on the human body also is more definitely observed by the administration of a single dose than by any other method.

bald nach der erstern, wieder eine zweite
Gabe derselben Arznei gegeben wird; auch
laſst sich bei Anwendung einer einzigen Gabe die Dauer der Wirkungszeit einer Arznei
im menschlichen Körper gewisser, als auf
irgend eine andre Art, beobachten.

109.

Wo man aber noch ohne Rücksicht
auf Wirkungsdauer, und Succession blos
die Symptomen vor sich, besonders einer
schwachkräftigen Arznei erforschen will;
da ist die Veranstaltung vorzuziehen, daſs
man jeden Tag eins erhöhete Gabe, auch
wohl des Tages mehrmahls eine solche reiche.
che. Dann wird der Effekt auch der mil-
desten, noch unbekannten Arznei an den
Tag kommen.

110.

Nicht alle einer Arznei eignen Symptomen kommen schon bei Einer zum Versuche gewählten Person, auch nicht alle
sogleich oder denselben Tag zum Vorscheine sondern bei der einen Person die-

G

§ 109

But if the purpose is to investigate the symptoms themselves, especially those of a medicine of weaker power, without regard to duration of action and succession of symptoms, then the better method is to give it every day in an increasing dose or several times a day in the same dose. In this way the effects of even the weakest medicine, perhaps not known till now, will become known.

§ 110

Not all the characteristic symptoms belonging to a medicine appear in one attempt in one person [**Ss:** the prover], nor yet do all appear at once or on the same day, but some appear in one person, others in another, yet in such a way that perhaps in a fourth or tenth person some or many of the symptoms which had been found in the second or sixth or seventh person may be visible; again, all will not appear exactly at the same hour.

se, bei der andern jene vorzugsweise;
doch so, dafs vielleicht bei einer vierten
oder zehnten Person wieder einige oder
mehrere von denen Zufällen, welche schon
etwa bei der zweiten oder sechsten, sie-
benten Person sichtbar geworden, sich
hervorthun; auch erscheinen sie nicht genau zu derselben Stunde wieder.

111.

Der Inbegriff aller Krankheitselemente, die eine Arznei hervorzubringen vermag, wird erst in vielfachen, an vielen
dazu tauglichen Personen angestellten
Beobachtungen der Vollständigkeit nahe
gebracht.

112.

Ie kleiner, bis zu einer gewissen Mase, die Gaben einer zu solchen Versuchen
bestimmten Arznei sind — indefs man
nur die Beobachtung durch die Wahl einer auf sich aufmerksamen, empfindlichen, in jeder Rucksicht gemasigten Person, so wie durch die gespannteste Auf-

§ 111

The totality of all disease-elements which a medicine is capable of producing is only brought near completeness by repeated observations on many suitable persons.

§ 112

For a certain measure of the dose of a given medicine for such an experiment, more so with ever smaller dose, careful observation can be only attained by the choice of person who in every regard is cautious, attentive and sensitive person, only then one can endeavour to get the clearer knowledge of Primary symptoms, and the Secondary symptoms will remain back.

merksamkeit zu erleichtern sich bestrebt —
desto deutlicher kommen fast blos die Primärsymptomen, als die wissenswurdig-
sten hervor, und die Sekundärsymptomen
bleiben zuruck.

113.

Bei übermäsig grofsen Gaben spielen
nicht nur die Sekundärsymptomen eine
grofse Rolle mit, sondern die Primärsymp-
tbmen treten dann auch in so verwirrter
Eile und so stürmisch auf, dafs sich nichts
genau beobachten läfst; der Gefahr derselben nicht zu gedenken, die dem, welcher Achtung gegen die Menschheit hat,
und auch den geringsten im Volke für seinen Bruder schätzt nicht gleichgültig
seyn kann.

114.

Die gewählten Personen mussen ihre
Empfindung bestimmt und deutlich auszudrücken fähig seyn.

G 2

§ 113

If very large doses are administered, not only do the secondary symptoms play a big role, but the primary symptoms appear in a more confused, sudden and aggravated manner so that they cannot be properly observed; we can not overlook the danger of the same, which cannot be a matter of indifference to any person who respects mankind and values the lowest of the people as his brother.

§ 114

The selected person (**Translator's note:** the prover) must be capable of expressing their feelings precisely and clearly.

115

Bei Erkundigung dieser Arzneisymptomen muſs alle Suggestion, eben so sorgfaltig vermieden werden, als nur irgend
bei Erforschung der Symptomen der Krankheiten. Es muſs groſstentheils nur frei-
willige Erzählung der zum Versuche ge-
nommenen Person seyn — nichts Erra-
thenes, nichts Vermuthetes, und so wenig
als möglich Ausgefragtes, — was man als
wahren Befund niederschreiben will; am
wenigsten aber Ausdrücke von Empfindungen, die man der Versuchsperson vorher schon in den Mund gelegt hatte, oder
worauf sie blos Ia, oder Nein antworten
könnte.

116.

Hier dient, um diese wichtigen Aussagen, möglichst zur Wahrheit zu erheben, noch der Rath, sich die schon nie-
dergeschriebnen Zufälle und Empfindungen von der zum Versuche dienenden Person zulezt nochmals wiederholen zu lassen, um das, worin sie auf einerlei Rede

§ 115

In the inquiry of the medicine-symptoms, as in the investigation of the symptoms of disease, all suggestions and opinions must be as carefully avoided. The major part of what is recorded as the genuine result of experiment must be the voluntary statements of the experimented persons (**Translator's note:** the provers); nothing must be conjectural, nothing as of guesses, and as little as possible of interrogation; nothing at all of the findings should written down which contain expressions relating to feelings with which they have been earlier prompted, or the results of questions that can be answered in *yes* or *no*.

§116

For the purpose of making these important statements as much truthful as possible is that as soon as any symptoms or sensations of the person undergoing the trial [**SS:** the prover] are written down, he should be asked to repeat his description once more, so that, when his second statement is identical with the first, it may be recorded in that form, and when his words are different from earlier he may be shown both and invited to choose and confirm the statement which is nearest to the truth, and thereby render true, pure and striking portrait of the medicinal disease which has been discovered through his help. The physician who is observing the experiment adds to the description of experimented person (**Translator's note:** the prover) every alteration in health which he himself has observed in him.

bleibt, als bestimmt anzuzeichnen, wo es
aber Varianten giebt, sie ihr vorzuhalten,
damit sie den der Wahrheit angemesse-
nern Ausdruck vorziehen und nochmals
bestätigen könne und das Bild der von
ihr empfundenen Arzneikrankheit wahr,
rein und treffend werde. Der beobachtende Arzt setzt hiezu die Veränderungen,
die er selbst an der Versuchsperson offenbar wahrnimmt.

117.

Die deutlichern, und auffallendern Zufälle werden, mit Bemerkung der nach
der Gabe verflossenen Stunden, der Tageszeit, ihrer Dauer und aller vorgefalle-
nen Nebenumstande in dem Verzeichnisse
aufgeschrieben; die öfterer auf gleiche Art
beobachteten werden als die bestätigtern
durch Vorzugsmerkmahle ausgezeichnet,
die zweideutigen aber mit Zeichen des
Zweifels belegt oder in Klammern einge-
schlossen bis auch sie vielleicht, nach
öfterer Bestätigung, dieser Zweideutigkeit
wieder entledigt werden.

§ 117

The record of the more distinct and striking symptoms must be accompanied by a note of the time that elapsed between the administration of the dose and the appearance of the symptoms, the time of day at which they appeared, their duration, and all accessory circumstances; those symptoms which are observed very often in the same way should be underlined, and those which are ambiguous should be marked by a sign of interrogation or enclosed in brackets until, perhaps, the ambiguity concerning them is removed by the confirmation in further experiments.

Die Versuche des fein beobachtenden, vorurtheillosen Arztes mit Arzneien an sich selbst bleiben die wichtigsten.

Wie man aber selbst in Krankheiten, besonders in den chronischen, unter den Symptomen der ursprunglichen Krankheit die Symptomen der Arznei ausfinden könne, ist ein Gegenstand höherer Kunst und blos Meistern in der Beobachtung zu überlassen.

Hat man nun eine ansehnliche Reihe Arzneien in gesunden Menschen so geprobt und alle die Krankheitselemente und Symptomen sorgfaltig und treu aufgezeichnet, die sie vor sich als künstliche Krankheitspotenzen zu erzeugen fähig sind, so hat man eine Materia medica — eine Sammlung der wahren, positiven Wirkungsarten der einfachen Arzneistoffe vor

§ 118

The experiments with medicines which are carried out by the minutely observing and unprejudiced physician upon himself are most reliable.

§ 119

Even in diseases, particularly in chronic ones, the symptoms of a medicine can be discovered amongst the symptoms of the original disease which is an object for the higher Art and should be left only to the masters in observation.

§ 120

When we have in this manner tested on healthy persons a considerable of medicines, and have carefully and reliably recorded all the disease-elements and symptoms which as artificial disease-powers are capable to produce, only then we have a Materia Medica – a collection of the true, irrefutable mode of action of simple medicinal-substances, a codex of Nature wherein is recorded considerable list of peculiar symptoms of each one of the investigated efficacious medicine and disease-elements, as they were discovered to the observer, among which shall be found the elements of several of the natural diseases which in future can be cured through the similarity established from these records.

sich, einen Kodex der Natur, worin von
jeder so erforschten, kräftigen Arznei eine
ansehnliche Reihe besonderer Symptomen
und Krankheitselemente, wie sie sich der
Aufmerksamkeit des Beobachters zu Tage
legten, aufgezeichnet stehen, in denen die
Elemente mehrerer natürlichen, dereinst
durch sie zu heilenden Krankheiten in
Aehnlichkeit vorhanden sind.

121.

In einer solchen Arzneimittellehre sei
nichts Vermuthetes, Behauptetes, Erdach-
tes, Fingirtes, sondern alles reine Sprache
der befragten Natur.

122.

Freilich kann nur ein ansehnlicher
Vorrath genau nach dieser ihrer positiven
Wirkungsart gekannter Arzneimittel uns
in den Stand setzen, für jeden der unendlich vielen natürlichen Krankheitsfälle ein
homöopathisches Heilmittel (ein vollstan-
diges Analogon von Gegenkrankheitspotenz) auszufinden.

§ 121

In such a Materia Medica[11] there is nothing conjectural, assertion, imagined, arbitrary; but everything is the pure language of Nature obtained by careful enquiry.

§ 122

In reality only a considerable supply of medicines thus exactly known with their irrefutable modes of action can serve our purpose, and enable us to discover a homoeopathic remedy (completely analogue or similar to the counter disease-force) for each one of the infinite number of cases of disease in nature.

Footnote: When thousands of accurate and reliable observers, instead of only one as till now, have been occupied in the investigation of *these first elements of the doctrine of medicinal substance*, which will not be the first in the whole extent of the endless disease-fields! Then the medical occupation will no longer be ridiculed at as a groundless Art of conjecture.

---

[11] **Translator's note:** Hahnemann here has used the German word *Arzneimittellehre* whose dictionary meaning is *Pharmacology*. However in the context of this aphorism it has been translated as Materia Medica. It is interesting to note that in the previous aphorism (No. 120) though he has used the word Materia Medica.

Anm. Wenn statt eines Einzigen, wie bisher
Tausende von genauen und zuverlässigen
Beobachtern sich mit Erforschung dieser
ersten Elemente einer rationellen Arzneistoff - Lehre beschäftigt
haben werden; was wird dann nicht erst
im ganzen Umfange des unendlichen Krank-
heits = Gebietes ausgerichtet werden können. Dann wird das Heilgeschäft (nicht
mehr als grundlose Vermuthungskunst (ars
conjecturalis) verspottet werden können.

123.

Indessen bleiben auch jezt — Dank
sei's der Vielheit von Symptomen und dem
Reichthume an Krankheitselementen, welche jede der kraftigen Arzneisubstanzen,
in ihrer positiven Wirkung am gesunden
Korper schon aufgewiesen hat — doch
nur wenige Krankheitsfalle ubrig für welche selbst aus diesem geringen Vorrathe*)

----

*) Fragmenta de viribus medicaminum, po-
sitivis, sive in sano corpore humano observatis, P. I. II. Lips. Barth. 8. 1805. Etwas
seitdem Vervollständigtes wird vielleicht noch von
mir erscheinen.

§ 123

Meanwhile, even now there remains - thanks to the multitude of symptoms and abundance of disease-elements, which ever one of the powerful medicinal-substance has already shown in its irrefutable effect on the healthy body – only few remaining cases of diseases for which, even out of this small supply[Fn], a suitable analogue of counter disease-force (i.e. a remedy) cannot be discovered which will restore the health gently, swiftly and permanently without any remarkable disturbances. In spite of limited choice among the incompletely known remedies incredibly better cures can be made by this method than by the so-called ordinary methods or any other of all the irrational, paralogistic (**Translator's note:** contrary to reason] non-homoeopathic methods.

Fn: Footnote: *Fragmenta de viribus medicaminum positivis, sive in sano corpore humano observatis*, P. I. II, Lips. Barth. 8. 1805 will perhaps be published by me after its completion. (**Translator's note:** it is interesting to note that title of the book, a copy of which this translator possesses has the title as *Fragmenta de viribus medicamentorum positivis, sive in sano corpore humano observatis*)

sich nicht ein erträgliches Analogon von Gegenkrankheitspotenz (ein Heilmittel) auffinden lassen sollte, was, ohne sonderliche Beschwerde, Gesundheit sanft, schnell und dauerhaft wiederbringt — wegen eingeschränkter Wahl zwar noch unvollkommene Hülfsmittel, wodurch aber unglaublich mehr und besser geheilt wird, als nach der sogenannten allgemeinen Methode, oder als nach allen irrationellen, paralogen, nicht homöopathischen Methoden.

184.

In welcher Symptomenreihe einer unter den so, nach ihrer positiven Wirkungsart durch Beobachtung am gesunden Körper befragten Arzneien man nun das meiste Aehnliche von dem Symptomenkomplexe einer gegebnen natürlichen Krankheit antrifft, das wird, das muſs die passendste Gegenkrankheit zur Vertreibung und Auslöschung jener natürlichen Krankheit seyn; das passendste, specifische Heilmittel ist in dieser Arznei gefunden.

§ 124

From amongst the symptom-array of its irrefutable mode of action of medicines observed on the healthy body can be found the most similar symptom-complex to that of a natural disease, which must be the best counter-disease for dislodging and annihilating the natural disease; the best, the specific remedy is found in that medicine.

Ist nun so die Gegenkrankheits - Potenz (Arznei) völlig passend nach der Symptomenähnlichkeit, das ist, homoopathisch ausgesucht worden, und wird sie gehörig angewendet, so vergeht die zu bezwingende natürliche, auch noch so schlimme, mit noch so viel Zufällen beladene Krankheit, wenn sie unlängst entstanden war, unvermerkt in einigen Stunden — wenn sie älter war, in einigen wenigen Tagen und man wird von den krankhaften Symptomen der Arznei, das ist von der künstlichen Gegenkrankheit fast nichts gewahr; es erfolgt in schnellen, unbemerklichen Uebergängen, nichts als Gesundheit, die natürliche und die Gegenkrankheit verlöschen schnell beide zusammen, ohne bemerkbare Reaktion, ganz in der Stille — eine wahre dynamische Vernichtung.

125.

Hier kömmt es nun auf den dritten Punkt der rationellen Heilkunde, auf die

§ 125

So, if, now, the counter disease-force (the medicine) selected is best suitable due to its symptoms-similarity, i.e., which is exactly homoeopathic, and if, it is properly administered then, the natural disease, however dangerous or severe, however complicated with too many symptoms, will go away almost unnoticed in a few hours, provided it has not been of long duration - if it is of longer duration, it disappears within a few days and in either case practically none of the pathogenic symptoms of the medicine, that is, of the artificial counter-disease can be observed; there comes only health in rapid and hardly noticeable sequence; the natural and the artificial disease both are quickly and mutually extinguished, without perceptible reaction - a true dynamic annihilation.

§ 126

Here we come to the *third point* in a rational system of treatment, the proper application of the homoeopathic remedy in diseases.

gehörige Anwendung des homöopathischen Heilmittels in Krankheiten an.

127.

Werden dem Arzte ein oder ein Paar geringfügige Zufälle geklagt, welche seit Kurzem erst bemerkt wurden, so hat er diefs für keine vollständige Krankheit anzusehen, welche arzneilicher Hülfe bedürfte. Eine kleine Abänderung in der Diät und Lebensordnung reicht gewöhnlich hin, sie zu verwischen. Sind es aber ein Paar heftige Beschwerden, die der Kranke klagt, so findet der forschende Arzt gewöhnlich noch nebenbei mehrere, obschon kleinere Zufälle, welche ein vollständiges Bild von der Krankheit geben, wie es gemeiniglich in chronischen Uebeln statt findet; wovon weiter unten.

128.

Ie schlimmer eine Krankheit ist, aus desto mehrern, aus desto auffallendern Symptomen ist sie dann gewöhnlich zusammen gesetzt; um desto gewisser läfst

§ 127

If one or two minor complaints have become manifested in a patient recently, the physician should not consider this as a complete disease requiring medicinal help. A slight alteration in diet and mode of life will be usually enough to remove such an illness. But if the patient complains of only one or two severe complaints, the physician on examination, will usually find, in addition, lesser ailments, which make up a complete portrait of the disease, which generally is the case with chronic disorders, of which more is below.

§ 128

The more severe a disease is, the more numerous and more striking are usually its symptoms of which it is usually composed of; and so more surely also is an appropriate remedy found for it, if a sufficient number of known medicines is available to us having tested their positive effect. Among the symptom-array for many medicines as a rule, it is not, difficult to find out one medicine whose particular disease-elements and symptom complex present a very similar counter-image to those of the natural disease, thereby constituting it an appropriate counter disease-agent; and then this is the this is the chosen remedy.

sich aber auch ein passendes Heilmittel
für sie auffinden, wenn eine hinreichende
Zahl nach ihrer positiven Wirkung gekannter Arzneien vorhanden ist. Unter
den Symptomenreihen vieler Arzneien
läfst sich nicht schwierig eine finden, aus
deren einzelnen Krankheitselementen sich
ein dem Symptomenkomplexe der naturlichen Krankheit sehr ähnliches Gegenbild,
eine passende Gegenkrankheitspotenz zusammensetzen läfst; und diese ist dann
das gesuchte Heilmittel.

129.

Bei dieser Aufsuchung eines homöopathisch specifischen Heilmittels, das ist,
bei dieser Gegeneinander - Haltung des Zei-
cheninbegriffs der natürlichen Krankheit
gegen die Symptomenreihen der vorhandnen Arzneien sind die auffallendern,
sonderlichen, charakteristischen
Zeichen der erstern vorzüglich fest ins Auge zu fassen; denn vorzüglich diesen
müssen sehr ähnliche in den Krankheitselementen der Symptomenreihen der gesuch-

§ 129

During this search for a homoeopathic specific remedy, that is, in this comparison of the symptoms-totality of the natural disease with the array of symptoms of available medicines, the *more striking, more peculiar, more characteristic* symptoms of the disease should be kept in view in the first place; for it is particularly to this list if symptoms that a very much similar must be found among the disease-elements of the medicine which is to be the most suitable remedy for effecting the cure. Whereas the more common symptoms, like anorexia, debility, discomfort, disturbed sleep, etc. are of little significance and deserve far less attention *when are not characterised by more detailed* indications, because they are found in the symptom-array of most medicines, thus also in most natural diseases.

ten Arznei entsprechen, wenn sie die passendste zur Heilung seyn soll — während
die allgemeinern Zeichen: Anorexie, Mattigkeit, Unbehaglichkeit, gestörter Schlaf,
u. s. w. in dieser Allgemeinheit, und wenn
sie nicht naher bezeichnet sind,
weit weniger Aufmerksamkeit verdienen,
weil sie wie in den meisten naturlichen
Krankheiten, so auch in den Symptomenreihen der meisten Arzneien angetroffen
werden.

130.

Enthält nun das aus der Symptomenreihe der treffendsten Arznei zusammen gesezte Gegenbild jene in der zu heilenden
Krankheit anzutreffenden charakteristischen Zeichen in der gröfsten Zahl und in
der gröfsten Aehnlichkeit, so ist diese
Arznei fur diesen Krankheitszustand die
passendste künstliche Gegenkrankheitspotenz, das specifische Heilmittel; die Krankheit wird (oft schon durch die erste Gabe
desselben während der Wirkungsdauer dieser Arznei) ohne Beschwerde gehoben und
ausgelöscht.

§ 130

Now, the counter disease-picture, constructed from the symptom-array of the medicine found to be most suitable, contains in the greatest number and closest similarity, these striking and characteristic symptoms of the disease which is to be cured, then *this* medicine affords the best artificial counter-disease for this case of disease, and is, in short, the specific remedy and the disease will be removed and annihilated (often even during the span of action of the first dose of this medicine) without difficulty.

131

Ich sage ohne Beschwerde. Denn
beim Gebrauche dieser passendsten Gegenkrankheitspotenz sind blos die, den Krankheitssymptomen entsprechenden Arzneisymptomen in Wirksamkeit (indem leztere
die erstern vernichten); die, oft sehr vielen, übrigen Symptomen in der Symptomenreihe der passenden Arznei aber, welche in dem vorliegenden Krankheitszustande keine Anwendung finden, schwei-
gen dabei ganzlich; es läfst sich fafst
nichts von ihnen in dem Befinden des sich
stundlich bessernden Kranken bemerken—,
vermuthlich weil sich die ganze Kraft des
specifischen Heilmittels auf seine der
Krankheit ähnlichen Symptome koncentrirt,
und seine ganze Kraft im Vernichten dieser ähnlichen Symptomen erschöpft.

> Anm. Indessen giebt es kein, auch noch so
> passend gewähltes, homoopathisches Arz-
> neimittel, welches nicht Eine, wenigstens
> ganz kleine, ungewohnte Beschwerde, ein
> kleines neues Symptom während seiner
> Wirkungsdauer bei sehr reitzbaren und
> feinfühlenden Kranken erregen sollte;

§ 131

I say, without difficulty. For in employing this most suitable counter disease-force, only those medicinal symptoms are brought into action which correspond to the disease-symptoms (and the first destroy the latter); the other and often very numerous symptoms found in the symptom-array of the suitable remedy remain entirely latent because they find nothing to correspond to them in the disease-condition; nothing of them will be found in the condition of the patient, which will improve from hour to hour; presumably because the whole power of the specific remedy is concentrated on those disease-symptoms which resemble its own and its whole power is consumed in annihilation of these similar symptoms.

Footnote: However, there is almost no homoeopathic remedy, suitably chosen, which in the course of its action on a very irritable and sensitive patient, may not produce at least one, probably very negligible, unusual complaint, some slight new symptom; because it is almost impossible that medicine and disease should cover each other in their symptoms as exactly as two triangles

weil es fast unmöglich ist, daß Arznei
und Krankheit in ihren Symptomen einander so genau decken sollten, wie zwei
Triangel von gleichen Winkeln und gleichen Seiten. Aber diese (in gutem Falle)
unbedeutende Aberration wird von der
eignen Energie des lebenden Organisms
mehr als zulänglich ausgeglichen, und
Kranken von nicht übermäsiger Zartheit
nicht einmahl bemerkbar; die Herstellung
geht dennoch vorwärts, wenn sie nicht
durch Fehler in der Lebensordnung oder
durch Leidenschaften gehindert wird.

132.

So gewiß es aber auch ist, daß ein passend homöopathisches Heilmittel ohne
Lautwerdung seiner übrigen, ihm eignen
Symptomen, das ist, ohne Erregung neuer
bedeutender Beschwerden die ihm analoge
Krankheit ruhig aufhebt und vernichtet,
so pflegt es doch gleich nach der Einnahme (in der ersten, oder in den ersten Paar
Stunden) eine Art kleiner Verschlimmerung zu bewirken, welche so viel Aehnlichkeit mit der ursprünglichen Krankheit
hat, daß sie dem Kranken eine Verschlim-

with equal angles and equal sides cover each other. Yet, these (in ample cases) unimportant differences are easily overcome by the individual energy of the living organism, and is not perceptible by patients not excessively sensitive; recovery goes steadily forward, unless obstructed by errors in the mode of life of the patient or due to hindered passions.

§ 132

Although it is definite that a suitably selected homoeopathic remedy gently destroys and removes disease, without arousing such characterising symptoms of its own as are not present in the patient, that is, without exciting similar diseases of a new and serious kind, yet it usually causes, as it were, a slight aggravation of the patient's condition (in the first one or two hour) after its administration. This aggravation so closely resembles the original disease that it seems to the patient to be a real worsening of his symptoms. But it is in reality no more than the onset of a very similar medicinal disease rather more powerful than the original disease. This slight homoeopathic aggravation during the first hours (which is, in fact, a very good prognostic indication that the acute disease will most probably yield to the *first* dose), is quite as it should be; because the drug-disease must naturally be somewhat stronger than

merung der Krankheit selbst zu seyn deuchtet, aber nichts andres ist, als die, die ursprüngliche Krankheit etwas an Starke ubertreffende, hochst ähnliche Arzneikrankheit. Diese kleine homoopathische Verschlimmerung in den ersten Stunden (eine sehr gute Vorbedeutung, daſs die akute Krankheit meistens von der ersten Gabe beendigt seyn wird) ist ganz in der Regel, da die Arzneikrankheit natürlich um etwas starker seyn muſs, als das zu heilende Uebel, wenn sie lezteres uberstimmen und ausloschen soll, so wie auch eine analoge Krankheit die andre nur wenn sie starker als die andre ist, aufheben und vernichten kann (§. 28). Ie kleiner die Gabe des homoopathischen Mittels, desto kleiner diese anscheinende Krankheitserhohung in der ersten Stunde. Da man jedoch die Gabe eines homoopathischen Heilmittels kaum je so klein bereiten kann, daſs sie nicht die ihr analoge Krankheit uberstimmen und bessern, ja völlig heilen und vernichten könnte (§. 244.), so wird es begreiflich, warum auch die kleinstmogliche Gabe passend homoopa-

the disease to be cured if it is to overcome and extinguish the natural disease; even as an analogous natural disease can only remove and annihilate another when it is the stronger (§ 28). The smaller the dose of the homoeopathic remedy, so much slighter will be this aggravation of symptoms appearing in the first hours. But the dose of a homoeopathic remedy can hardly be made so small that it will not over power and ameliorate its analogous disease, rather completely cure and banish it (§ 244). Therefore, we can easily understand that even the very smallest dose of a homoeopathic remedy always causes a light homoeopathic aggravation of this kind, although a very mild one, in the first hours after its administration.

Footnote: This aggravation resembling an increase of the medicinal-symptoms over its analogous disease-symptoms has also been observed by other physicians who applied a homoeopathic remedy. *Viola tricolor* when used in the beginning caused an aggravation in the rash of the face for which it is curative (Leroy, *Heilk. für Mütter,* p. 406).

thischer Arznei immer noch in der ersten
Stunde nach der Einnahme eine, obgleich
sehr kleine homöopathische Verschlimmerung dieser Art zuwege bringt.

Anm. Diese, einer Verschlimmerung ähnliche
Erhöhung der Arzneisymptomen über die
ihr analogen Krankheitssymptomen haben
auch andre Aerzte, wo sie ein homoopathi-
sches Mittel anwendeten, beobachtet. Den
Gesichtsausschlag, den die viola tricolor
heilete, hatte sie beim Anfange ihres Gebrauchs verschlimmert (*Leroy*, Heilk. für
Mütter, S. 406.)

133.

Zuweilen findet sich bei der noch
eingeschränkten Zahl genau nach
ihrer positiven Wirkung gekannter Arzneien, dafs von den Symptomen der zu heilenden Krankheit nur ein
mehr oder weniger grofser Theil in der
Symptomenreihe einer der noch am besten
passenden Arzneien angetroffen wird, folglich diese unvollkommne Gegenkrankheitspotenz in Ermangelung einer vollkomm-
nern angewendet werden mufs.

H

§ 133

Sometimes it so happens that *because the still limited number of medicines exactly tested in regard to their positive effect,* only a smaller or greater part of the symptoms of a case of disease can be found in the symptom-array of the most appropriate medicine, hence this imperfect counter-disease force must be employed because of lack of a more perfect one.

134

In diesem Falle läfst sich freilich von
dieser Arznei keine vollständige, unbe-
schwerliche Heilung erwarten. Vielmehr
treten da bei ihrem Gebrauche mehrere
Zufälle am Kranken hervor, welche vorher in der Krankheit nicht zu finden waren. Diese hindern zwar nicht, dafs ein
betrachtlicher Theil des Uebels von dieser
Arznei getilgt werde, und dadurch ein
ziemlicher Anfang der Heilung entstehe,
aber doch nicht ohne jene Nebenbeschwerden.

135

Die geringe Zahl bei der nach bester
Einsicht gewählten Arznei anzutreffender
homoopathischer Symptome thut jedoch
der Heilung wenig oder keinen Eintrag,
wenn diese wenigen Symptomen
gröstentheils von charakteristischer, die Krankheit besonders
auszeichnender Art waren; sie erfolgt dann dennoch bald und ziemlich unbeschwerlich.

§ 134

In this case a complete, undisturbed cure by this medicine is naturally not to be expected for after its use many more morbid symptoms may appear in the patient than were previously present due to the disease. This will not prevent eradicating a considerable part of the disease, nor the establishment of an appreciable beginning of cure; but even then, not without appearance of those accessory complaints.

§135

The small number of homoeopathic symptoms shown by the best-selected medicine is little or no obstacle to the cure, *if these few symptoms are mainly of characteristic type and are especially distinctive to the disease,* almost undisturbed cure then follows shortly.

136.

Ist aber von den auszeichnenden, charakteristischen Symptomen der Krankheit wenig in der Symptomenreihe der gewählten Arznei vorhanden und entspricht sie der Krankheit meistens nur in den allgemeinen Krankheitszufällen (Uebelkeit, Mattigkeit, gestörter Schlaf, Unbehaglichkeit, u. s. w.) und findet sich keine homoopathisch passendere unter den gekannten Gegenkrankheitspotenzen, so hat der Heilkunstler sich keinen unmittelbar vortheilhaften Erfolg von ihrer Anwendung zu versprechen.

137.

Indessen ist dieser Fall auch bei der jezt noch so beschränkten Zahl nach ihren positiven Wirkungen gekannter Heilmittel selten, und seine Nachtheile mindern sich, sobald ein folgendes Heilmittel passender gewählt werden kann.

138.

Entstehen nämlich beim Gebrauche dieser zuerst gewählten unvollkommen ho-

H 2

§136

If, however, in the symptom-array of the selected remedy, few only resemble the distinctive, characteristic symptoms of the disease and if it corresponds to the disease mainly in such common[12] symptoms (nausea, exhaustion, disturbed sleep, discomfort, etc.), and in little else; then, if no remedy more suitably homoeopathic can be found among known counter-disease forces, the physician will look in vain for immediate favourable effect from the use of this unhomoeopathic medicine.

§ 137

However, such a case, is rare even with the still very limited number of remedy known in their positive affects; and the bad effects occurring due to such a remedy are diminished as soon as a more suitable remedy can be selected.

§ 138

If after the use of the first selected medicine, which is not perfectly homoeopathic, accessory symptoms of some

---

[12] **Translator's note:** Hahnemann has used the german word *allgemeinen* in the 1st as well as in all other editions including 5th edition to denote *undefined and vague symptoms*. However, Dudgeon and most of the translators have opted to translate this as '*General*' which has resulted in the confusion in many homoeopaths especially when they come across Kent's classification of symptoms and his use of the term '*General*' in a totally different context. This can very easily be avoided if *allgemeinen* is translated as *common* which is more appropriate and befitting in the context.

moopathischen Arznei Nebenbeschwerden
von einiger Bedeutung, so läfst man diese
erste Gabe nicht völlig auswirken, und
überläfst den Kranken nicht der vollen
Wirkungsdauer des Medicaments, sondern
untersucht den geänderten Krankheitszustand aufs Neue, das ist, den Rest der
ursprunglichen Symptomen bringt man
mit den neu entstandnen zusammen in
Verbindung, um ein neues Krankheitsbild
zu entwerfen.

139.

Nun wird man leichter ein diesem
entsprechendes Analogon aus den gekannten Arzneien ausfinden, dessen selbst ein-
mahliger Gebrauch die Krankheit wo nicht
gänzlich vernichten, doch der Heilung um
Vieles näher bringen wird. Und so fahrt
man wenn auch diese Arzneo zur Herstellung der Gesundheit nicht völlig hin-
reichen sollte, mit abermahliger Untersuchung des noch übrigen Krankheitszustandes und der Wahl einer darauf möglichst
passenden, neuen homoopathischen Ge-

significance appear, this first dose should not be allowed to exhaust its action and nor the patient should be exposed to the full duration of its action; rather the altered disease-state should be examined again, and a new portrait of disease be made from the combination of the remaining original symptoms and those that have newly developed.

§ 139

Now, we shall be then able to find more easily from among our known medicines a fitting analogue to the new disease-picture just presented, and a single dose of this remedy, completely will bring recovery much nearer even if it does not annihilate the disease. And even if this remedy is not quite sufficient to bring a restoration of health, we proceed similarly with the repeated investigating the disease-state again and again and the repeated selection of the most suitable, new homoeopathic counter-force till our object of completely restoring the health of the patient is attained.

genkrankheitspotenz fort, bis die Absicht,
den Kranken in den vollen Besitz der Gesundheit zu setzen, erreicht ist.

140.

Wenn man bei der ersten Untersuchung einer Krankheit und der ersten Wahl
der Arznei finden sollte, daſs der Symptomeninbegriff der Krankheit nicht zurei-
chend von den Krankheitselementen einer
einzigen Arznei gedeckt werde — eben
der unzureichenden Zahl gekannter Arzneien wegen —; daſs aber zwei Arzneien
um den Vorzug ihrer Paſslichkeit streiten,
so daſs für den einen Theil des Symptomenkomplexes mehr die eine, für den andern Theil aber die zweite passend sei, so
läſst sich weder anrathen, die eine Arznei
unbesehens nach der andern zu brauchen,
noch auch beide zugleich anzuwenden,
weil niemand voraussehen kann, wie sehr
die eine die andre in der Wirkung hindern und umstimmen würde (§. 235. 236).

141.

Weit besser ist es hier, die für vor-
züglicher unter beiden zu achtende Gegen-

§ 140

If on the first examination of a disease and the first selection of a remedy it is observed that the totality of the symptoms of the disease cannot be sufficiently covered from the symptom-element of a single medicine - because of the insufficient number of known medicines - and if further it is found that two medicines appear to be equally merited, the one resembling more closely to one part of the symptom-complex and the other more suitable to second part of the disease then it is not advisable to apply one medicine after the other without further closer examination, nor to give both at the same time, as no one can anticipate how the one may impede and disturb the action of the other (§ 235- 256).

§ 141

It is much better here to give first only the counter-disease force (**SS note:** medicine) which on the whole appears to be more suitable. It will not only give certain amelioration to the part of sickness but in addition will also produce newer symptoms.

krankheitspotenz zuerst allein zu geben.
Sie wird freilich die Krankheit zum Theil
mindern konnen, aber dagegen einen Zusatz neuer Symptomen hervorbringen.

142.

In diesem Falle kann nach den Gesetzen der Homöopathie keine zweite Gabe
dieser ersten Arznei gereicht werden; aber
auch die bei der anfanglichen Indikation
fur die zweite Halfte der Symptomen passend gefundne Arznei kann hier nicht unbesehens an ihrer Stelle, und ohne wei-
tere Untersuchung in dem Zustande angewendet werden, den die erstere Arznei
ubrig gelassen hat.

143.

Vielmehr mufs auch hier, wie uber-
all, wo eine Aenderung des Krankheitszustandes vorgegangen ist, der gegenwärtige, noch ubrige Symptomenkomplex aufs
neue ausgemittelt, und ohne Rucksicht
auf die anfanglich passend geschienene
zweite Arznei, eine dem neuen jetzigen

§ 142

When it happens, the homoeopathic law does not permit second dose of the first medicine to be given; but at the same time the other medicine, which seemed suitable upon the initial indications for the other half of the symptoms, must not be given without consideration and a further examination into the state remaining after the use of the first medicine.

§ 143

Not only in this case, rather, always when a alteration has come in the disease-state, the presently remaining symptom-complex must be considered afresh and without thinking of the second medicine which at first seemed partly suitable, so that if possible a new counter-disease force (**SS note: medicine**) most appropriate to the present new condition may be selected without prejudice.

Zustande möglichst angemessene Gegenkrankheitspotenz von Neuem ausgewählet
werden.

144.

Es trifft sich nicht oft, daſs die anfänglich als zweit - beste projektirte Arznei
nun noch passen sollte; fände sich dieſs
aber gleichwohl nach der neuen Untersuchung, daſs sie auch jezt noch wenigstens
eben so gut, als irgend eine andre Arznei
paſste, so wird sie um desto mehr das Zu-
trauen verdienen, vorzugsweise angewendet zu werden.

145.

Nur in einigen Fällen alter, keiner
sonderlichen Veränderung unterworfener,
chronischer Krankheiten, welche gewisse
feststehende Grundsymptomen haben, lassen sich zuweilen zwei fast gleich homöopathisch passende Heilmittel mit Erfolg ab-
wechselnd brauchen; so lange der Vorrath
der in ihrer positiven Wirkung am gesunden
Körper geprüften Arzneien keine ganz voll-

§ 144

It happens not often that the medicine which initially was projected to be the second best will now be indicated; but nevertheless, if after a fresh examination, this very remedy appears really fitting, at least as suitable as any other, then it deserves our greater confidence and should be administered in preference.

§ 145

It is only in some cases of long standing chronic disease, not subject to any important change, which possess certain fixed fundamental symptoms, that sometimes two suitable medicines almost equally homoeopathic can be used alternately with advantage; as, long as the supply of medicines proved as to their positive effects on healthy body does not offer any perfect counter-disease force, in whose array of symptoms the group of phenomena of the chronic malady is completely or almost completely represented, in which case it would give satisfaction and cure it speedily and permanently without difficulty.

kommene Gegenkrankheitspotenz darreicht, in deren Symptomenreihe die Gruppe von Zufällen des chronischen Uebels völlig oder fast völlig anzutreffen ist, die ihr dann allein Genüge leistet, und sie schnell und dauerhaft heilt, ohne Beschwerde.

146.

Eine ähnliche Schwierigkeit im Heilen entsteht von der allzu geringen Zahl der Krankheitssymptome —, ein Umstand, der unsre sorgfältige Beachtung verdient, da durch seine Beseitigung fast alle Schwierigkeiten, die die Heilkunde (außer dem Mangel homöopathisch gekannter Arzneien) nur darbietet, gehoben sind.

147.

Blos diejenigen Krankheiten scheinen nur wenige Symptomen zu haben, und deshalb Heilung schwieriger anzunehmen, welche man einseitige nennen kann, weil nur ein, oder ein Paar Hauptsymptome hervorstechen, welche fast den ganzen

§ 146

A similar difficulty in the way of curing arises in cases where the disease-symptoms are too few in number - a condition which demands the most careful attention, for if the difficulty which it creates is now removed, then almost all the difficulties (except the lack of homoeopathically known remedies) which hinder the therapeutic art are eliminated.

§ 147

The only diseases which seem to possess few symptoms, and so are more difficult to cure, are those which may be called *one-sided*, because they present only one or two chief symptoms, which obscure almost all the remaining symptoms. They belong mostly to the class of chronic diseases.

Rest der ubrigen Zufälle verdunkeln. Sie gehoren gröſstentheils zu den chronischen.

148.

Ihr Hauptsymptom kann entweder ein inneres Leiden (z. B. ein vieljähriges Kopfweh, ein vieljähriger Durchfall, eine vieljährige Kardialgie, u. s. w.) oder ein mehr aufseres Leiden seyn. Letztere pflegt man vorzugsweise Lokalkrankheiten zu nennen.

149.

Bei den einseitigen Krankheiten ersterer Art liegt es oft blos an der Unaufmerksamkeit des ärztlichen Beobachters, wenn er die Zufälle, welche zur Vervollständigung des Umrisses-der Krankheitsgestalt vorhanden sind, nicht vollzählig aufspurt.

150.

Indeſs giebt es doch einige wenige Uebel, welche, nach aller anfänglichen Forschung (§. 63 — 81. §. 178 — 182.), aufser einem Paar starker heftiger Zufälle,

§ 148

Their chief symptom may either be an internal suffering (as for example, headaches of many years duration, diarrhoea of many years, cardialgia which has been there for many years, etc.); or it may be an affection more of an external kind. The latter class are preferably called local diseases.

§ 149

In one-sided diseases of the first kind, it is often due to the inattentiveness of the medical observer that the symptoms which are actually present and which sketch the complete disease-picture are not entirely discovered.

§ 150

There are, nevertheless, a few illnesses which, after all preliminary examinations (§ 63 - 81, § 178 - 182), present but one or two intense and violent complaints while all others are indistinctly noticeable.

die übrigen nur undeutlich bemerken lassen.

151.

Um nun auch diesem, obgleich sehr
seltnen Falle mit Glück zu begegnen
wählt man zuerst, nach Anleitung dieser
wenigen Symptomen, die hierauf nach be-
stem Ermessen ausgesuchte Gegenkrankheitspotenz.

152.

.Es wird sich zwar wohl zuweilen treffen, daſs diese mit sorgfältiger Beobachtung des homöopathischen Gesetzes gewählte Arznei auch wirklich die passende
Gegenkrankheit zur Vernichtung des gegenwärtigen Uebels darreiche, welches um
desto eher möglich war, wenn diese wenigen Krankheitssymptomen sehr auffallend,
besonders und charakteristisch sind.

153.

Im häufigern Falle aber kann die hier
zuerst gewählte Arznei nur zum Theil, das

§ 151

To encounter successfully with such cases which luckily are *rare* the first instruction is to hereupon choose the counter disease-force (**Translator's note:** medicine) which is best indicated by these few symptoms.

§ 152

Well, , indeed, it will, surely, happen sometimes that this medicine, chosen by most careful observation in accordance with the homoeopathic law, even though from few symptoms, will actually prove to be the suitable counter-force required to annihilate the existing disease, and this is will be possible when these few disease-symptoms are very striking, notable and characteristic.

§ 153

But more frequently, the medicine so selected firstly, in this case, will prove only partially and is not exactly suitable, since there was no complex of many symptoms to guide to an appropriate choice.

ist, nicht genau passen, da kein Komplex
von mehrern Zeichen zur treffenden Wahl
leitete.

154.

Da wird nun die zwar so gut wie
möglich gewählte, aber dennoch nur unvollkommen homöopathische Arznei bei
ihrer Gegenwirkung gegen die ihr nur zum
Theil analoge Krankheit (eben so wie in
obigem Falle, wo die Armuth an Gegenkrankheitspotenzen die Wahl unvollstän-
dig liefs) Nebenbeschwerden erregen, und
mehrere Zufälle aus ihrer eignen Symptomenreihe in das Befinden des Kranken ein-
mischen, die zugleich bisher noch nicht ge-
fühlte Beschwerden der Krankheit selbst
sind; es werden Zufälle sich entdecken,
oder sich in höherm Grade entwickeln, die
der Kranke vorher gar nicht, oder nicht
deutlich wahrgenommen hatte.

155.

Man werfe nicht ein, dafs die jezt
erschienenen Nebenbeschwerden und neuen

§ 154

Then, in the above case, though chosen as exactly as possible, nevertheless, the medicine being only imperfectly homoeopathic, will cause accessory symptoms to appear while counteracting a disease to which it is only partially analogous. A similar sequence of events has been already noted as likely to occur when the choice of a remedy is incomplete from lack of sufficient counteracting forces. The accessory symptoms and phenomena, which appear in these circumstances out of the characteristic symptom-array of the medicine or some totally new symptoms, are intermingled with those of the patient's complaints, but are at the same time themselves to be regarded as symptoms of the disease, although they were not felt at all before the administration of the medicine or at least never perceived to this higher degree.

§ 155

The accessory complaints and newly appearing symptoms of disease must not be attributed entirely to the remedy in use. They originate from it[Fn], but they are always and only such symptoms as this disease is capable to produce in this body, symptoms which the medicine, as an agent having a similar tendency, merely elicited and caused to appear. In a word, the whole of now visible symptom-complex is to be regarded as that of the disease itself, as its true existing state, and to be treated farther as such.

Symptomen in dieser Krankheit auf Rechnung des eben gebrauchten Arzneimittels kämen. Sie kommen von ihm *), es sind aber doch immer nur solche Symptomen, zu deren Erscheinung diese Krankheit und in diesem Körper auch vor sich schon fähig war, und welche von der gebrauchten Arznei — als Selbsterzeugerin ähnlicher — blos hervorgelockt und zu erscheinen bewogen wurden. Man hat, mit einem Worte, den ganzen jezt sichtbar gewordnen Symptomenkomplex für den der Krankheit selbst zugehörigen, für den gegenwärtigen wahren Zustand anzunehmen und hienach ferner zu behandeln.

156.

So leistet die hier fast unvermeidlich unvollkommne Wahl des Arzneimittels

---

*) Wenn nicht der nahe unvermeidliche Todeskampf sie erregte, wenn keine wichtigen Fehler in der Lebensordnung, keine Ausbrüche heftiger Leidenschaften sie erzeugten, oder keine stürmische Evolution des Organismus durch Ausbruch oder Abschied der Monatszeit, Empfängniß, Niederkunft, u. s. w. dazwischen getreten sind.

Footnote: If they are excited by the nearing of an unavoidable death struggle, if there are no significant mistakes in lifestyles, no outbreak of severe passion or stormy evolution of the organism through the beginning or end of the monthly-period, conception, child birth, etc. have in between stepped in.

§ 156

Therefore the choice of the remedy provided in this case is almost inevitably imperfect, which however serves to make the symptom-complex complete and so to facilitate the finding of a second more exactly suitable homoeopathic counter disease-force.

dennoch den Dienst einer Vervollständigung des Symptomenkomplexes und erleichtert so die Ausfindung einer zweiten treffendern, homöopathischen Gegenkrankheitspotenz.

157.

Es muſs also nach vollbrachter Wirkung der einzelnen Gabe der ersten Arznei (wenn die neu entstandnen Beschwerden
ihrer Heftigkeit wegen nicht eine schleuni-
gere Hulfe heischen) wieder, ein neuer Befund der Krankheit aufgenommen, es muſs
der status morbi, wie er jezt ist, aufgezeichnet, und nach ihm ein zweites homöopathisches Mittel gewählt werden, was
gerade auf den heutigen, auf den jetzigen Zustand passet; welches nun um desto
angemessener gefunden werden kann, da
die Gruppe der Symptomen zahlreicher
und vollständiger geworden ist.

158.

Und so wird ferner, nach vollendeter Wirkung jeder Arzneigabe, der Zu-

§ 157

Therefore, after the effect of the single dose of the first medicine is completed (if not the severity of the newly appearing complaints demand more speedy aid) a new examination of the disease must be undertaken; so the *status morbi*, as it now is, must be recorded, and a second homoeopathic remedy chosen according to it, which shall be exactly suitable to the current state and is more appropriately found because the group of symptoms has become more numerous and more complete.

§ 158

Moreover, after completion of every dose of the medicine, the remaining symptoms of the disease is considered afresh and based on these group of symptoms a suitable counter disease-force is selected and to be proceeded in this way till recovery.

stand der noch übrigen Krankheit nach
den noch übrigen Symptomen jedesmahl
von neuem aufgenommen, und nach dieser gefundnen Gruppe von Zufällen eine
abermahls passende Gegenkrankheitspotenz
ausgesucht, und so fort bis zur Genesüng.

159.

Unter den einseitigen Krankheiten,
nehmen die sogenannten Lokalübel eine
wichtige Stelle ein.

160.

Diejenigen Lokalübel, welche nicht
seit kurzem blos von einer äufsern Beschä-
digung entstanden sind, hangen stets mit
einem innern, durch den ganzen Organism
verbreiteten Uebelbefinden zusammen, und
ihre ärztliche Behandlung muss deshalb
auch auf das Ganze gehen, wenn sie ver-
nunftig (rationell), konsequent und hülfreich seyn soll.

161.

So wie kein aus innern Ursachen entstehendes und an einer besondern Stelle

§ 159

Among one-sided diseases the so-called *local-maladies* hold an important place.

§ 160

That local-malady, which if not have originated only shortly from an external lesion, *always* depend upon an inner malady imbued throughout the whole organism; and their medicinal treatment, therefore, also have regard to the whole organism, if it is to be prudent (rational), consistent, and effective.

§ 161

So-called local malady resulting from internal causes and persisting in a particular spot can not be thought to be produced without the accordance of the rest of the general health, and without the participation of the other sensitive and irritable parts and all vital organs of the body; so how the healthful changes and even complete cures of maladies which

verharrendes sogenanntes Lokalübel ohne
Zustimmung des ganzen übrigen Befindens,
und ohne die Theilnahme aller übrigen em-
pfindenden und reitzbaren Theile und aller
lebenden Organe des Körpers gedacht werden kann, so kann es auch blos durch die
gemeinsame, in allen Theilen des lebenden
Körpers für die arzneikräftigen Potenzen
rege und wache Perception, blos durch diese den ganzen Körper beseelende Theilnahme an der Arzneikraft möglich und erklär-
bär werden, wie durch wenige, blos an
die Zunge oder in den Magen gebrachte,
homöopathisch angemessene Arznei selbst
auf die an den entferntesten Stellen der
Haut befindlichen, anscheinend isolirten
Lokalübel heilsame Veränderungen und
selbst die vollständigsten Heilungen er-
zielet werden können.

162.

Diefs geschieht am zweckmäsigsten,
wenn bei Eruirung des Krankheitsfalles,
nächst der genauen Beschaffenheit des Lo-
kal-Leidens, zugleich alle im übrigen Be-

appear isolated on the most distant parts of the skin, by means of a small dose of a remedy homoeopathically suitable, placed on the tongue or introduced into the stomach, can only be caused and explained by the ever-ready general sensitiveness to medicinal powers inherent in all parts of the living body and the susceptibility to medicinal powers which permeate through all the parts of the living organism and by the same cure of the apparently local maladies can be achieved.

§ 162

Such best purpose of cures are effected when, in the investigation of the case of disease, besides the precise character of the local-sufferings, all the noticeable changes and symptoms in the patient's health, are taken in conjunction to sketch a complete disease-picture before searching the whole group of symptoms of suitable counter disease-force amongst the known medicines, so that the selection may be perfectly homoeopathic.

finden bemerkbaren Veränderungen und Symptome in Vereinigung gezogen werden zum Entwurfe eines vollständigen Krankheitsbildes, ehe man ein dieser ganzen Gruppe von Zufällen entsprechende Gegenkrankheitspotenz unter den gekannten Arzneien sucht, um eine vollständig homöopathische Wahl zu treffen.

163.

Durch diese blos innerlich eingegebne Arznei wird dann der gemeinsame Krankheitszustand des Körpers mit dem Lokalübel zugleich aufgehoben und lezteres mit erstern zugleich geheilt, zum Beweise, daſs das Lokal-Leiden von einer Krankheit des übrigen Körpers abhängt und nur als ein Theil des Ganzen, als eins der gröſsten Symptome der Gesamtkrankheit anzusehen ist.

Die Wahrheit, die wir alle nöthig haben,
die uns als Menschen glücklich macht,
ward von der weisen Hand, die sie uns zugedacht,
nur leicht verdeckt, nicht tief vergraben.
GELLERT.

Dieſs ist so wahr, daſs selbst jedes blos äuſserlich aufgelegte Lokalmittel, wenn es allein geholfen und Gesund-

§ 163

Owing to this medicine, administered only internally the disease-state of the organism is abrogated together with the local-sufferings, and the first and the last are cured at the same time, proving that the local-sufferings depended solely on a disease of the body as a whole, and should only be regarded as one of the most striking symptoms of the whole disease.

§ 164

It is so true that, if any local-remedy has ever cured without other aid and has restored *health* (as it has rarely done), it has only been able to do so not without exercising a homoeopathic a healing influence upon the internal disease-state, and it would have cured equally well had it been administered only internally and not at all externally.

heit (wie selten) wiedergebracht hatte,
dieſs nicht vermochte, ohne zugleich auf
den innern Krankheitszustand einen homoopathisch heilenden Einfluſs bewirkt
zu haben, und auch dieselbe Heilung zu
Stande gebracht haben würde, wenn es
blos innerlich und gar nicht äuſserlich gebraucht worden wäre.

Anm. So werden einige Flechten durch äu-
　　ſserliche Auflegung der Kanthariden, und
　　einige andre Hautausschläge durch aufge-
　　legte Quecksilberpräcipitate, wohl ober-
　　flächlich vertrieben, aber nicht so geheilt,
　　daſs allgemeiner Gesundheit drauf folgt,
　　wenn diese äuſsern Mittel den vom Lo-
　　kalübel unzertrennlichen, innern, krank-
　　haften Zustand nicht zugleich zu heben
　　vermocht, und nicht bei ihrer Auflegung
　　den ganzen Organism mit ihrer Heilkraft
　　afficirt hätten.

165.

Es scheint zwar, als wenn die Heilung solcher Uebel beschleunigt würde,
wenn man das für den ganzen Krankheits-
komplex als homöopathisch richtig erkann-

I

Footnote: Thus some eczemas are superficially removed by the external use of Cantharides (**Translator's note:** Cantharis vesicateria) and some other eruptions by a similar use of mercurial preparations; but none of them are cured so as to restored the general health, unless these external remedies had also the power at the same time to remove the internal disease-state inseparably mixed with the local-affection and by their local applicable have, therefore, affected the whole organism with their curative power.

§ 165

In fact, it would appear as if the cure of such affections would be quickened, if the remedy selected as correctly homoeopathic to the whole disease-complex were not only administered internally but also applied externally; seeing that the local-affection generally tries to isolate itself completely, although it can never do this completely in the living organism,

te Arzneimittel nicht nur innerlich anwendete, sondern auch äußerlich auffe-
gete; in Hinsicht daß das Lokalübel sich
gewöhnlich zu isoliren strebet, ob es sich
gleich im lebenden Körper nie völlig isoliren kann, und da man wahrgenommen
hat, daß die Arzneien auf dem Orte ihrer Anwendung eine schnellere Wirkung
als auf die entferntern Theile bewirken.

> Anm. Die Einspritzung des Kirschlorbeer-
> wassers in den After der Thiere macht
> seine spastische Wirkung zuerst an den
> untern Extremitäten bemerklich, später
> an den obern Theilen, und so umgekehrt
> an den obern Theilen zuerst, wenn es
> oben eingegossen wird.

166.

Indeß hat die neben dem innern
Gebrauche gleichzeitige topische
Anwendung des Heilmittels bei Krankheiten, welche ein statiges Lokalübel zum
Hauptsymptome haben, den großen Nachtheil; daß durch die örtliche Auflegung
desselben dieses Hauptsymptom (Lokal-

and as if that medicines have been found to produce more rapid, effect on the part to which they are applied than to more distant parts.

Footnote: The injection of cherry-laurel water into the anus of animals shows its spasmodic action first of all in the lower extremities, later in the upper parts, and in the reverse order on the upper parts first of all, if it is swallowed.

§ 166

Nevertheless, this *simultaneous application of topical application* and internal use of a remedy in diseases where the local-sufferings are the more marked, has this great disadvantage, that through the local application these chief symptoms (the local-sufferings) will be annihilated sooner than the internal disease, and because of its similarity with perfect cure it will be difficult and impossible in many cases to determine from the premature disappearance of local symptoms if the total-disease is annihilated by the simultaneous use of the internal medicine.

übel) schneller als die innere Krankheit vernichtet wird, und uns nun die Beurtheilung, ob auch die Totalkrankheit durch die innere Kur vernichtet sei, durch die vorzeitige Verschwindung dieses lokalen Symptoms erschwert und in manchen Fallen unmoglich macht.

167.

Einen ähnlichen, wo möglich noch großern Nachtheil bringt in den meisten Fallen die blos örtliche Auflegung jeder wirksamen, selbst der homöopathisch heilkräftigen Arznei auf das örtliche Hauptsymptom (Lokalübel) hervor, wenn sie nicht vorher von innen bis zur Bewirkung der gänzlichen Vernichtung der allgemeinen Krankheit angewendet worden war. Denn dann wird es noch weit unwahrscheinlicher, daß die blos örtlich aufgelegte Arznei unter der Hebung des Lokalsymptoms, zugleich auf den innern Organism so eindringlich und vollständig heilkräftig eingewirkt haben sollte, daß die Totalkrankheit aufgehoben und ver-

I 2

§ 167

A similar but, possibly a greater disadvantage follows in most of the cases by local application of every effective medicine, even if homoeopathically curative, to the local chief symptoms (local sufferings) it has been employed earlier internally to bring about the complete annihilation of the total disease. Because then it is even more unlikely that the remedy when only locally applied should have simultaneously acted so urgently and completely on the inner organism as to remove and annihilate the total disease and at the same time abrogate the local symptoms. This favourable result will only occur in the very rare cases in which perhaps the inner disease is minor and recent and the external suffering is on a large scale, therefore, the topical application will have spread over a considerable surface of the body.

nichtet worden wäre. Diefs wird nur in aufserst seltenen Fällen geschehen, etwa wo die innere Krankheit sehr gering und neu, das aufsere Uebel aber von grofsem Umfange war und daher das Topikum sehr weit auf der Oberfläche des Körpers sich ausbreitete.

168.

In allen andern Fällen wird das in einem kleinen Umfange blos aufserlich aufgelegte Mittel viel zu wenig Einwirkung auf den innern Organism aufsern, als dafs die oft alte und wichtige innere Krankheit dadurch vernichtet werden könnte. Wenn nun seine uberwiegend schnellere Heilkräftigkeit als Topikum das auffallendste Symptom der innern Krankheit, das Lokalubel, vorzeitig hinweg nimmt, so bleibt das innere Uebel dennoch und der Fall ist schlimmer als vorher,

169.

Denn, ist das Lokalubel blos örtlich und einseitig aufgehoben worden, so

§ 168

In all other cases the simple external application of a small quantity of the remedy will not produce upon the inner organism an effect nearly powerful enough to annihilate often the chronic and serious inner disease. Now, even if its predominantly faster medicinal action of the topical application removes the local-sufferings prematurely, which is merely the most striking symptom of inner disease, the inner malady still persists and the case has become worse than before.

§ 169

Because, the local-suffering is made to eliminate by this local and one-sided treatment, the internal treatment vital for the complete cure of the total disease remains in uncertain obscurity; for now only the other (fainter) symptoms remain, symptoms which are less constant and persistent than the local complaints, and often are not characteristic enough to represent an intelligible and complete outlines of the portrait of the disease.

bleibt nun die zur völligen Herstellung
unerläfsliche innere Kur der Totalkrankheit im ungewissen Dunkel; dann sind
nur noch die andern (schwachern) Symptomen übrig, welche nicht so statig und
permanent, als das Lokalleiden, und oft
zu wenig charakteristisch sind, als dafs
sie noch ein Bild der Krankheit im deutlichen und vollständigen Umrisse darstellen sollten.

170.

Der Heilkünstler wird im Verfolge
der innern Kur immer zweifelhaft bleiben,
ob das selbst anerkannt homöopathische
Heilmittel die Totalkrankheit völlig ohne
Rückstand gehoben und vernichtet habe,
da das wichtigste und permanenteste
Hauptsymptom, da das Lokalübel, schon
vorzeitig seinen Augen entzogen worden
ist. Er wird so halb im Dunkeln wirkend,
des Medikaments entweder zu wenig oder
zu viel geben, und es entweder nicht bis
zum völligen Heilpunkte, oder es allzu lange brauchen, zum Verderben des Kranken.

§ 170

The physician in his search for a suitable internal treatment must remain always doubtful if the selected homoeopathic remedy has completed annihilated and removed the total disease without any remained; for the most important and most persistent chief symptom, the local-suffering, has already prematurely vanished from his vision. He will have to work in semi-darkness, and thus will either give too much or too little of the medicine, or he will employ it not the point of complete cure or too long than needed; and thus will ruin the patient.

171.

Wenn nun vollends das der Krankheit angemessene Heilmittel zu der Zeit noch nicht gefunden war, als das örtliche Symptom durch ein beizendes oder austrocknendes Topikum oder durch den Schnitt vernichtet ward, so wird der Fall wegen der allzu uncharakteristischen und unstäten Erscheinung der noch übrigen Symptome noch schwieriger, weil, was die Wahl des treffendsten Heilmittels und seine innere Anwendung bis zum Punkte der Totalheilung noch am meisten hätte leiten und bestimmen können, das äußere Hauptsymptom unsrer Beobachtung entzogen worden ist.

172.

Ware es noch da, so würde seine bleibende Gegenwart zeigen, daß die innere Kur noch nicht vollendet ist; heilete es aber bei der blos innern Kur, so bewiese dies überzeugend, daß das Uebel bis zur Wurzel ausgerottet und die Genesung von der Totalkrankheit bis zum er-

§ 171

Now, if the remedy which is completely appropriate to the disease not been discovered at the time before the local symptoms have been destroyed either by some destructive or desiccating topical application or by the knife, the case necessarily becomes more difficult on account of the indefinite appearance and all too uncharacteristic nature of the remaining symptoms; because the external chief symptoms, which would have led most surely to the choice of the exact remedy and its internal application till the point of complete healing, have been removed from our observation.

§ 172

If the external phenomena were still present, then their failure to disappear would show that the internal treatment was not yet completed; if, on the contrary, they disappeared under internal medication alone, that would constitute a convincing proof that the disease was eradicated from root and that the desired recovery from the total disease was achieved—an invaluable advantage.

wunschten Ziele gediehen ist. Ein un-
schatzbarer Vortheil!

173.

Die blos örtliche Wegnahme des Lokalsymptoms wird von der Natur fast stets
durch Vergröfserung und Erweckung der
schon neben ihm bestandnen, nur noch
schlummernden übrigen Symptomen und
durch Erzeugung neuer Zufälle, das ist,
durch eine Erhöhung der übrigen Gesamtkrankheit ersetzt, (wo man dann unrich-
tig zu sagen pflegt, das áufsere Uebel sei
durch das Topikum auf die Nerven, oder
in die Säftmasse zurück getrieben worden).

174.

In einigen Krankheiten geschiehet
dieses Aufwachen der übrigen Symptome
nach Hinwegräumung des Lokalübels nur
allmáhlig, so dafs die Verschlimmerung
erst nach geraumer Zeit in die Augen fällt.

Anm. 1. Das sprechendste Beispiel von diesen Sätzen liefert die venerische Krankheit. So bald der Schanker einige Tage

§ 173

The local removed of local symptoms by local treatment is almost always replaced by Nature by the increasing the internal suffering and intensification the remaining symptoms which existed in a latent state although recognizable, and by the appearance of new disease-phenomena, that is to say, there is an increase of the total disease. This result of a etocal application is usually expressed though *incorrectly* that the external sufferings has been driven inward upon the nerves or into the "body fluid".

§ 174

In some diseases this intensification of the remaining symptoms occurring after removal of the local sufferings, only takes place *gradually*, so that the aggravation is observed only after a considerable time.

Footnote No. 1: The most common example of these maxims is provided by the venereal disease. The chancre becomes visible only after a few days of infection which gives a complete proof that the whole body in general has become venereal. Soon after, there appears a clear sign of the general

nach der Ansteckung sich sichtbar ausgebildet hat, giebt er auch den vollen Beweis daſs der ganze Körper schon (durch ihn) allgemein venerisch geworden ist. Schon dann erscheinen bei vielen Personen deutliche Zeichen des allgemeinen Uebelbefindens, die jedoch bei Einigen weniger deutlich und nur mit Mühe auszuforschen sind. Aber auch im leztern Falle, wo die allgemeinen Symptomen nicht so offenbar sind, wird die Allgemeinheit der Krankheit dadurch unwiderleglich daſs selbst die Ausschneidung des noch frischen Schankers die Krankheit nicht entfernt und das Emporkommen der nachgängigen venerischen, über den Körper sich verbreitenden Symptomen nicht verhütet. Sie brechen dennoch nach mehreren Monaten hie und da aus, zum Zeichen daſs der Schanker nicht ein bloses isolirtes Lokalübel war — so wenig es deren überhaupt giebt — sondern ein bloses auffallendes Zeichen der Existenz der venerischen Krankheit im ganzen Körper.

So lange der Schanker noch auf seiner Stelle steht, bleibt er das, die innere allgemein venerische Krankheit zum gröſsern Theile vertretende Hauptsymptom, und verhindert durch seine ungestörte Gegenwart, daſs die übrigen Symptome vor sich

indisposition in many persons, which however is less clear and is found with much effort. However, in the last case where the general symptoms are not quite visible, thereby making the generality of the diseases almost irrefutable by it, the excision of the newly developed chancre does not prevent the development and spread of the venereal symptoms throughout the body. After several months, however, it breaks out here and there as a sign that the chancre is not merely an isolated local-complaint – as, actually, there are few - but only a striking sign of the existence of the venereal disease throughout the whole body.

As long as the chancre remains in its position, it remains the chief symptom, representing to a greater extent the internal general venereal disease, and, as long as it is left undisturbed in the present condition, it prevents more or less by its presence the outbreak of other troublesome symptoms – it continues in the same position— if it is not expelled locally– till the end of life, even in the most strongest of the body, demonstrating thereby the importance of the internal disease. If it had not an independent great internal disease for its foundation, of which it acts as the chief symptom, how easily would an ulcer, so small at first, be cured naturally!

wenig oder gar nicht ausbrechen können. —
Unverruckt beharrt er auf derselben Stelle — wenn er nicht örtlich vertrieben
wird — bis ans Lebensende, auch bei dem
vollkräftigsten Körper, und zeugt so von
der Wichtigkeit der innern Krankheit.
Wie leicht würde er als ein so kleines Ge-
schwur durch die eigne Energie der Natur
heilen, wenn ihm nicht eine so selbstsän-
dige, grosse, innere Krankheit, für die er
als Hauptsymptom vikarirt, zum Grunde
läge!

Verführt man nun nach gewöhnlicher
Art und beizt den Schanker weg, oder
legt sonst ein, dieses Lokalsymptom blos
örtlich zerstörendes und vertreibendes Mittel, oder selbst das schwarze Quecksilber-
oxyd auf, so wird zwar gewöhnlich, auf
der Stelle, dieses Lokalsymptom des innern venerischen Leidens vernichtet; aber
zum Schaden des Kranken.

Der allgemeine Zustand bleibt dann nicht
nur eben so venerisch, als während der
Schanker noch zugegen war, sondern die
innere und allgemeine, venerische Krankheit ersetzt nun auch den Mangel dieses,
die Heftigkeit der innern Uebel bisher
gleichsam ableitenden und mildernden
Hauptsymptoms durch allmählige Belebung
und Verstärkung der übrigen, neben ihm

Till now the ordinary physician still treats in the usual way, and cauterises the chancre away, or this local symptom of the internal venereal complaints is destroyed and removed by locally destructive or expulsive means or by black mercuric oxide, but only at the cost of great harm to the patient.

The general condition remains not only just as venereal as when the chancre was still present, but the internal general venereal disease, which, as its nature is, goes on gradually but constantly increasing, now replaces the loss of the chancre; this chief symptom, which till now deflected, as it were, and lessened the severity of the internal malady by gradual stimulation and developing the rest of the dormant symptoms, and through the production of new symptoms which are much worse than the dispelled chancre. Now the sufferings of the general disease breaks out soon (inguinal buboes) or late (often only after several months) as ulceration of the tonsils, papular eruptions, or red spotted rashes, flat, painless, smooth, round, cutaneous ulcers, rough growths on the uvula or on the side of the nose; or nocturnally painful swellings of periosteum, etc.

schon schlummernden Symptome, und
durch Erzeugung neuer Zufälle, welche
weit beschwerlicher als der vertriebne
Schanker sind. Es brechen nun die Leiden des allgemeinen Uebels über kurz (Bu-
bonen) oder über lang (oft erst nach vielen
Monaten) als Tonsillenverschwärung, als
pustulöser oder Fleckenausschlag, als fla-
che, schmerzlose, runde Geschwüre, als
krause Auswuchse am Zäpfchen oder an
den Nasenflügeln, als nächtlich schmerzhafte Beinhautgeschwulst, u. s. w. hervor.

Alle diese nachgehends überhand neh-
menden Symptomen sind jedoch nie so
deutlich und feststündig, als der vertriebne Schanker war, vergehen leicht beim
innern Gebrauche des Quecksilbers, um
von Zeit zu Zeit entweder selbst wieder zu
kommen, oder andern venerischen Symptomen unter dieser oder jener Gestalt Platz
zu machen, und man ist nun fast nie der
Heilung, der völligen Austilgung der allgemeinen Krankheit sicher. Giebt man zu
wenig von der Arznei, oder unheilkräftig.
Präparate derselben, so wird die Krankheit keinesweges vernichtet, sondern bricht
mit der Zeit wieder hervor; giebt man
aber diese Merkurialpräparate in langer
Zeit fort, um dem Körper viel davon allmählig beizubringen, weil die Schärfe die-

All these continually increasing symptoms are, however, never so distinct and persistent as the chancre which have been driven-off. They readily disappear for a time by the administration of mercury internally, but either come back from time to time in its own form or in the form of other venereal symptoms of one kind or another; in short, one is never quite sure of its cure and complete annihilation of the general disease. If after the local destruction of the chancre we give very little medicine or preparations with no healing powers, the disease will not be annihilated, but will recur with the passage of time. But if one gives the mercurial preparation with longer gaps in between, in order to help them get acquainted with it gradually, because the strength of this preparation when administered in large and successive doses would very soon destroy the strength, we shall not attain our end, and considering the unstable character of these symptoms we shall never know *when and if* the illness has been eradicated.

ser Präparate in grofsen, schnellen Gaben
die Kräfte allzu schnell zerstören würde,
so weifs man doch bei der Unstätigkeit dieser Symptome nie, wann und ob man
das Uebel ausgetilgt hat.

Indefs wird durch den langwierigen Gebrauch einer so mächtigen Krankheitspotenz als das Quecksilber ist; eine schleichende Quecksilberkrankheit zu dem alten
Uebel gefügt, und beide verschmelzen zu
einer komplicirten, zu einer neuen, dritten Krankheit (gemeiniglich verlarvte
venerische Krankheit genannt), die
sich nun nicht mehr weder durch Quecksilber, noch durch Schwefelleber heilen
läfst, sondern sich durch das eine, so wie
durch das andre verschlimmert.

War hingegen das wichtige Lokalsymptom (das permanenteste aller venerischen
Zeichen, der Schanker) noch ursprünglich
und unverlezt bei der innern Kur vorhanden und nicht örtlich behandelt worden
(durch eigne Hülfe der Natur kömmt es
zuweilen auch nach seiner örtlichen Vertreibung wieder zurück auf seine alte Stelle als Schanker, oder wenn dieser nur
zum Theil weggebeizt war, in jener aus-
geärteten Gestalt wieder hervor, die man
Feigwarzen nennt, welche nun glücklicherweise wieder als Lokalsymptome, d. i. als

But by the long-continued use of such a powerful disease producing power as mercury is an insidious mercurial disease is added to the old malady, and the two unite to form a complicated, a new, third disease, commonly called *masked venereal disease*, which cannot be cured, either by mercury or by hepar sulphuris but is aggravated by the each other's influence.

However, if the most important local symptom (the most permanent of all venereal signs, the chancre) remain undisturbed during the internal treatment, and be not treated locally and had not been treated locally (with the help of nature it comes back at times to its old place as chancre even after its local removal or when it has been cauterized to a great extent in a more degenerated form which is named as fig-warts which fortunately now can be considered as a local symptom i.e. as the sure sign leading to the point of total cure), it is heals up perfectly of itself during the appropriate only internal use of the most powerfully antisyphilitic mercurial preparation, but ofcourse not

das sicher leitende Zeichen, den Punkt der
Totalheilung bei einer blos innern Kur entscheiden konnen); so heilt er beim moglichst schnellen, blos innern Gebrauche
des angemessensten, und antisyphilitisch
kraftigsten Merkurialpräparats, vollständig; doch nie eher, als wenn eben die Totalkrankheit völlig vernichtet ist. Ist durch
die blos innere Behandlung endlich
selbst der Schanker oder die Feigwarze geheilt; und an ihre Stelle gesunde Haut gekommen, so ist dann ohne Widerrede die
Gesamtkrankheit ausgetilgt.

Eben so geartet sind die Krankheiten,
welche, wie *Bruningshansen* beobachtete, nach Ausschneidung alter Speckge-
schwülste sich hervorthaten; so die Krankheiten, welche alten Schenkelgeschwüren
jederzeit zum Grunde liegen, und
wenn dieses bedeutende Lokalsymptom
durch ein austrocknendes oder beizendes
Topikum einseitig weggenommen wird,
nun allmählig als ein allgemeines, oft das
Leben befahrdendes Leiden sich entwickeln — und so noch eine ungeheure
Menge andrer, deren Lokalsymptomen
blos durch die innere Kur der Gesamtheit des Uebels ohne Topikum geheilt
werden sollten —, wenn man rationell
verfahren wollte —, durch innere Au-

untill before the total disease has been completely annihilated and cured. If the chancre or fig-wart has been completely cured and the new healthy skin has developed in place part covered with sound skin by *internal treatment only*, only then can we say without slightest doubt that the entire disease has been eradicated.

Similar type of the diseases are those which as *Brüningshausen* observed recur even after excision of the old steatomatous ulcers. So also the diseases that *always* remain at the base of old ulcers of the thighs, and if this significant local symptom is suppressed by a desiccating topical application, a general malady often dangerous to life develops itself. And so it is with an immense number of other diseases whose local symptoms should be cured only by treating the entire disease with internal treatment, without the employment of any external remedy, if we desire to cure in a rational manner and consonant with nature, namely, by the internal administration only of a medicinal agent corresponding in exact similarity to the symptom-complex, which, by the complete annihilation of the entire disease, naturally cures at the same time also its chief symptom, the so-called local malady.

wendung einer dem ganzen Symptomenkomplexe mit treffender Aehnlichkeit entsprechenden arzneilichen Krankheitspotenz, welche durch Vernichtung der Totalkrankheit natürlich auch ihr Hauptsymptom, das anscheinende Lokalübel
zugleich heilt.

Anm. 2. Die mechanischen und physischen
Beihülfen bei alten Lokalübeln (zu Ende
der innern Behandlung der Totalkrankheit), um den Ton der erschlafften Theile
zu unterstützen, z. B. kalte Fußeintau-
chungen oder die Cirkularbinde als Mit-
hülfe bei den, der Heilung nahen Schenkelgeschwüren und mehrere solche un-
schädliche äußere Veranstaltungen über-
gehe ich hier.

175.

Andre Krankheiten mit Lokalsymptomen hingegen erhöhen, wenn durch ein
Topikum das wichtige Lokalsymptom vernichtet worden ist, ihre übrigen größten-
theils innern Leiden und Zufälle oft
plötzlich und akut zu einer furchterli-
chen Höhe, oft bis zum schleunigen Tode.

Footnote No. 2: It is sometimes advantageous to support the place where the old local injury (till the end of the internal treatment of the entire disease) has been healed with mechanical and physical assistance, and to raise the tone of the weakened parts, *e.g.* by cold foot-baths, circular bandages, the cure of femoral ulcers and many such harmless external arrangements.

§ 175

At the same time, some other diseases with local symptoms, often show an *abrupt* and *acute* development upto frightful extent of the greater part of the inner sufferings and symptoms, often to the immediate death, when the important local manifestation has been removed by topical applications. Here the sufferings of local nature not only serve the end of hindering the development of the internal symptoms, as in a chronic and insidious disease, but also seem to be intensified to the prominence of the chief symptom, the symptom which, as it were, for the time absorbs the *intensity and danger* of the total disease and prevents their fatal development. The saddest experience teaches how irrational it is in such disease, as in the others, to remove in one sided manner the relatively advantageous local symptoms by a purely local treatment.

Hier scheint das Lokalleiden von der Natur nicht blos, wie bei erstern, denen eine chronische, schleichende Krankheit zum Grunde liegt, in der Absicht, um die Hervortretung der innern Symptomen uberhaupt aufzuhalten, sondern auch deshalb zum Hauptsymptome erhoben worden zu seyn, damit es die Große und Lebensgefährlichkeit der ubrigen Symptome der Totalkrankheit gleichsam absorbire und zum Theil ihre Stelle gefahrloser vertrete. Wie irrationell auch in solchen Krankheiten (wie in erstern) die einseitige Vernichtung des (relativ wohlthätigen) Lokalsymptoms sei, lehren die traurigsten Erfahrungen.

Anm. Die oft höchst akuten, schrecklichen Folgen der blos örtlichen Tilgung mehrerer, vorzuglich alter Falle verschiedner Arten von Krätze, des Grindkopfs, langwieriger Schwinden, Schenkelgeschwüre, u. s. w. zeigen, wie groß und wichtig die diesen Lokalsymptomen zu Grunde liegenden innern Krankheiten (die Kratzkrankheit, die Grindkopfkrankheit u. s. w.) seien, wenn man ihnen das die Gefährlichkeit ihrer ubrigen Symptomen ab-

Foot note: The often highly acute and terrible consequences of the merely local annihilation of many, especially old cases of scabies, ringworm of the scalp, chronic tetters, ulcers of the legs, etc., show, how great and important these local symptoms are in relation of the internal disease (the scabies, ringworm of the scalp, etc.) if one robs them of the local symptoms and dangers of the remaining symptoms without having the internal disease cured. Then the remaining symptoms which were till now dormant and could not be easily noticed except by a very keen observation, often appear suddenly in their true original form and severity. The mental weakness, which was so far not clearly visible increases to a kind of mania, the slight cough, which was little conspicuous breaks out fast as suffocating pulmonary ulceration or as acute pulmonary consumption, the slight oedema of the feet which was almost unnoticeable rapidly passes into genral dropsy, a rarely occurring weakness of sight and hardness of hearing turn, almost before we are aware of it, into amaurosis and deafness, that is to say, these disease appear now in the form and intensity they originally possessed when they no longer have the local affection that lessened their severity.

sorbirende grofse Lokalsymptom raubt, ohne die innere Krankheit selbst vorher geheilt zu haben. Da treten dann die bisher nur schlummernden, ohne scharfsichtige Beobachtung nicht leicht bemerkbaren, ubrigen Symptomen oft plötzlich in ihrer wahren ursprunglichen Gröfse und Heftigkeit auf; die bisher nur undeutlich bemerkte Geistesschwäche erhöhet sich auf einmahl zur Manie; der geringe Husten, die wenig auffallende Brustengigkeit bricht als schnell erstickendes Lungengeschwür, oder als akute Lungeneiterung aus, das bisher fast unmerkliche Anlaufen der Fufse wird schnell zur allgemeinen Wassergeschwulst, die bis dahin geringe Blödsichtigkeit und das etwas stumpfere Gehör, ehe man sichs versieht, bis zur Amaurosis und Taubheit erhöhet — das ist, diese Krankheiten erscheinen nun in ihrer eigenthumlichen Gestalt und Gröfse, wie sie ursprunglich sind, wenn ihnen das ihre Heftigkeit mildernde Lokalleiden fehlt.

Man kann auch gar nicht zweifeln, dafs alte Lokalsymptome dergleichen enorme innere Krankheiten schon zum Grunde haben.

Es ist Aberglaube, dergleichen auf Unterdrückung des Lokalübels erfolgende heftige Krankheiten von einem sogenannten

One can in no way doubt that the old local symptoms have as its cause an internal disease that is equally serious.

It is a superstition that the suppression of the local sufferings of the effecting severe diseases is derived from a so called recession of morbid matter in the inside of the body, through which the first disease had emerged. No ! It was already existing as the local symptoms and was still going on in the external parts, only it was restrained from bursting forth and risking life. 'A candidate for the ministry with a robust appearance, who had to preach in a few days, and thus wanted to free himself from scabies of long standing, applied an ointment for scabies one morning and within few hours he was seized with anxiety, dyspnoea and tenesmus immediately after midday and died in a few hours. The post mortem examination showed the whole lung filled with liquid pus. '(which could not possibly have been produced in these few hours, but must have been there previously, but hitherto kept subdued

Zurucktritt des Krankheitsstoffes in das Innere des Körpers herzuleiten, wodurch nun erst die innere Krankheit entstunde und sich anspinne. Nein! sie war schon vorhanden, wie das Lokalsymptom noch im Gange war, nur in ihren Ausbruchen und ihrer Lebensgefährlichkeit von dem Lokalsymptome bisher aufgehalten worden. Ein robust scheinender Kandidat der die nachsten Tage predigen und sich deshalb von seiner Kratze befreien wollte, bestrich sich den einen Morgen mit Kratzsalbe und binnen wenigen Stunden war er unter Aengstlichkeiten kurzem Odem und Stuhlzwang gleich nach der Mittagszeit verschieden; die Leichenofnung zeigte, dafs die ganze Lunge von flussigem Eiter ausgedehnt war (welches sich in diesen wenigen Stunden unmoglich erzeugt haben konnte, sondern schon vorher, nur durch das Lokalsymptom des Ausschlags bisher gemildert, da gewesen seyn mufste) m. s. *Unsers Arzt,* CCC St. S. 598.

Hinwiederum zeigt die starke Beharrlichkeit, oft auch grofse Schmerzhaftigkeit des Lokalsymptoms, welche oft dem jugendlichsten, und kraftvollesten Korper zum Trotze, auf seiner Stelle zuweilen Iahre lang qualet und wuthet wie ent-

and rendered harmless only by the local symptom, the eruption spread over the skin). M.s. *Unzers Arzt,* CCC St., p. 508.

Again, the great persistency, often also the extreme painfulness of the local symptom which often over rides the strong and young bodies, which frequently torments the patient for many years and grows bigger and becomes worse, shows how terrible and frightful the internal disease must be, for which it serves as a repulsive palliative substitute on the least dangerous part of the organism, the external parts.

Are the often life-endangering acute or chronic malady that appear after the removal of plica polonica anything else than the plica disease previously present, although hitherto latent, and seldom manifesting itself during the continuance of the local symptoms? The former were only fully intensified

setzlich und furchterlich das innere Uebel
seyn muſs, dem es zum ableitenden, mildernden Stellvertreter an der wenigst gefährlichen Gegend des Organismus — an
den äuſsern Theilen — dient.

Sind die oft lebensgefährlichen, theils
akuten, theils chronischen Leiden, welche
sich nach Abschneidung des Wichtelzopfes
hervorthun, etwas andres, als die vorher
schon vorhandne, obgleich bisher nur
schlummernde, allgemeine Wichtelzopf-
krankheit? die blos wieder erwachte, als
der palliative Beschwichtiger des innern
Gesamtleidens, das vikarirende groſse Lokalsymptom der Wichtelzopf (jenes Zu-
sammenwachsen der in ein empfindliches
Afterorgan von ihrer Wurzel an ausgear-
teten Haare) ihr geraubt worden war.
Dieselbe allgemeine Krankheit des Körpers geht auch vorher, ehe sich der Wichtelzopf hervorthut sie mildert sich, wenn
sich der Wichtelzopf ausbildet, und uber-
tragt alle ihre Heftigkeit auf dieses Lokalsymptom; doch, auch noch so lange Zeit
durch die ungestörte Gegenwart dieses vi-
karirenden Afterorgans beschwichtiget, er-
wacht sie gleichwohl mit aller Heftigkeit
aus ihrem bisherigen Schlummer, wenn
ihr dieſs ihre Stelle zum groſsen Theile
vertretende Hauptsymptom geraubt, wenn

K

when they were deprived of the palliative dormancy of the internal general disease, the vicarious local symptom, the plica polonica (those tuft of hair which matted together on the sensitive organ and have degenerated from their roots). The same general disease precedes the outbreak of the plica, it becomes milder when the latter develops itself and transfers all its intensity and dangerous character to this local symptom. But however long it may be kept in abeyance by the undisturbed presence of this vicarious abnormal organ; the internal disease wakes from the latent state, in which it has hitherto existed, with great violence, when robbed of this chief symptom that has served as its substitute to a great extent, when the plica closely attached to the head is cut off.

176.

Zum Glucke bringt die eigne Thatigkeit des Organismus das durch Kunst vernichtete Lokalsymptom zuweilen von selbst an seinem Orte wieder zum Vorscheine; kunstliche Hulfe zu seiner Wiedereinsetzung ist diefs weniger im Stande. Auch die Einimpfung ist oft unzureichend, weil man gewöhnlich nicht dasselbe Lokalleiden einimpfet, sondern ein andres, blos dem Anscheine nach ahnliches.

177.

Alle solche Krankheiten können blos durch die innere Anwendung einer ihrem ganzen Symptomeninbegriffe (in welchem das Lokalsymptom als das am meisten charakteristische obenan stehet) homöopathisch anpassenden, arzneilichen Gegenkrankheitspotenz rationell geheilt werden, bei deren innerm Gebrauche und einer überdiefs zweckmäsigen Lebensordnung,

§ 176

Fortunately sometimes the activity of the organism itself causes the reappearance of the local symptom to appear again which has been artificially annihilated; it is not proper to reinstating this by artificial assistance, because even such inoculation is usually insufficient as the local-suffering inoculated is not the original one, but merely bears just a superficial semblance.

§ 177

The rational cure of all such diseases depends completely on the internal use of a counter & medicine disease-force, suitably adapted by its homoeopathicity to the whole symptom-complex, (in which the local symptom is but the most characteristic sign among a number of others). If this remedy is given internally, and if in addition a suitable regimen is ordered, the topical application of the specific remedy will be found useless and will hardly ever be needed.

die topische Auflegung desselben specifischen Heilmittels kaum je nebenbei nöthig seyn wird.

Anm. Hierin verlangen wenigstens die verschiednen Krankheiten verschiedne Masregeln. Am zweckwidrigsten ist z. B. die Anwendung topischer Mittel auf Schanker, die oft grofse Neigung haben, vor der Zeit den Lokalmitteln zu weichen. Sicherer ist die äufsere Anwendung des Schwefels bei fast schon ganz durch innere homöopathische Kur geheilter Wollarbeiter-Krätze — und die topische Anwendung des Arseniks in einigen Arten Gesichtskrebs, wenn die innere Anwendung desselben Mittels sich in dem gegenwärtigen Falle schon hülfreich erwiesen hat und durch sie die Heilung des Lokalsymptoms schon weit gediehen ist.

178.

Die Schwierigkeit der homöopathischen Heilung dieser einseitigen Krankheiten, zu denen die sogenannten Lokalkrankheiten vorzüglich gehören, besteht, wie gesagt, hauptsächlich darin, dafs an ihnen nicht viel mehr als ein einziges starkes

K 2

Footnote: In this different diseases require respect different measures. For example the most suitable is, , the topical application of remedies on chancre, which often have a great tendency to go away before its schedule with local-medicine. More certain than the external use of sulphur is the internal homoeopathic treatment for complete cure of wool-worker's scabies; and the topical application of Arsenics in a some varieties of facial-cancer, if the internal usage of the same medicine in the present cases has already been proved helpful and the local-symptoms has been cured by its use.

§ 178

Homoeopathic cure of these *one-sided* diseases, including the so-called local diseases which belong to this class, is much difficult as it depends mainly, as has been already said, on the fact that they rarely present more than one striking, prominent symptom, with which the remaining symptoms, usually remain unrecognisable in the background and escape the attention of common observers, completes the outline of the disease-picture.

kes Symptom hervortritt, wogegen die
übrigen Symptomen, welche zur Vervollständigung des Umrisses der Krankheitsgestalt gehören, sich in den Hintergrund zurück ziehen, und dem Auge des gewöhnlichen Beobachters unkenntlich werden.

179.

Diese Schwierigkeit wird durch ge-
schärftere, sorgfältigere Beobachtung und
Nachforschung gehoben.

180.

Zu dieser Absicht, wenn ein solcher
Kranker seine wenigen grofsen Beschwerden geklagt und vor der Hand nichts weiter anzuführen weifs, verschiebt der Arzt
am besten das Urtheil über seine Heilbar-
keit und seine Heilverordnungen, da es
fast immer chronische *) Krankheiten sind,

---

*) Fast nur diejenigen Lokalkrankheiten sind akut,
welche man Metastase nennt — d. i. ein örtli-
ches, gröfseres Symptom, welches die Natur in
akuten Krankheiten sich bestrebt, mehr nach auf-

§ 179

This difficulty can only be overcome by more attentive and more careful observations and investigations.

§ 180

For this purpose, if such a patient complains only of a few severe complaints and can give no more at the first examination, the physician does best to defer his judgment as to the curability of the disease and its curative treatment. Such diseases are nearly always chronic* in nature and will not suffer for a long time from delay of a few more days, during which all deviations from health in the patient, great or small, can be more attentively investigated until each one, even the trivial and hitherto unnoticed symptoms, has been elicited and precisely described.

Footnote: Local diseases are hardly ever acute except when there are *Metastases* – i.e. a local severe symptom which by nature appears in acute diseases on an outward and the least dangerous and less vital area of the

welche unbeschwerlich Aufschub leiden,
mehrere Tage hinaus, und trägt dem Kranken auf, indeſs noch genauer auf alle kleine und gröſsere Abweichungen seines Befindens vom gesunden Zustande die sorg-
fältigste Aufmerksamkeit zu richten, um
alle, auch die kleinern, bisher unbeachte-
ten Zufälle angeben und genau beschreiben
zu können.

181.

Hier wird er seine Aufmerksamkeit
von seinem Lokalleiden indeſs abziehn,

---

sen zu, an die mindest gefährlichen Stellen des Organismus zu verlegen, um auf dasselbe die Gröſse
und Lebensgefährlichkeit des innern Allgemeinlei-
dens zum gröſsern Theile überzutragen. Auch hier
vikarirt dieses Lokalsymptom für die übrigen Symptome, welche leztere aber in diesem Falle leichter
aufzufassen sind aus ihrer Beschaffenheit gleich vor
Entstehung der Metastase, und mit dem Lokalsymptome zusammengenommen, das Krankheitsbild liefern, den Symptomeninbegriff, auf welchen das blos
Innerlich anzuwendende homöopatische
Heilmittel passen muſs, wenn die Heilung gründlich und rationell seyn soll. Auch hier ist die blos
örtliche Vertreibung des Lokalsymptoms mehr zum
Schaden.

organism in an attempt to save the inner life in general from the suffering to a great extent and from the danger that threatens it. Here also, the local symptoms act vicariously for the remaining symptoms, yet, in such cases, the remaining symptoms are more easy to discover due to the condition which preceded the metastasis, and taken together with the local symptoms the entire symptom-complex and disease-picture can be obtained and when an appropriately selected homoeopathic remedy be *administered internally only*, cure then proceeds rationally and radically. Here removing the local symptoms by local application only is very harmful.

§ 181

Here the attention may be diverted from the local-sufferings to take note of the smaller accessory complaints and in this way peculiar symptoms, till now unremembered, will be observed, which the patient had not perceived on account of the pressing nature of the greater sufferings.

und sie auf die, selbst kleinern Nebenbe
schwerden und Zufalle richten und auf
diese Art besondre Symptomen wahrneh
men, die er, unerinnert, neben seinem
grofsern Uebel nicht bemerkt haben wurde

Anm. Ware der Kranke jedoch starrig, behaup-
tete er nichts weiter bemerken zu konnen,
und wollte sich keinen Aufschub in der
Kur gefallen lassen, so dient es, ihn statt
Arznej eine unarzneiliche Flussigkeit mehrere Tage lang einnehmen zu lassen und
ihm hierbei genaue Aufmerksamkeit auf
alle und jede Veranderungen in seinem
Befinden, auf alle in gesundem Zustande
nicht gewohnliche Zeichen, Zufalle und
Ereignisse einzuscharfen — eine unschul-
dige Tauschung, die die meisten seiner
Krankheit eignen Symptomen an den Tag
bringen wird.

182.

Diese kleinern und grofsern Beson-
derheiten in seinem ubrigen Befinden werden dem Arzte nun den Krankheitsumrifs
vervollstandigen helfen; und behutsame
Fragen uber den Zustand der verschied-

Footnote: If the patient, however, stubbornly maintains not to be any further observed and wants treatment without delay, it is advisable to serve him an un-medicinal fluid for a few days instead of medicine, in order to gain time for the discovery, by further accurate attention, of all and every alterations from his healthy state, any sign, conditions, occurrence or intensity that is not usual. It is a harmless deception which will bring to light most of the characteristic symptoms of his disease.

§ 182

Besides, these smaller and great special-features peculiarities of the state of health which will help the physician to complete the disease-picture; and careful queries into the condition of different functions, a close observation of the sensation and entire behaviour of the patient, together with any information furnished by friends, questioned in private, if necessary, will be the necessary additions and confirmations to the already recorded facts for successful treatment.

nen Funktionen, genaue Beobachtung seines Aeufsern und seines ganzen Benehmens, so wie die Auskunft, welche die
Angehörigen, selbst ingeheim ausgefragt,
über ihn geben können, werden die nöthigen Zusätze und Bestätigungen zu dem
schon Niedergeschriebenen liefern.

183.

So kann es nicht fehlen, dafs dem
Heilkunstler der vollständige Zeicheninbe-
griff der auch noch so versteckten chronischen Krankheit offenbar werde, um fur
ihn nach den Krankheitselementen, welche
die am gesunden Menschen gepruften Arzneien enthalten, eine ihr möglichst ähnliche, das naturliche Uebel folglich zu uberstimmen fahige Gegenkrankheitspotenz homoopathisch auswahlen zu konnen. Auch
hier mussen vorzuglich die besondern und
charakteristischen Symptomen der Krankheit in der Symptomenreihe des Heilmittels anzutreffen seyn.

§ 183

Thus, the physician will not fail to complete the symptom-complex of any chronic disease however hidden it may be, in order to find the disease-elements among the remedies that have been tested on healthy human beings and select the counter disease-force as similar as possible to the natural disorder, that is, the chosen homoeopathic remedy. Likewise, here the most peculiar and characteristic symptoms of the disease must, above all others, be found in the list of symptom of the appropriate remedy.

184.

Ist die zuerst gewählte Arznei wirklich die den Krankheitszufällen in ihrem Umfange angemessene, so muſs sie das Uebel heilen; hatte sie aber aus dem unzulänglichen Vorrathe nach ihren positiven Wirkungen am gesunden Körper gekannter, arzneilicher Krankheitspotenzen nicht hinreichend homöopathisch gewählt werden können, so wird die Arznei neue Symptomen erregen, die zur fernern Wahl des zunächst nöthigen und dienlichen Heilmittels Anleitung geben werden.

185.

Die nächste Hauptschwierigkeit in der Heilung, scheinen die Gemuthskrankheiten darzubieten. Sie sind aber in der That nicht schwieriger zu heilen, als die andern einseitigen Krankheiten, zu denen sie gezählet werden können.

186.

Auch machen sie gar keine, von den übrigen scharf getrennte Klasse von Krank-

§ 184

If the medicine first chosen really corresponds to the disease-state in its entirety it must cure it. But if, due to the inadequate number of medicines whose full positive effects on healthy organisms are known and the thus restricting our choice, the medicinal disease-force selected may not be able to sufficiently homoeopathic, then the medicine will produce new symptoms which will, in their turn, guide us to the next serviceable remedy.

§ 185

In the next category of diseases difficult to cure comes the *mental diseases*. They are known as kind of one-sided diseases and are actually not much more difficult to cure than others of similar kind.

§ 186

Moreover, in reality they are not a sharply separated class of disease from other diseases because in every kind of diseases the mind and state of the disposition is *always* altered in some way and in *all* curable cases of diseases the state of mind of the patient is the chief symptoms to be included in

heiten aus, da in jeder der ubrigen Krankheiten auch die Gemuths - und Geistesver-
fassung allemahl geandert ist, und in
allen zu heilenden Krankheitsfällen, von
welcher Art sie auch seyn mogen, der Gemuthszustand des Kranken als ein Hauptsymptom unter den ubrigen, mit in den
Inbegriff der Krankheitssymptomen aufzunehmen ist, wenn man acht rationell und
homoopathisch heilen will.

Anm. Wie oft trifft man nicht z. B. in den
schmerzhaftesten, mehrjahrigen chronischen Krankheiten ein mildes, sanftes Gemüth an, ab dafs der Heilkünstler Achtung und Mitleid gegen die Kranken zu
hegen sich gedrungen fühlt. Besiegt er
aber die Krankheit und stellt die Kranken wieder her (wie nach homoopathischer Art nicht selten in kurzer Zeit möglich ist), da staunt und erschrickt er oft
uber die schauderhafte Veranderung des
Gemuths. Da sieht er oft Undankbarkeit,
Hartherzigkeit, raffinirte Bosheit, und die
die Menschheit entehrendsten, emporend-
sten Launen hervortreten, welche gerade
den Kranken in ihren ehemahligen gesunden Tagen eigen waren.

the totality of the disease-symptoms for achieving a rational and homoeopathic cure.

Footnote: It is not often that one meet, for example, a mild, calm nature in the patients of most painful chronic diseases of several years, so that the physician closely feels attentive and compassionate towards him. In case he overcomes the disease and recovers again (as it is possible often in a short time according to homoeopathic method) he is astonished and dismayed to note the horrifying change of mind. He often sees the emergence of ingratitude, hard heatedness, malice and the most disgraceful and outrageous moods, which were quite peculiar to his earlier days of health.

Patience in times of well-being, but when diseased one often finds furious, violent, hasty as well as unreasonable stubbornness and on the other hand impatience or despair. One frequently finds the bright headed to be stupid, the usual moron to be almost cleverer, more sensible and not rarely those with slower reflection, with greater presence of mind and quick witted, and so on.

Den in gesunden Zeiten Gedultigen findet, man oft in Krankheiten stürmisch,
heftig, hastig, auch wohl unleidlich, eigen-
sinnig, und wiederum auch wohl unge-
dultig, oder verzweifelt. Den hellen Kopf
findet man nicht selten stumpfsinnig, den
gewöhnlich Schwachsinnigen hinwiederum
gleichsam kluger, sinniger und den von
langsamer Besinnung nicht selten mit Gei-
stesgegenwart und schnell entschlossen.

187.

Diefs geht so weit, dafs bei der Wahl
einer arzneilichen Gegenkrankheitspotenz
der Gemuthszustand des Kranken oft hauptsächlich den Ausschlag giebt, als charakteristisches Zeichen, was dem genau beobachtenden Arzte unter allen am wenigsten
verborgen bleiben kann.

188.

Auf dieses Hauptingredienz aller
Krankheiten, den veränderten Gemuths-
und Geisteszustand hat auch der Schöpfer
der Heilpotenzen vorzüglich Rucksicht ge-

§ 187

The fact is so over powering that it is not too much to state that the choice of a medicinal counter - disease-force is mainly determined by the mental state of patient as they are the characteristic signs an accurately observing physician can not succeed by overlooking it.

§ 188

These alterations in the state of mind and disposition are the chief feature of every disease which has been excellently considered by the Creator of medicinal-powers, for there is no powerful medicinal-substance in the world which does not produce in healthy persons very appreciable changes in the state of mind and disposition, which are *different for every medicine.*

nommen, indem es keine kraftige Arzneisubstanz auf der Welt giebt, welche nicht
im gesunden Menschen, den Gemüths- und
Geisteszustand sehr merkbar veränderte,
jede Arznei anders.

189.

Man wird daher nie rationell und homöopathisch heilen lernen, wenn man
nicht bei jedem Krankheitsfalle mit auf das
Symptom der Geistes- oder Gemüthsverän-
derung siehet, und nicht zur Hülfe eine
solche Gegenkrankheitspotenz unter den
Heilmitteln auswählt, welche einen ähnlichen Gemüths- oder Geisteszustand vor
sich zu erzeugen fähig ist.

> Anm. So wird bei einer stillen, gleichför-
> mig gelassenen Gemüthsart der Napell-
> sturmhut nie eine, weder schnelle, noch
> dauerhafte Heilung bewirken, eben so
> wenig als die Krähenaugen bei einem mil-
> den, phlegmatischen, die Kuchenschelle
> bei einem frohen, heitern, oder die Ignatz-
> bohne bei einem gesetzten, unwandelba-
> ren, weder zu Schreck noch zu Aerger-
> niß geneigten Gemüthszustande.

§ 189

We shall, therefore, never learn to cure rationally and homoeopathically, unless we do not consider in every case of disease these symptoms of intellect and mental changes, and with their help do not select a counter disease-force amongst the remedies which is capable of producing a similar state of mind and disposition.

Foot Note: Thus *Aconite* will *never* bring about a rapid and permanent cure in a patient of gentle, consistently calm nature; *Nux vomica* is of little service in mild, phlegmatic patients, *Pulsatilla* of little use for the gay and cheerful, *Ignatia* as little to those whose mental state are not disinclined either to fear, fright or to vexation.

190.

Was ich also über die Heilung der
Geistes-und Gemuthskrankheiten zu sagen
habe, wird sich auf Weniges beschränken
können, da sie auf dieselbe Art als alle
übrige Krankheiten, das ist, durch ein
Heilmittel, was eine möglichst ähnliche
Krankheitspotenz in ihren (an Leib und
Seele des gesunden Menschen zu Tage gelegten) Symptomen darbietet, zu heilen
ist, und gar nicht anders geheilt werden
kann.

191.

Die sogenannten Geistes-und Gemuthskrankheiten sind fast durchaus nichts
anders als Körperkrankheiten, bei denen
das gewöhnliche Symptom der Geistes-und
Gemuthsumstimmung sich unter Vermin-
derung der Körpersymptomen schneller
oder langsamer erhöhet, oft bis zur auffallendsten Einseitigkeit, fast wie eine Lokalkrankheit.

§ 190

Thus all that I have to say concerning the cure of diseases of the intellect and mind can be restricted to a few words, for they can be cured in the same was as all other types of diseases, that is, by a remedy, by a disease-force producing symptoms on the body and soul of healthy persons as similar as possible, and in no other way can they be cured.

§ 191

The so-called emotional and mental diseases are, for the most part, no more than the corporeal diseases wherein the usual symptoms of mind and disposition have more or less quickly increased, while the corporeal symptoms have diminished, until a most striking one-sidedness is attained, almost like that of a local disease.

192

Die Falle sind nicht selten, wo eine den Tod drohende sogenannte Korperkrankheit — eine Lungenvereiterung oder die Verderbnifs irgend eines andern edeln Eingeweides, oder eine akute gefahrliche Krankheit z. B. im Kindbette u. s. w. durch schnelle Erhohung des bisherigen Gemuthssymptoms, in Wahnsinn, Melancholie oder Raserei ausartet, und alle Todesgefahr der Korpersymptomen verschwindet; diese bessern sich indefs fast bis zur Gesundheit, oder verringern sich vielmehr bis zu dem Grade, dafs ihre dunkel fortwahrende Existenz nur von dem beharrich und fein beobachtenden Arzte noch erkannt werden kann. Sie arten mit einem Worte zur einseitigen Krankheit, gleichsam zu einer Lokalkrankheit aus, in welcher das in der ursprunglichen Krankheit gegen die ubrigen Symptomen bisher nur verhaltnifsmasige, gelinde Symptom der Gemuthsumstimmung zum Hauptsymptome sich vergrofsert; welches dann zum grofsern Theile fur die ubrigen Symptome vikarirt, und ihre Heftigkeit palliativ be-

§ 192

It is not rare that the cases where a so-called corporeal disease in which death is imminent—a lung-suppuration, or the deterioration of some other important organs, or a dangerous acute disease, *e.g.,* in childbed, etc.—becomes transformed into insanity, melancholia or into mania by a quick increase of the mental symptoms that were previously present, whereupon all the fatal dangers of the corporeal symptoms disappears; these latter improve almost to perfect health, or rather they decrease to such grade that their obscured continued existence can only be recognised by the persistent and finely observant physician. Similarly, in other words, they become one-sided disease, almost a local disease, in which the symptoms of the disposition which were originally mild and unimportant increase until they become the chief symptoms and, then they take the place, to a large extent, of the remaining (corporeal) symptoms, which they palliate by their own intensity; as was seen in the chief symptoms of the so called local disease.

schwichtiget, wie wir bei den grofsen
Hauptsymptomen der sogenannten Lokalkrankheiten gesehen haben.

193.

Deshalb gehort wie zur Ausforschung
des Symptomenkomplexes der leztern
(§. 180. 181.), eine ähnlich grofse Beharr
lichkeit, ein ähnlich feiner Beobachtungs-
geist, eine gleich sorgfältige Unterschei-
dung, und eine eben so behutsame Er-
kündigung zur Ausforschung der übrigen
Symptome des körperlichen Befindens bei
Gemüthskranken, nächst der genauen Auf-
fassung des eigentlichen Charakters ihres
individuellen, vorwaltenden Geistes - und
Gemüthszustandes, um zur Auslöschung
des Gesammtzustandes dieser Totalkrankheit, eine Gegenkrankheitspotenz unter den
gekannten Heilmitteln auszufinden, ein
Heilmittel, welches in seiner Symptomenreihe nicht nur diesen Geistes - und Ge-
müthszustand, sondern auch möglichst allen
übrigen Körpersymptomen enthält.

§ 193

In these diseases (§ 180, 181), therefore, to discover the bodily symptoms in mental diseases, the investigation of the symptom-complex demands a great perseverance, finer observation, most careful differentiation and a careful inquiry; the precise perception of the actual characters of each individual, change in emotion and mental states, in order to discover, for the purpose of extinction of the entire state of total-disease, a counter disease-force among the known remedies, whose symptom-array contains, not only the emotion and mental states but also as far as possible the corporeal symptoms also.

194.

Zur Ausforschung der leztern dient vorzüglich eine genaue Beschreibung der sämtlichen Zufälle der vormahligen sogenannten Körperkrankheit, ehe sie zur einseitigen Erhöhung des Gemüthssymptoms, zur Geistes- und Gemüthskrankheit ausartete.

195.

Die Vergleichung dieser ehemahligen Krankheitssymptome mit den davon jezt noch übrigen obgleich unscheinbarer gewordenen, wird zur Bestätigung der fortdauernden Gegenwart der leztern dienen, um ein charakteristisches Symptomenbild der Krankheit entwerfen zu können.

196.

Ist die von Körperleiden entstandne Gemüthskrankheit noch nicht völlig ausgebildet, und es fände noch einiger Zweifel statt, ob es nicht vielmehr Erziehungsfehler, schlimme Angewöhnung, oder verderbte Moralität, Aberglaube oder Unwis-

---

§ 194

The fine and a precise description of all the phenomena previous to the so-called corporeal disease, before the one-sided increase of mental symptoms and its degeneration into emotional and mental disease serves to the investigation.

§ 195

The comparison of these previous disease symptoms with the existing symptoms, although inconspicuous, will serve to confirm that they are still present, so that a characteristic symptom-picture of the disease will be possible to be drawn.

§ 196

If the mental disease be not fully developed, and if there is some kind of doubt whether it has not arose from a corporeal affection, or did not rather result from faults of education, evil practices, tainted morality, superstition or ignorance; the mode of deciding this point will be, that if it arose from one or other of the latter causes it will diminish and be improved by sensible exhortations, consolation, sensible advice and serious

senheit sei, da dient als Zeichen, dafs
durch verständigendes, sorgsames Zureden, Vernunftgründe, Trostgrunde oder
ernstlrafte Vorstellung leztere nachgeben,
wahre Gemuthskrankheit aber schnell dadurch verschlimmert, Melancholie noch
zuruckgezogener, boshafter Wahnsinn dadurch noch mehr erbittert, und thorichtes
Gewasche offenbar noch unsinniger wird.

197.

Doch giebt es Gemuthskrankheiten,
welche nicht blos aus Korperkrankheiten
dahin ausgeartet sind, sondern, in umge-
kehrter Ordnung, bei geringer Kranklich-
keit, vom Gemuthe aus Anfang und Fort-
gang nehmen durch anhaltenden Kummer,
Krankung, Aergernifs, und grofse Veranlassung zu Furcht und Schreck. — Diese
Art Gemuthskrankheiten verderben dann
mit der Zeit auch den korperlichen Ge-
sundheitszustand, oft in hohem Grade.

198.

Blos diese von aufsen herein durch
die Seele zuerst angesponnene Art von

representations and sensible advice; whereas a true mental disease would have quick exacerbation, the melancholic become more reclusive, malicious mania becomes more bitter, and the chattering fool would become more nonsensical.

§ 197

But, there are certain mental diseases which have not simply developed from corporeal diseases, but, in the reverse order, these the minor corporeal sickness, originate and are maintained from mental causes, such as continued grief, insult, chagrin and exposure to fear and fright – these types of mental diseases ruins to a higher grade, in due course of time, the state of corporeal health.

§ 198

It is only such types of mental diseases, which were first caused and subsequently kept up by the soul, while they are still new and before they have greatly destroyed the corporeal state, are precisely those which can be quickly transformed

Gemüthskrankheiten lassen sich, so lange
sie noch neu sind, und den Körperzustand
noch nicht allzu sehr zerrüttet haben, blos
durch psychische Mittel, Zutraulichkeit,
gütliches Zureden, Vernunftgründe, am
meisten, aber durch wohl verdeckte Täu-
schungen schnell in Wohlbefinden der
Seele (und des Leibes) verwandeln.

Anm. Bei den durch Körperkrankheit entstandnen Geistes- und Gemuthskrankheiten,
welche einzig durch angemessene, homöopathische Arzneien zu heilen sind, muſs
allerdings auch, als beihülfliche Seelen-
diät, ein passendes psychisches Verhalten
der Angehörigen und des Arztes gegen
den Kranken sorgfältig beobachtet werden.
Dem wüthenden Wahnsinn setzt man
stille Unerschrockenheit, und kaltblüti-
gen festen Willen — dem peinlich kla-
genden Iammer stummes Bedauern in Mienen, dem unsinnigen Geschwätz nicht ganz
unaufmerksames Stillschweigen, ekelhaf-
tem und gräuelvollem Benehmen und
Reden völlige Unaufmerksamkeit entgegen. Den Verwüstungen und Beschädi-
gungen beugt man blos vor, und verhütet sie ohne Vorwürfe und richtet alles
so ein, daſs durchaus alle körperliche

L

into healthy state, of soul (and of body), by psychical means, such as a display of confidence, amicable persuasion, sensible advice, and often by well-concealed deceptions, and can be cured by such measures, however, and only while they are yet recent and the bodily conditions little disturbed by them.

Foot Note: In mental and emotional diseases arising from diseases of body, which can only be cured by an appropriate homoeopathic medicine and by way of mind-regimen always requires a carefully observed decent psychical behaviour towards the patient on the part of attendants and that of the physician.

Furious mania must be opposed by calm courage, and cold-blooded, firm will—to doleful, querulous regret, a mute expression of sympathy, to nonsensical chattering, a silence but not inattention, and to disgusting and abominable conduct and speech, total inattention. Destructions and injuries must be prevented without reproaches to the patient, and everything must be

Züchtigungen wegfallen. Denn da keine
Imputation bei Gemuthskranken, nach allen menschlichen Rechten, statt findet,
so kann auch keine Strafe statt finden.
Diefs geht um desto leichter an, da bei dem
Einnehmen (dem einzigen Falle, wo noch
Zwang durch Entschuldigung gerechtfertigt
werden konnte) in der homöopathischen
Heilart die kleinen Gaben hülfreicher Arznei dem Geschmacke nie auffallen und
dem Kranken nur unbewufst in Getränken gegeben werden können, wo dann
ebenfalls aller Zwang wegfällt. Wider-
spruch, eifrige Verstandigungen, heftige
Zurechtweisungen, und Harte sind so wie
schwache, furchtsame Nachgiebigkeit am
unrechten Orte, sind gleich schädliche Be-
handlungen ihres Geistes und Gemuths.
Am meisten jedoch werden sie durch Hohn,
Betrug und Tauschungen erbittert und
in ihrer Krankheit verschlimmert. Immer mufs man den Schein annneh-
men, als ob man ihnen Vernunft
zutraute. Dagegen suche man alle Art
von Stöhrungen ihrer Sinne und ihres Gemuths von aufsen zu entfernen; es giebt
keine Unterhaltungen, keine wohlthatigen
Zerstreuungen, keine Belehrungen, keine
Besänftigung fur ihre in den Fesseln des
kranken Korpers schmachtende oder em-

arranged in such a way to avoid any corporal punishment. For as in mental diseases there can be no imputation, so by all human justice there should be no punishments. This is so much the more easily effected, (the only case in which the employment of coercion could be justified) in the homoeopathic healing system the small doses of the helpful medicine never offend the taste, and may consequently be given to the patient without his knowledge in his drink, so that all coercion is unnecessary. Contradiction, eager explanations, rude reprimand and cruelty are as out of place as weak, timid yielding in the to such patients and are harmful in treatment of their mind and in emotion. Most of all, cynicism, deceit and fraud exacerbate their condition. One must always assume an appearance to believe them to be capable of reason. However, all kinds of external disturbing influences on their senses and disposition should be removed; there are no amusements, no salutary diversions, no training, no mollification, for the sick soul is languishing in the shackles of the diseased body; it is only when the bodily health is changed for the better by a suitable remedy that again ease of their mind returns.

pörte Seele, als die, welche durch ihr
vom angemessenen Heilmittel zum Bessern
umgestimmtes Körperbefinden auf ihren
Geist zurückstrahlt.

Ist das für den individuellen Fall der
Geistes - oder Gemüthskrankheiten (denn
ihre Zahl ist Legion!) gewählte Heilmittel dem treulich entworfenen Bilde ihres
Krankheitszustandes ganz homöopathisch
angemessen — welches um desto leichter
ist, da ihr Gemüths - und Geisteszustand
als Hauptsymptom sich zugleich so unver-
kennbar als charakteristisch zu Tage legt —
so ist oft die kleinstmögliche Gabe hinreichend, die auffallendste Besserung in der
kürzesten Zeit hervorzubringen, was durch
die stärksten und gehäuftesten Gaben aller
übrigen unpassenden Arzneien oft bis an
den Tod nicht zu erreichen war; ja, ich
kann behaupten, daß sich der erhabne
Vorzug der homöopathischen Heilkunde
vor allen denkbaren Kurmethoden nirgend
in einem triumphirendern Lichte zeigt,
als in alten Gemüths - und Geisteskrank-
heiten, welche aus Körperleiden ursprünglich, oder auch nur gleichzeitig mit ihnen,
entstanden sind.

When for any individual case of mental or emotional disease (there are legion of its number!) an exact homoeopathically selected remedy has been chosen according to the faithfully traced picture of the disease-condition - which is easier from the unmistakable characteristic of the mental symptoms, as the emotional and mental state, constituting the chief symptom of such a patient - then even the smallest possible dose will be sufficient to produce the most striking improvement in the shortest time, an improvement denied to the strongest and often repeated doses of all other unsuitable medicines taking the patient to the extent of death. Yes, I assert that the advantageous of the homoeopathic system of medicine, over all the other conceivable treatment methods is nowhere shown in more triumphant a light as in the relief of long-standing mental and emotional diseases which have originated from bodily diseases or developed simultaneously with them.

199.

Alle ubrigen Krankheiten bedurfen zur Heilung keiner besondern Erinnerung. Sie folgen samtlich dem ewigen, ausnahmelosen Gesetze der Homoopathie.

200.

Nachdem wir also bisher gesehen haben, auf welche Umstande der Krankheiten uberhaupt und der abweichendsten insbesondre Rucksicht bei der Wahl des homoopathischen Heilmittels zu nehmen sei, so gehen wir nun zu den speciellern Gesetzen der rationellen Heilkunde, in Absicht der Gebrauchsart der Heilmittel, uber.

201.

Iede merklich fortgehende, und immer, obschon nur um Weniges zunehmende Besserung in einer akuten oder in einer chronischen Krankheit ist ein Zustand, welcher, so lange er anhalt, durchaus jede fernere Anwendung irgend einer

§ 199

No special directions are required for curing all other diseases. All of them follow, without exception, the eternal law of homoeopathy.

§ 200

Till now, thus, we have seen those general conditions of the disease which have the greatest bearing upon the choice of the homoeopathic remedy, *we now move over to the special laws of rational medicine in the mode of use* of the remedy.

§ 201

Every appreciable improvement, however small it be, provided it is *progressive improvement*, in an acute or a chronic disease is a condition which always absolutely forbids any further application of any medicine as long as it lasts because all the good of the previous medicine is not yet exhausted and is still not complete. Each new dose of any medicine would interfere with the process of recovery.

Arznei ausschliefst, weil alles das Gute,
was die vorige Arznei auszurichten indefs
fortfahrt, noch nicht vollendet ist. Iede
neue Gabe irgend einer Arznei wurde das
Besserungswerk storen.

202.

Diese Erinnerung ist um so wichti-
ger, da wir noch fast von keiner Arznei
die genauen Gränzen ihrer Wirkungsdauer mit Gewifsheit bestimmen konnen.
So lange also die fortschreitende Besserung auf eine zulezt gegebne Arznei dauert, so lange ist auch anzunehmen, dafs,
wenigstens in diesem Falle, die Wirkungsdauer der helfenden Arznei anhalte.

Anm. Einige Arzneien haben schon in 24
Stunden beinahe ausgewnkt (die kurzeste
Wirkungsdauer unter allen mir bekannten
Arzneien, die nur bei sehr wenigen angetroffen wird); andre vollenden erst in einigen, andre erst in mehrern Tagen, einige wenige sogar erst nach mehrern Wochen ihren Lauf.

§ 202

This reminding is the more important because nearly no one knows nor can he ascertain with certainty the precise duration of action of any medicine. Thus, as long as the improvement continues, so long must we accept that, at least in this case, the duration of action of the medicine is continuing and has not stopped.

Footnote: Some remedies seem to almost exhaust their effect in about twenty-four hours (very few have been affected by the short duration of action amongst all the medicine familiarised by me), others take a few days, few also take several weeks, to complete its course.

203

Hiezu kommt, dafs, wenn das Mittel angemessen homoopathisch wirkte, der
gebesserte Zustand auch noch nach verflos-
sener Wirkungsdauer merklich bleibt. Das
gute Werk wird nicht gleich unterbrochen,
wenn auch erst mehrere Stunden (ja, bei
chronischen Krankheiten, erst mehrere Tage) nach Verflufs der Wirkungsdauer der vorigen Arzneigabe, eine zweite Gabe gereicht wird. Der schon vernichtete Theil
der Krankheit kann sich indefs nicht wieder erneuern, und die Besserung würde
auch ohne neue Arzneigabe immer noch
eine betrachtliche Zeit auffallend sichtbar
bleiben.

204

Wenn die fortgehende Besserung von
der ersten Gabe der homoopathisch angemessenen Arznei sich nicht in vollige Gesundheit auflosen will (— wie doch nicht
selten —), so wird ein Zeitpunkt des Still-
standes (gewohnlich zugleich der Granz-
punkt der Wirkungsdauer der vorher ge-

§ 203

Hence it follows that, when the appropriately homoeopathic remedy has acted, the improved state will persist even after its duration of action is expired. The good work will not be discontinued even if a second dose is not given until several hours (in chronic diseases, actually not until several days) have elapsed after the duration of action of the previous medicinal dose has exhausted. The part of the disease already annihilated will not be renewed again, and improvement will remain clearly visible for a considerable time even without the administration of a new medicinal dose.

§ 204

When the continuous improvement that follows the first dose of the medicine homoeopathically appropriate to the disease does not go on to the complete restoration of health (as, not rarely, it will), the standstill period (usually immediately before the exhaustion of the duration of action of the medicine) that ensues and to repeat the dose of the medicine before its appearance is without foreseeable benefit, without sensible ground (irrational), and is harmful.

gebnen Arznei) eintreten, vor dessen Erscheinung es ohne absehbaren Nutzen, ohne vernünftigen Grund (irrationell) gehan-
delt, ja schädlich seyn wurde, eine abermahlige Gabe Arznei zu reichen.

205.

Selbst eine Gabe derselben, bis dahin
so hülfreich sich bewiesenen Arznei wird,
eher wiederholt, als die Besserung in allen
Punkten still zu stehen anfing (als Potenz
von Gegenkrankheit welche in der Mase,
als wir von einer neuen Gabe erwarten konnen, nicht mehr nothig ist) blos verschlimmern; denn bei einer leicht veranderbaren,
nicht ganz chronischen Krankheit wird die
vorige Gabe der best gewählten Arznei
nach Verfluss ihrer eigenthümlichen Wirkungsdauer schon alles das Gute, schon alle die zweckmasigen Veranderungen ausge-
fuhrt haben, als die Arznei überhaupt f u r
j e z t vermochte — eine Art von ihr fur
jezt erreichbarer Gesundheit —, und eine
abermahlige Gabe derselben wird diesen gu-
ten Zustand andern, also verschlimmern

432

§ 205

Till now one dose of the remedy which has proved so helpful by may do nothing but harm if repeated before improvement has come to the point of standstill (*when the force of opposing disease* is no more necessary in such measure which is expected of a new dose), mere aggravation, in any mild changeable and not fully chronic disease, the first dose of the best selected medicine will have already caused in the course of its own duration of action all the good, already all the desired alterations which the physician is really in apposition to achieve for the moment —a types of its health achievable for now - second dose of the same medicine given before the duration of action of the first is exhausted would change this good condition, and therefore must do harm, causing a medicinal disease to be mixed with the remaining disease-symptoms, a kind of complicated and exaggeration of the disease.

mussen, und eine Arzneikrankheit mit dem
Reste der Krankheitssymptomen gemischt,
eine Art verwickelter und vermehrter Krankheit hervorbringen, um desto mehr, wenn
die zweite Gabe noch vor Verfluss der
Wirkungsdauer der erstern gereicht wird.

Anm. Die Vernachlassigung dieser Regel bestraft sich allgemein durch Verschlimmerung der Krankheiten, vorzuglich derer
von gefährlicher Art, oder doch durch
verspatigte Genesung.

206.

Wenn die bis dahin nur vorwarts gegangene, nicht zur vollen Heilung gediehene Besserung Stillstand nimmt, wird
man auch bei genauer Untersuchung der
bis auf den gegenwartigen Augenblick gebesserten Krankheit eine so veranderte,
wenn auch kleine Symptomengruppe antreffen, auf welche eine neue Gabe der vorigen Arznei jezt durchaus nicht mehr homoopathisch passen kann, sondern immer
eine andre, diesem Reste von Zufallen angemessenere Gegenkrankheitspotenz.

434

Foot Note: Neglecting this rule is punished by an aggravation of the disease on the whole, which either becomes more threatening or slower in recovery.

§ 206

When these thriving improvements, which has steadily continued but not to the complete cure, comes a stand-still, a careful investigation of the present improved condition of the disease will show a small modified symptom-group, to which a second dose of the previous medicine would no more be suitably homoeopathic, but, this remnant state will always indicate another counter disease-force.

207.

Hat daher die erste Gabe des moglichst
gut gewahlten Arzneimittels die vollige
Herstellung der Gesundheit innerhalb ihrer
Wirkungsdauer nicht vollenden konnen
(wie sie es doch in den meisten Fallen schnell
entstandner neuer Uebel kann); so bleibt
für den dann noch ruckstandigen, obgleich viel gebesserten Krankheitszustand
offenbar nichts Besseres zu thun ubrig,
als eine Gabe eines andern, fur den jetzigen Rest von Symptomen moglichst passenden Arzneimittels zu reichen.

208.

Nur wenn vor Ablauf der Wirkungsdauer einer Arzneigabe der Zustand einer
dringenden Krankheit sich im Ganzen um
nichts gebessert, vielmehr sich (wenigstens um etwas) verschlimmert hat —, die
Arznei folglich nicht nach ihren positiven
Wirkungen homoopathisch fur den Fall gewahlt war —, muss auch noch vor Verlauf
der Wirkungsdauer der zulezt gegebnen
Arznei eine Gabe der fur den nunmehri-

§ 207

Therefore, the first dose of a well selected remedy cannot complete the restoration of health within its duration of action (as it can in most cases of rapid and recent maladies), obviously nothing better remains to be done for the remainder symptoms, though much improved disease state than to give a dose of another remedy as suitable as possible to the rest of the symptoms.

§ 208

Only when in the course of duration of action of a medicinal dose a threatening disease shows no improvement rather has exacerbated (at least somewhat) - the medicine consequently has not manifested its positive homoeopathic effect against the given case – a dose of the particularly suitable medicine adapted for this disease findings must be given before the end of the course of the duration of effect of previous medicine.

gen Krankheitsbefund genauer passenden Arznei gereicht werden.

Anm. Da nach allen Erfahrungen fast keine Gabe einer specifisch passenden, homöopathischen Arznei bereitet werden kann, welche zur Hervorbringung einer deutlichen Besserung in der ihr angemessenen Krankheit (etwa die venerische ausgenommen) zu klein wäre (§. 132. 244.), so würde man zweckwidrig und schädlich handeln, wenn man bei Nicht-Besserung, oder einiger, obschon kleiner Verschlimmerung dieselbe Arznei wiederholen, oder sie wohl gar an Gabe noch verstärken wollte. Iede Verschlimmerung durch neue Symptomen — wenn in der übrigen Geistes-oder Körper-Diät nichts böses vorgefallen ist — beweiset stets nur Unpafslichkeit der vorigen Arznei in diesem Krankheitsfalle, deutet aber nie auf Schwäche der Gabe.

209.

Um so mehr, wenn dem scharfsichtigen, genau nach dem Krankheitszustande forschenden Heilkunstler sich in dringenden Fallen schon nach Verfluſs von 6, 8,

Footnote: In all experiences almost no dose of a specifically suitable homoeopathic medicine can be so small (§ 132, 244) to produce a clear improvement of its appropriate disease (excepting a few venereal diseases); when the same medicine is repeated it would act inappropriately and harmfully and produce no-improvement or some kind of slight aggravation, then it would be better if the dose is still more strengthened. Every aggravation of new symptoms, when in remaining part of the mind and body, nothing bad is liked in diet, only proves that the indisposition of the earlier medicine in this case of disease indicate nothing but weakness of the dose.

§ 209

When it is evident to the keenly observant physician after the lapse of only six, eight or twelve hours, who has carefully investigated the disease-condition in threatening cases that last given medicine was his mis-choice, and that the patient's condition is growing distinctly worse, however slightly, from hour to hour, it is not only permitted to him, but it is his duty to correct his mistake by choosing and administration of a remedy again which shall be not merely bearably suitable, but the most appropriate possible for the existing disease-condition (§ 138).

12 Stunden offenbarte, dafs er bei Wah-
lung der zulezt gegebnen Arznei eine Mis-
wahl getroffen und der Zustand des Kranken sich deutlich von Stunde zu Stunde,
obgleich immer nur etwas verschlimmere,
ist es ihm nicht nur erlaubt, sondern
Pflicht gebeut es ihm, den begangenen
Misgriff durch Wahl und Reichung eines
nicht blos ertraglich passenden, sondern
des dem gegenwartigen Krankheitszustande möglichst angemessenen Heilmittels
wieder gut zu machen (§. 138.).

210.

Selbst in chronischen Krankheiten ist
es selten der Fall, dáfs, zumahl Anfangs,
nichts Besseres zu thun ware, als zweimahl nach einander dasselbe Arzneimittel
— obgleich erst nach Verflufs der Wirkungsdauer der zulezt gereichten Gabe —
zu verordnen.

211.

Wo demnach nicht sogleich ein durchaus angemessenes, einzig specifisches Mit-

§ 210

Even in rare cases of chronic diseases, especially since duration of action of the first dose has exhausted, it is better not to prescribe the same remedy a second time.

§ 211

Therefore, when an absolutely appropriate and single specific remedy cannot immediately be found, usually next best medicine is chosen on the ground of one or two characteristic original symptoms of the disease (always to this state or the former disease condition) which are used alternately with the main medicine, although insufficient in themselves to achieve a cure, yet forward it more surely than does the repetition once or twice of the original medicine, which, being chosen in accordance with the original character

tel zu finden ist, wird es gewöhnlich noch
eine oder ein Paar für die charakteristischen Ursymptomen der Krankheit nächst
beste Arzneien geben, deren (nach dem jedesmahligen Zustande der Krankheitszufälle entweder diese, oder jene) als Zwi-
schenarznei jezt am besten passen wird,
und deren mit der Hauptarznei abwech-
selnder Zwischengebrauch die Herstellung
obgleich nicht eigends bewirket, doch
weit sichtbarer fordert, als die für den
Urcharakter des Uebels anfänglich zwar
nicht vollkommen, doch unter den vorhandnen noch am angemessensten befun-
dene Hauptarznei zweimahl oder mehr-
mahl hinter einander, allein gebraucht.

212.

Fände sich aber, das leztere in un-
unterbrochner Folgereihe einzig und allein
fortzugeben, das beste Verfahren wäre (in
diesem Falle würde ihre Gegenkrankheitspotenz dem chronischen Uebel sehr ähnlich entsprechen), so wird man sich gleichwohl überzeugen, daß auch dann nur je-

of the sufferings, was most reasonably held to be the most suitable, and yet proved not so completely adapted to the case as to cure it alone.

§ 212

However, if it should be found that the best process is the uninterrupted administration of the first-selected medicine (as may be the case when the counter disease-force is very similar to the chronic sufferings), then, while each successive dose is left to act for the whole period of its duration of action, only a small and smaller dose should be given each time, so as not to disturb the improvement, but rather to guide the case along the shortest way to the desirable line of cure.

desmahl eine kleinere und kleinere Gabe
— nach jedesmahligem Verflufs der Wirkungsdauer — gereicht werden durfe, um
die Besserung nicht zu storen und die Heilung auf dem geradesten Wege zum er-
wünschten Ziele zu führen.

213.

Sobald aber die chronische Krankheit
gewichen ist durch ein einziges, völlig passendes (für den Fall specifisches), oder
durch ein dem specifischen nahe kommen-
des Heilmittel (unter eben bemerktem Zwischengebrauch einer zunächst besten Arznei); so mufs, wenn das Uebel von altem
Datum, etwa 10, 15 oder 20 Iahr alt war,
noch wohl ein viertel oder halbes Iahr hindurch, in Zwischenzeiten von einigen und
zulezt von mehrern Wochen eine Gabe von
dem Hauptmittel gereicht werden — aber
immer eine kleinere und kleinere — bis
alle Neigung des Organismus zu dem chronischen Siechthum vollends verschwunden
und ausgelöschet ist.

§ 213

As soon as the chronic disease, an old suffering of ten, fifteen or twenty years, has yielded to a single completely suitable remedy (specific to the case), or to a remedy as nearly specific to the case as possible (aided perhaps by the temporary intermediate use of the next most suitable medicine), then, after 3 or 6 months, a dose of the man remedy must again be given at intervals first of one week and later of several weeks, each successive dose being smaller than its immediate predecessor, until all tendency of the organism to relapse into its chronic disease has completely disappeared.

Footnote: The negligence of this care can bring even the best treatment a bad reputation.

Anm. Die Vernachlassigung dieser Fürsorge kann auch die beste Kur in ubeln Ruf bringen.

214.

Der aufmerksame Beobachter merkt den zur Wiederholung der Gabe bestimmten Zeitpunkt an dem leisen Erscheinen einiger Spuren des einen oder andern Ursymptoms der ehemahligen Krankheit.

215.

Merkt man aber, dafs diefs nicht hinreichend ware, und dafs der Kranke eine gleich grofse, auch wohl erhohete und oftere Gabe des ihm immer wohl bekommenden homoopathischen Heilmittels fortbrauchen mufste, um keinen Ruckfall zu leiden, so ist diefs ein gewisses Zeichen, dafs die die Krankheit erzeugende Ursache noch fortwahrt, und dafs sich in der Lebensordnung des Kranken oder in seinen Umgebungen ein Umstand befindet, welcher abgeschafft werden mufs, wenn die Heilung dauerhaft zu Stande kommen soll.

§ 214

The attentive observer notices the exact moment for the repetition of the dose and the particular time of mild appearance of the track of one or another of the chief symptoms of former disease.

§ 215

If it is noticed that this procedure is not sufficiently effective, and that the patient is only kept from a relapse of the sufferings by the use of increased and frequent doses of the best selected homoeopathic remedy, then, although these doses are still followed by good results, it is a sure sign that the cause that keeps up the disease still persists, and that there is some circumstance in the mode of life or his surroundings which must be removed before a state of permanent cure can come.

216

Unter den Zeichen, die in allen, besonders akuten Krankheiten eine kleine, nicht jedermann sichtbare Besserung oder Verschlimmerung lehren, ist der Zustand des Gemüths und des ganzen Benehmens des Kranken das sicherste und einleuchtendste. Im Falle der auch noch so kleinen Besserung: eine gröfsere Behaglichkeit, eine zunehmende Selbstgelassenheit und Freiheit des Geistes; eine Art wiederkehrender Natürlichkeit. Im Falle der, auch noch so kleinen Verschlimmerung hingegen, das Gegentheil hievon: ein befangener, genirter, mehr Mitleid auf sich ziehender Zustand des Gemüthes, des Geistes, des ganzen Benehmens und aller Stellungen und Verrichtungen, was bei genauer Aufmerksamkeit sich leicht sehen oder zeigen, nicht aber in einzelnen Worten beschreiben lafst.

217.

Die übrigen theils neuen, theils erhoheten oder verminderten Zufälle werden

§ 216

Among the signs that, in all, particularly in acute disease, show of a slight improvement or aggravation that is not perceptible to every one, the state of mind and the whole behaviour of the patient are the surest and most illuminating. In the case of even so slight an improvement a greater ease, an increased calmness and freedom of the mind, a kind of return of the natural state is observed. In the case of ever so small aggravation, however, the exact opposite of this - an increased self-conscious, helpless, pitiable state of the mind and intellect, of the whole behaviour, and of all gestures, postures and actions - may be more easily noted by particularly careful observation, than it can be specifically described in words.

§ 217

Moreover, the other new or increased symptoms, or, on the contrary, the ameliorated state will soon leave no doubts to

dem scharf beobachtenden und forschenden Heilkunstler an der Verschlimmerung
oder Besserung bald keinen Zweifel mehr
ubrig lassen; indessen giebt es doch Personen, welche theils die Besserung, theils
die Verschlimmerung entweder anzugeben
unfahig, oder sie zu gestehen, nicht geartet sind.

218.

Dem ungeachtet wird man hieruber
leicht zur Ueberzeugung gelangen, sobald
man weifs, dafs, wenn beim Gebrauche
der lezten Arznei sich keine neuen Beschwerden hervorthaten, und der Kranke
keine neuen, in seiner Krankheit vorher
ungewohnlichen Zufalle klagen kann, die
Arznei auch durchaus reelle Besserung hervorgebracht haben mufs, oder wenn die
Zeit zu kurz dazu war, bald hervorbringen mufs. Auf der andern Seite, wenn
der Kranke diese oder jene neu entstandnen Zufalle und Symptomen von Erheb-
lichheit erzahlt (als Merkmahle der nicht
homoopathisch passend gewahlten Arznei),

the carefully observing and investigating physician with regard to the aggravation or amelioration; but, there are persons who are either incompetent to give an account of this amelioration or aggravation, or are unwilling to confess it.

§ 218

Despite, easy belief of people that if no new complaints of disease appear immediately after the use of the medicine, and if the patient complain of no new or unusual occurrences, then the medicine must either have brought about an absolutely real improvement, or be about to cause such a change when more time is allowed to develop it. On the other hand, if the patient relates this or that new occurrence or important symptom (the indication that it is not the proper homoeopathically suitable medicine), then, although he may assure us in a good-natured way that he feels better, however, we must not put any confidence in this assurance, but must study this exacerbated state, and likewise this will soon be evident as well.

so mag er noch so gutmuthig versichern: er befinde sich in der Besserung; so hat man ihm in dieser Versicherung dennoch nicht zu glauben, sondern seinen Zustand als verschlimmert anzusehen, wie es denn ebenfalls der Augenschein bald lehren wird.

219.

Da einige Symptomen der Arzneien am gesunden menschlichen Körper (wie man bei Beobachtung ihrer positiven Wirkungen abnehmen kann) um mehrere Stunden, ja wohl mehrere Tage später, als andre erscheinen, so können die in Krankheiten ihnen entsprechenden Symptomen, wenn auch die übrigen schon vernichtet waren, doch nicht eher, als um diese Zeit der Kur auslöschen; welches daher nicht befremden darf.

Anm. Z. B. das Quecksilber, was seine Neigung, runde Geschwüre mit hohem, entzündetem, schmerzhaftem Rande zu erregen, erst nach mehrern Tagen, bei gewissen Körpern aber erst nach einigen Wochen zum Vorscheine bringt, kann

M

§ 219

Then, some symptoms of medicines, when tested on healthy human body (for taking down the observation of its positive effect), appear several hours or even several days later than other symptoms, so they cannot annihilates the corresponding symptoms in disease except after a corresponding lapse of time, a fact which need not surprise us.

Foot Note: For example, the tendency of mercury to cause deep, round ulcers with inflamed and painful edges does not appear on healthy bodies not until several days, even weeks; in the same way, its internal use in venereal disease does not immediately remove the chancre and may need the treatment until several days to cure it.

auch beim innern Gebrauche in der venerischen Krankheit, die Schanker nicht
gleich in den ersten Tagen der Kur heilen.

220.

Hat man die Wahl, so sind zur Heilung chronischer Krankheiten, Arzneien
von langer Wirkungsdauer, hingegen zur
Heilung schneller, akuter Fälle, das ist,
in solchen Krankheiten, die schon vor sich
zu öfterer Veränderung ihres Zustandes
geartet sind, Arzneien von kurzer Wirkungsdauer vorzuziehen.

221.

Der rationelle Arzt wird es zu vermeiden wissen, sich Arzneien vorzugsweise zu Lieblingsmitteln zu machen, deren Gebrauch er, zufälligerweise, vielleicht
öfter mit Passendheit und gutem Erfolge
anzuwenden Gelegenheit gehabt hatte. Dabei werden seltner angewendete, welche
angemessener waren, oft hintangesezt.

§ 220

If we have the choice, we should prefer medicines of long duration of action for healing of chronic diseases; however, healing of the more rapid acute cases, that is, for diseases which tend to often change its condition, can preferably be done by medicines of shorter duration of action.

§ 221

The rational physician will take care to avoid making favourite-remedies of medicines by giving them preference, whose use, by chance, perhaps found often suitable, and which he has had opportunities of using with good success. If he does so, he will often neglect some medicines of rarer use, which otherwise would have been more capable.

So wird der rationelle Arzt auch die, wegen unpassender Wahl hie und da mit Nachtheil angewendeten Arzneien nicht aus mistrauischer Schwache beim Heilgeschäfte hintansetzen, und ohne achte Grunde (irrationell) vermeiden, eingedenk der Wahrheit, dafs immer blos diejenige unter den Gegenkrankheitspotenzen Achtung und Vorzug verdient, welche, in dem jedesmahligen Falle, dem Symptomenkomplexe am treffendsten entspricht, und dafs keine kleinlichen Leidenschaften sich in diese ernste Wahl mischen durfen.

223.

Bei der so nothigen als zweckmasigen Kleinheit der Gaben im homoopathischen Verfahren läfst sich leicht denken, dafs bei der Kur alles übrige aus der Diat entfernt werden musse, was nur irgend arzneilich wirken konnte, damit die feine Gabe nicht durch fremden Reiz uberstimmt oder verloschet werde.

M 2

§ 222

Moreover, the rational physician will not in his practice with mistrustful weakness of judgement disregard any medicine that he may have applied with disadvantage because of unsuitable selection (from his own fault, therefore), or may have avoided them without any good cause (irrationally), he should be being mindful of the truth that amongst the counter diseases force (SS: remedy) that alone always deserves privilege and preference which corresponds most aptly to the symptom-complex of any given case, and that no trifling passion should influence his sincere choice of the best medicine for his purpose.

§ 223

Considering the necessary and effective smallness of the doses required in homoeopathic action it is easy to understand that during treatment any substance having medicinal influence must be removed from the diet, so that the minute dose shall not be overpowered or extinguished by any foreign irritant.

Fur chronische Kranke ist diese sorg-
faltige Aufsuchung solcher Hindernisse der
Heilung, um so nothiger, da ihre Krankheit gewohnlich durch dergleichen Schäd-
lichkeiten und andre krankhaft wirkende,
oft unerkannte Fehler in der Lebensordnung theils entstanden war, theils verlän-
gert zu werden pflegt.

> Anm. Koffee, chinesischer und andrer Thee,
> Biere, mit arzneilichen für den Zustand
> des Kranken unangemessenen Kräutern an-
> gemacht, sogenannte feine, mit arzneilich
> wirkenden Gewürzen bereitete Liqueure,
> gewurzte Schokolade, Riechwasser und
> Parfümerien mancher Art, hochgewürzte
> Speisen und Saucen, gewürztes Backwerk,
> Gemuse, aus Krautern und Wurzeln, wel-
> che Arzneikraft besitzen, alter Kase und
> Thierspeisen, welche verdorben sind, oder
> arzneiliche Nebenwirkungen haben, sind
> eben so sehr von ihnen zu entfernen, als
> jede Uebermaße der Genüsse, Misbrauch
> geistiger Getranke uberhaupt, Stubenhitze,
> sitzende Lebensart in eingesperrter Luft,
> Kindersaugen, langer Mittagsschlaf (in
> Betten), Nachtleben, Unreinlichkeit, un-

§ 224

Therefore, in chronic patient this careful investigation into such obstacles to cure is much more necessary, because their diseases usually originate in the noxiousness of a similar kind and often in the morbid influence of unrecognised but harmful errors of regimen which partly nurture and prolongs it.

Footnote: Coffee, Chinese & other tea, beer prepared with medicinal herbs unsuitable for the patient's state, so called fine liquors prepared with medicinal spices, spiced chocolates, aromatic waters, and many types of perfumes, Highly spicy vegetables and sauces, spiced pastry, herbs & roots which possess medicinal strength, old cheese and non-vegetarian dishes which are putrid or have medicinal side-effects, are to be kept away from the patient, as they should avoid every excess consumption of food, misuse of spirituous drinks, heated rooms, sedentary life in an enclosed room, prolonged breast feeding, long afternoon siesta (in beds), night life, uncleanliness, unnatural lust, weakness of reading obscene writings, subjects of anger, grief, annoyance, passion for game, dwelling in swampy vicinity, damp buildings, excessive

naturliche Wohllust, Entnervung durch
Lesen schlupfriger Schriften, Gegenstände
des Zornes, des Grames und Aergernis-
ses, leidenschaftliches Spiel, sumpfige
Wohngegend, dumpfige Gebäude, uber-
masige Anstrengung des Geistes und Korpers, karges Darben, u. s. w. Alle diese
Dinge mussen moglichst vermieden oder
entfernt werden, wenn die Heilung nicht
gehindert oder unmoglich gemacht werden
soll.

225.

Die beim Arzneigebrauche in chronischen Krankheiten zweckmasigste Lebensordnung beruht auf Entfernung solcher
Genesungs-Hindernisse und dem Zusatze
des hie und da nothigen Gegentheiles:
Aufheiterung des Geistes, Bewegung in
freier Luft, angemessene unarzneiliche
Speisen und Getränke u. s. w.

226.

In akuten Krankheiten hingegen (den
Zustand des vollen Deliriums ausgenommen) entscheidet der feine untrugliche

straining of mind and body, meagre living, etc. All these things must be avoided or removed as far as possible for they might hinder or make the process of healing impossible.

§ 225

The most useful regimen along with the application of medicine in chronic diseases is based in the removal of such obstacles to recovery and supplementing such opposite conditions where necessary: cheering-up of mind, exercise in the fresh air, appropriate food and drink of unmedicinal nature, etc.

§ 226

In acute diseases, however (except in conditions of complicate delirium), the awakened finer and accurate life-preserving instinct determine so clearly and certainly that the physician need only to tell the family members and attendants to offer no obstacle in the way of this voice of nature either by refusing the patient anything that he strongly desires or offering him or persuading him to take anything harmful.

Takt des hier erwachten Lebenserhaltungs-Triebes so deutlich und bestimmt, dafs der Arzt blos die Angehörigen und die Krankenwärter zu bedeuten hat, dieser Stimme der Natur kein Hindernifs in den Weg zu.legen durch,Versagung des Gefoderten oder durch schädliche Anerbietungen, oder Ueberredungen.

227.

Zwar geht das Verlangen des akut Kranken an Genüssen und Getränken auf blos palliative Erleichterungsdinge; sie sind gewöhnlich aber nicht eigentlich arzneilicher Art, und blos einer Art Bedürfnifs angemessen. Die geringen Hindernisse, welche diese in masigen Schranken gehaltene Befriedigung etwa der gründlichen Entfernung der Krankheit in den Weg legen könnte, wird durch die homöopathisch passende Arznei und die durch sie entfesselte Lebenskraft reichlich wieder gut gemacht, und überwogen.

228.

Der rationelle Heilkünstler mufs die vollkräftigsten, ächtesten Arzneien in den

§ 227

Indeed, the desires of the patient suffering from an acute disease are for such delicacies and drink that give palliative relief; however, they are usually not of a real medicinal nature, and they merely supply a kind of suitable need. The slight obstacle that the satisfaction of these desire, within moderate limits, could oppose to the radical removal of the disease, but, will be generously counteracted and overcome by the suitable homoeopathic medicine and by the life-force (**SS note:** Vital Force) thereby liberated.

§ 228

The rational physician must have in his hand the strongest and most genuine medicines before he can rely on them as counter disease-forces (remedies). He must know himself of their genuineness.

Handen haben, wenn er sich auf sie als
Gegenkrankheitspotenzen (Heilmittel) will
verlassen konnen. Er mufs ihre Aechtheit
selbst kennen.

229.

Es ist Gewissenssache, in jedem Falle
untruglich uberzeugt zu seyn, dafs der
Kranke die wahre rechte Arznei eingenommen hat.

230.

Der Krafte der einheimischen oder
frisch zu erhaltenden Pflanzen bemachtigt
man sich am vollstandigsten und gewis-
sesten, wenn ihr ganz frisch ausgeprefster
Saft sogleich mit gleichen Theilen Weingeist gemischt wird; so erhalt sich ihre
ganze Kraft vollstandig und unverdorben
auf immer, in wohlverstopften Glasern
vor dem Sonnenlichte bewahrt.

Anm. Obwohl gleiche Theile Weingeist und
frisch ausgeprefster Saft gewohnlich das
angemessenste Verhältnifs ist, um die Ab-
setzung des Eiweifsstoffes zu erleichtern,

§ 229

It should be a matter of conscience with him to infallibly convince himself, in every case, that the patient receives the suitable and genuine medicine.

§ 230

The most complete and the most certain method to obtain the powers of those plants which are local (indigenous) or those which can be obtained in a fresh condition is to express their juice and mix it *immediately* with an equal part of spirit of wine; such preparations retain their total and unimpaired strength always if they are kept in a place devoid of sunlight and in well-stoppered glass bottles.

Foot Note: Although equal parts of spirit of wine and freshly expressed juice usually form the best proportion for effecting the precipitation of albuminous matter (and preventing all possible fermentation and deterioration

(und alle mögliche Gährung ~~und Zerstörung~~
bung auf immer unmöglich ~~zu machen~~)
so hat man doch für Pflanzen ~~welche~~
viel zähen Schleim oder ein Uebermaß ~~an~~
Eiweisstoff enthalten (z. B. Beinwellwurzel, Freisamveilchen, Hundsdillgleiß,
Schwarznachtschatten, u. s. w.) gewöhnlich ein doppeltes Verhältniß an Weingeist zu dieser Absicht nöthig. — Von
dem, nach Tag und Nacht in verstopften
Gläsern abgesetzten Eiweißstoffe wird das
Helle abgegossen zum Verwahren für den
arzneilichen Gebrauch.

231.

Die übrigen, nicht frisch zu erlangenden und ausländischen Gewächse, wird der
rationelle Arzt nie in Pulverform auf Treu
und Glauben annehmen, sondern sich von
ihrer Aechtheit in ihrem rohen, ganzen
Zustande vorher überzeugen, ehe er die
mindeste arzneiliche Anwendung von ihnen macht.

Anm. Um sie als Pulver zu verwahren, bedarf man Vorsicht. Die auch völlig trocknen, ganzen, rohen Gewächssubstanzen
enthalten doch noch immer innerhalb ih-

466

which had been impossible), yet for plants which contain much thick mucus or an excessive albumen (e. *g.* Symphytum officinale, Viola tricolor, Aethusa cynapium, Solanum nigrum, etc.) a double proportion of spirit of wine is usually needed; when this has stood in a close-stoppered glass bottle for a day and a night the precipitated albuminous material can be filtered off and the clear preparation kept for medicinal use.

§ 231

Moreover, the exotic plants or those which cannot be obtained fresh, the rational physician should never believe them on trust and not accept them in pulverised form but before making even their least medicinal application should first himself be convinced of their genuineness in their crude, intact state.

Foot Note: In order to preserve them in the form of powder, certain precautions are necessary. The powders of whole and raw vegetable

rer Substanz Feuchtigkeit, welche zwar
die ganze, ungepulverte Drogue nicht hindert, in einem so trocknen Zustande zu
existiren, als zu ihrer Unverderblichkeit
hinreicht, für eben dieselbe aber, im Zustande des feinen Pulvers viel zu viel ist.
Wird dieses nun nicht von der durch
diese Zerkleinerung überschussig gewordnen
Feuchtigkeit befreiet, so muß es durch
sie in Schimmel und Verderbniß gerathen. Deshalb kann selbst die älteste, im
ganzen Zustande auch noch so trockne ve-
getabilische und animalische Drogue nicht
so gerade zu, ohne inneres Verderbniß
zu leiden, in Gestalt eines Pulvers in verstopften Gefäßen aufgehoben werden,
wenn sie von ihrer, durchs Zerkleinen
überschussig gewordnen Feuchtigkeit nicht
vorher befreiet worden ist. Dieß geschiehet am besten, wenn die Pulver im
Wasserbade so weit getrocknet werden,
daß alle kleinen Theile desselben (nicht
mehr klumperig zusammenhängen, sondern)
wie trockner feiner Sand sich leicht von
einander entfernen und leicht verstieben.
In diesem Zustande lassen sie sich, auf
immer unverderblich, in versiegelten Gläsern aufbewahren in ihrer ursprünglichen
vollen Arzneikraft, und ohne je mietig
oder schimmlicht zu werden. In nicht

substances, though perfectly dry, yet contain, a certain quantity of moisture, not sufficient indeed prevent the unpulverized drug from remaining in as dry a state as is requisite to preserve it from decomposition, but which is quite too much for the finely pulverized state. When powdered they will decompose and become mouldy unless this moisture is driven off. Therefore, the animal or vegetable substance which in its entire state was perfectly dry, furnishes therefore, when finely pulverized, a somewhat moist powder, can yet not be preserved in corked bottles if not previously freed from this extra moisture. This is best done by drying the powder over a water-bath till all the small pieces of it are as easily separated from each other (no longer stick together in lumps, but) as fine sand and are readily converted into dust. In this condition it can be kept forever incorrubtibly in sealed bottles preserving all their original complete medicinal power. All vegetable and animal medicinal substances not preserved in air-tight vessels gradually lose more and more of their medicinal power.

luftdicht verschlossenen Behältnissen verlieren alle vegetabilischen und thierischen Arzneisubstanzen an ihren Kräften immer mehr und mehr.

232.

Da jede Arznei am bestimmtesten und vergleichbarsten in Auflosung wirkt, so wendet der rationelle Heilkunstler in Auflosung alle Arzneien an, deren Natur nicht ausdrucklich verlangt, in Pulverform angewendet zu werden. Alle andre Formen, aufser diesen, machen die Vergleichung der Beobachtungen und die Gabe jeder kräftigen Arznei unsicher.

Anm. Die Auflosung der blos trocken zu erlangenden, gepulverten Thier-und Gewachs-Substanzen in geistigen Flussigkeiten, namentlich in Weingeiste von bestimmter, gleicher Stärke ist die einzige, nicht durch Gährung verderbliche; sie erhält die Arzneikrafte derselben am vollständigsten. Blos die mehligen Samen aus der Gras-und Schmetterlingsblumen-Familie lassen ihre Arzneikräfte durch Weingeist am wenigsten ausziehn, und sind als Pulver anzuwenden. Einige wenige Sub-

§ 232

As every medicine work most certainly and in most comparable manner in solution, so the rational physician will administer all medicines in solution, except those whose nature demand that they be given in the pulverised form. All other forms except these make the comparison of observations difficult and the estimation of the dose of every powerful medicine unreliable.

Footnote: The dissolution of powdered animal & plant substances obtainable in dry form in spirituous fluids, especially in pure spirit of wine of definite, equal strength is the only one that is not spoilt through fermentation and contains its most complete medicinal strength. The powdered seeds of grass & papilionaceous-flower family allow its medicinal strength to be extracted by least amount of spirit of wine. A few substances for dissolution require sweetened salt-peter spirit or naphtha.

stanzen verlangen zur Auflösung durchaus versüssten Salpetergeist oder Naphthe.

233.

Die Metall - die Salz - und andern Bereitungen dieser Art, deren Aechtheit nicht
gleich beim ersten Anblicke, einleuchtet
und unverkennlich ist, lafst der rationelle,
gewissenhafte Heilkünstler. blos unter seinen eignen Augen entstehen.

234.

In keinem Falle von Heilung ist es
nöthig, mehr als eine einzige, einfache Arzneisubstanz auf einmahl anzuwenden.

235.

Es ist nicht einzusehen, wie es nur -
dem mindesten Zweifel unterworfen seyn
könne, ob es rationeller und vernünftiger
sei, einen einzelnen gekannten Arzneistoff in einer Krankheit zu verordnen,
statt eines Gemisches von mehrern.

§ 233

Metals, salts, and other preparations of this kind, whose authenticity is not evident and cannot be recognized immediately at first sight, should only be used by the rational and conscientious physician unless they have been prepared before his eyes.

§ 234

In none of the case is it necessary for cure to apply more than *one, single, simple, medicinal substance* at one time.

§ 235

It is not conceivable how the least doubt could exist that it is more rational and sensible to prescribe a mixture of several instead of a single well-known medicinal substance at one time in a disease.

236

Da der rationelle Heilkunstler in ganz
einfachen, einzeln angewendeten Arznei-
stoffen schon findet, was er nur irgend
wunschen kann: kunstliche Krankheitspotenzen, welche die naturlichen Krankheiten durch homoopathische Kraft zu uberstimmen, auszuloschen und dauerhaft zu
heilen vermogen, so wird es ihm nach dem
allgemeinen Weisheitsspruche: quod fieri
potest per pauca, non debet fieri per plura
nie einfallen, je etwas andres, als einen
einzelnen, einfachen Arzneistoff als Heilmittel zu geben, auch schon deshalb, weil
es völlig unbekannt ist, wie sich zwei und
mehrere zusammengesezte Arzneistoffe einander in ihren Wirkungen auf den menschlichen Korper hindern und abandern mögen, und weil hingegen ein einfacher Arzneistoff bei seinem Gebrauche in Krankheiten, deren Symptomenkomplex genau
bekannt ist, selbst in dem schlimmsten
Falle, dafs er nicht homoopathisch angemessen gewahlt werden konnte und also
nicht hulfe, doch dadurch nuzt und die
Heilmittel - Kenntnifs befordert, dafs die

§ 236

Thereupon, the rational physician finds all that he can desire in quite simple and uncombined medicines administered singly, artificial disease-forces, which by their homoeopathic powers can overcome, extinguish and permanently cure natural diseases. Thus, he will always act according to the universal wise maxim: '*quod fieri potest per pauca, non debet fieri per plura*[12]; and he will never use as remedies anything but single, simple medicinal matters. It is wholly unknown, therefore, how two or more medicinal matter mixed together may hinder and alter one another in their effect on the human body; and because, on the other hand, a simple medicinal substance when used in diseases whose symptom-complex is accurately known, will cure, if it is exactly and homoeopathically selected; and in the worst case, if it is not rightly chosen and cannot therefore

---

[12] **Translator's note:** Hahnemann here uses an age-old Latin maxim which means: *Any attempt to employ complex means is wrong when simple means are sufficient.*

in solchem Falle von ihm erregten neuen
Beschwerden diejenigen Symptomen bestätigen helfen, welche dieser Arzneistoff
sonst schon in Versuchen am gesunden
menschlichen Korper gezeigt hatte.

> An m. Bei der treffend homöopathisch für
> den wohl überdachten Krankheitsfall ge-
> wählten und innerlich gegebnen Arznei
> nun noch einen aus andern Arzneistoffen
> gewählten Thee trinken, ein Kräutersäck-
> chen oder eine Bähung aus mancherlei
> Kräutern auflegen, oder ein andersartiges
> Klystir einspritzen zu lassen, wird der ra-
> tionelle Arzt der irrationellen Empirie
> überlassen.

237.

Giebt man eine allzu starke Gabe
einer für den gegenwärtigen Krankheitsfall
auch völlig homöopathisch, völlig angemessen und specifisch gewählten Arznei, so
wird sie zwar allerdings für die ursprüngliche Krankheit wohlthätig seyn, doch abgerechnet den hier unnöthigen, überstar-
ken Eindruck, den sie auf den Organismus
macht durch allzu grofse Menge und Heftigkeit.

be useful, its application can yet add to our knowledge of remedial agents, because, by the new sufferings excited by it in such a case, those symptoms which this medicinal substance had already shown in experiments on the healthy human body are established.

Foot note: The rational physician gives up to irrational empiric when the patient along with the appropriate homoeopathic medicine for a case of well shrouded disease, which had been chosen and internally administered, still drinks tea of otherwise medicinal substances, takes a herbal pack or applies fomentation of various herbs or is injected with different clysters.

§ 237

If *too strong a dose* of a medicine is given, even if it is fully homoeopathic to the case of disease, is totally suitable and is specifically chosen, then it will without doubt favourably act on the original disease, even if given in too large a quantity; but there will be an unnecessary and too strong impression made on the organism because of its large quantity and intensity.

258

Denn, wird diese von der allzu vielen Arznei herruhrende starkere, obgleich der ursprunglichen Krankheit sehr ahnliche Umstimmung des Organisms allzustark durch die starker als nothig gewählte Gabe — so erfolgt aufser der erhoheten homoopathischen Verschlimmerung (§. 132) wenigstens eine unnothige Entkräftung nach Verflufs der Wirkungsdauer des Medikaments, und wenn die Gabe ganz ubermasig war, so erfolgen aufser den erhoheten primaren Arzneisymptomen (§. 132) noch Symptomen ihrer Nachwirkung, eine Art Arznei Nachkrankheit, der erstern an Art entgegen gesezt.

259.

Da nun noch uberdem fast keine Arznei so vollkommen homoopathisch gewahlt werden kann, dafs sie dem Symptomeninbegriffe der Krankheit in allen und jeden Punkten mathematisch genau (§. 131 Anm) und vollkommen entsprache, so steigen die, bei angemessen kleinen Gaben unbe

§ 238

Because if the alterations in the organism produced by the excessive quantity of the medicine, as it was very similar to the original disease, be too stronger than was necessary, then besides the increase in the homoeopathic aggravation (§ 132) there follows an unnecessary weakening of the patient after the active period of the medicament has expired, and, if the dose was very excessive, then after the increased primary symptoms of medicine (§ 132) there ensue symptoms of its after-disease (**SS note: Secondary action**), a kind of medicinal after-disease of an opposite character to the first.

§ 239

Now, then, hardly any medicine can be selected that is so completely homoeopathic to the totality of the symptoms of sickness as to correspond to it with mathematical exactitude and completely in each and every point (§ - 131, note), so the new symptoms, which were inconsiderable when a suitable small dose was given, are increased into severe sufferings of various kinds when the quantity of medicine is excessively large.

deutenden neuen Symptomen zu hohen
Beschwerden mancherlei Art, wenn die
Menge Arznei so ubermasig grofs ist.

240.

Nach diesen und vielen andern Be-
weggrunden wird der rationelle Heilkunstler (welcher stets nur das Beste zur Richt-
schnur seines Verfahrens befolgt, weil
es das Beste ist, und sich davon nicht
durch blinde Observanz abhalten läfst) die
dem Uebel blos so eben nur angemessene
Gabe des angemessenen Heilmittels wahlen, die kaum einen Anschein von Krank-
heitsverschlimmerung ($. 132.) zu erregen,
das ist, kaum im mindesten seine Gegenkrankheitspotenz uber die zu heilende
Krankheit zu erheben vermag.

241.

Man darf diese anscheinende Verschlimmerung und Erhohung der gegenwartigen Krankheit durch das homoopathische Mittel kaum merken, und diefs

480

§ 240

Because of these and for many other reasons the rational physician (who always follows the best principle in practice *because it is the best*, and refuses to depart from it at the dictates of blind observance) will choose only the most suitable dose of the indicated remedy, so that hardly a semblance of disease-aggravation will be activated (§ 132); that is, will choose a dose which as a counter disease-force only just exceeds the disease-force which is to be cured.

§ 241

This apparent aggravation and increase of the existing disease as a consequence of the use of the homoeopathic remedy should be hardly perceptible, and then only in the first hour or two after its administration.

auch nur in den ersten Paar Stunden nach
der Einnahme. —

242.

Eins der Hauptgesetze der homoopathischen Heilkunde besteht namlich darinn:
die zur Aufhebung einer naturlichen Krankheit moglichst angemessen gewahlte Gegenkrankheitspotenz (das Heilmittel) nur so stark
einzurichten dafs sie nur so eben
zur Absicht hinreiche, und durch
unnothige Starke den Korper nicht
im mindesten angreife.

243.

Da nun die kleinste Menge Arznei den
Organismus, naturlich, am wenigsten an
greift, so wurde man die allerkleinsten
Gaben zu wahlen haben, wenn sie nur stets
der Krankheit gewachsen waren.

244.

Hier zeigt nun die Erfahrung durch-
gangig, dafs auf homoopathischem Wege

§ 242

One of the chief laws of homoeopathic therapeutics consists of, namely, the following: *the counter disease-force (the remedy), suitably chosen as exactly as possible for the removal of a natural disease should be sufficient enough so that it will only be of minimum strength to just attain its purpose and will do the body no harm in any way through unnecessary force.*

§ 243

Now, because the organism is, naturally, least deranged by the minimum quantity of medicine, we should choose the very smallest doses, provided always that they are equal to that of the disease.

§ 244

Here, universal experience has proved that the smallest doses of medicine chosen for their homoeopathic ways to diseases are a match each for the similar disorder. Since,

die kleinsten Gaben der Krankheit jederzeit
gewachsen sind. Denn liegt der Krankheit
nicht offenbar eine betrachtliche Verderbnifs eines wichtigen Eingeweides zum Grunde, so kann fast keine Gabe des homoopathisch gewahlten Heilmittels so klein seyn, dafs sie nicht
starker als die naturliche Krankheit ware, und sie nicht besiegen
konnte.

245.

Wie sehr sich in Krankheiten die Empfindlichkeit des Korpers gegen Arzneien,
vorzuglich die homoopathisch angewendeten erhohe, hievon hat nicht der gewohnliche, nur der genaue Beobachter hat hievon einen Begriff. Sie ubersteigt allen
Glauben, wenn die Krankheit einen hohen
Grad erreicht hat.

> Anm. Ein gefuhllos da liegender, komatöser
> Typhuskranker mit brennend heifser Haut
> von Schweifse bedeckt, mit schnarchen-
> dem, stofsweise unterbrochnem Athem aus

N

the disease does not obviously arise from a serious morbid change in some important organ, *therefore nearly no dose of the homoeopathically selected remedy can be so small as not to be stronger than the natural disease and that it shall not be able to overcome it.*

§ 245

The sensitiveness of the body, in diseases, towards medicines especially those employed homoeopathically is very much increased, of which the ordinary observer has no idea, but is known only to the accurate observer. It is more than any one can believe in the disease which has highly advanced.

Footnote: A patient suffering from typhus, lying insensible and comatose, with burning hot skin covered with perspiration, accompanied with stertorous respiration through his open mouth in a jerky interrupted manner, etc. is restored to consciousness in no time and can be completely recovered in a

offen stehendem Munde, u. s, wenn sie von
der kleinsten Gabe Mohnsaft binnen weni
gen Stunden zur Besinnung gebracht und
binnen noch einigen Stunden zur Gesund
heit wieder hergestellt, wenn auch die
Gabe millionmahl kleiner war, als sie je
ein Arzt auf der Welt verordnete. Die
Empfindlichkeit des kranken oder kränk-
lichen Korpers steigt in vielen Fallen so
hoch, dafs aufsere Potenzen auf ihn zu
wirken und ihn zu erregen anfangen deren Existenz sogar oft geleugnet ward
weil sie auf den gesunden, festen Korper
und in manchen dazu nicht geeigneten
Krankheiten keine in die Augen fallende Wirkung zeigen, wie z. B. der
thierische Magnetism (Animalism)
jene bei gewissen Arten der Beruhrung oder
Fast - Beruhrung von einem lebenden Korper auf den andern influirende Kraft, welche in schwachlichen, zartlichen und empfindlichen Personen beider Geschlechter
eine erstaunenswürdige Erregung hervorbringt. Wie unbegreiflich klein werden
hienach die immer noch materiellen Gaben
homöopathischer Arznei bereitet werden
konnen, um doch noch in dem so empfindlichen kranken Körper erstaunenswurdige
Erregung hervorzubringen!

few hours by the smallest dose of opium, even if it be a million times smaller than what was administered by any physician in the world. The sensitivity of the patient or diseased body attains such a height in many cases that it is acted on and excited by external forces, the existence of which is often denied because no *visibly obvious* effect on healthy robust bodies was displayed and in many disease for which the dose is not suitable; as for example *Animal Magnetism* (Animalism), that peculiar power that one living body exercises over another by certain conscious ways of touching or almost touching, which produces astonishing excitement in weak, delicate and sensitive persons of both gender. It is incomprehensible how small still always material doses of the homoeopathic medicine could be prepared, in order to generate astonishing excitement in the body of the extremely sensitive patients!

246

So ist auch jeder Kranker besonders
im Punkte seiner Krankheit von den passenden arzneikraftigen Potenzen höchst
umstimmbar; und es giebt keinen, selbst
noch so robusten, auch nur mit einem
chronischen oder sogenannten Lokalübel
behafteten Menschen, welcher in dem lei-
denden Theile nicht bald die erwünschteste
Veränderung spürte, wenn er die hülfreiche
und homöopathisch passende Arznei in
der erdenklich kleinsten Gabe eingenommen, welcher mit einem Worte nicht weit
mehr dadurch umgestimmt werden sollte,
als der einen Tag alte, aber gesunde Saug-
ling.

Anm. Man setze dieser Wahrheit nicht die
oft ungeheuern Gaben von Arzneien in der
gemeinen Praxis entgegen. Diese stehen
namlich (um hier nur einige Grunde anzugeben, da ich weiter unten noch etliche
anzuführen, Veranlassung habe,) höchst
selten in Homöopathie mit der Krankheit
(in welcher die Arzneien unendlich wirk-
samer, als auf andre Art gebraucht, das
Befinden umändern) und werden immer

N 2

§ 246

Thus, each patient is highly susceptible to properly applied medicinal powers, and there is no person, however robust, even if suffering from only a chronic or so-called local affections, who will not soon feel the desired change in the affected part if he takes the helpful and homoeopathically suitable medicine even in the smallest imaginable dose— who will not, in a word, be much more affected by this means than would an one day-old healthy baby.

Footnote: Let not the often enormous doses of medicines given in common practice be argued against this truth. These medicines (I will further specify below in order to indicate a few reasons) have rarely any homoeopathic

entweder blos in Zusammensetzung mit
andern starken Arznoien, oder so gebraucht, dafs noch daneben und dazwischen andre Arz, jen von heftiger {Wir-
kung eingegeben werden, in welcher Mischung nicht mehr jedes nach seiner eigenthümlichen Art wirkt, sondern abge-
ändert durch die Wirkung des zweiten,
dritten, oder vierten Ingredienzes. Die
Kräfte der mehrern Arznoien in einer Mischung heben einander zum gröfsten Theilo
auf, so dafs sie oft ohne grofsen Erfolg
eingenommen werden. Ein einzelnes dieser heftigen Ingredienzen, wenn es acht
und vollkräftig ist, wurde in derselben
Gabe, allein gereicht, sehr oft den Tod
bringen; ein furchterlicher Umstand, welcher die Aerzte stillschweigend, und wie
durch Instinkt mit dazu bewogen zu haben scheint, die nach ihren positiven Wirkungen bisher ungekannten Arzneien durch
vielfältige Zusammenmischung in Eine For-
mel weniger gefährlich zu machen. (eine
Veranstaltung, die ihnen bei dem Aus-
drucke corrigentia undeutlich vorgeschwebt
zu haben scheint) In dieser Rucksicht
ist es fast ein Glück zu nennen, dafs viele
Arzneien in der gemeinen Praxis, besonders die Extrakte durch die bisherige Ver-

relation to the disease (in which the medicines were infinitely effective than when used in other forms and state of health remains unchanged) and, moreover, they are always given either in combination with other strong medicines, or other violently acting medicines are administered besides or in between the doses of the first, in which mixture, each medicine can no longer exercise its peculiar effect, but is altered by the action of the second, third, or fourth ingredient. The strength of the different medicines in a mixture virtually neutralise one another to a great extent, so that they can often be taken without producing any great effect. Just one of these very powerful ingredients, if it be genuine and in full possession of its powers, is given *alone* in the same dose would be often sufficient to cause death; a dreadful possibility, on which the physicians remain and as if by instinct they were led to render the unknown medicines of whose positive action they are ignorant and is less dangerous by mixing a number of them together in one prescription. (An event seems to be inarticulately indicated by the expression '*corrigentia*'). Considering this, it may be called almost a good luck that in ordinary practice many medicines, especially the extracts, become almost absolutely powerless by the mode of preparing them used till date.

fertigung fast völlig kraftlos zu werden
pflegten.

247.

Um nun acht rationell zu verfahren,
wird der wahre Heilkunstler seine wohl-
gewahlte homoopathische Arznei genau
nur in so kleiner Gabe verordnen, als zur
Ueberstimmung und Vernichtung der gegenwartigen Krankheit zureicht — in einer Kleinheit von Gabe, welche, wenn ihn
die menschliche Schwache je verleitet hatte,
eine unpassendere Arznei gewahlet zu haben, den Nachtheil ihrer Unpassendheit in
der Krankheit bis zur Geringfugigkeit vermindert, welcher von der moglichst kleinsten Gabe auch viel zu schwach ist, als dafs
er durch die eigne Energie der Natur und
durch schnelle Entgegensetzung des nun
angemessener gewählten, homoopathischen
Heilmittels, ebenfalls in kleinster Gabe,
nicht alsbald wieder ausgeloscht und gut
gemacht werden konnte.

Anm. Wenn ich von moglichster Kleinheit
der Gabe in der homoopathischen Heil-

§ 247

Now, the true physician will pursue the rational course and prescribe the well-selected homoeopathic medicine in exactly such small dose which is sufficient to overcome and annihilate the existing disease - possibility of any injury caused because the human weakness being misled to selection of unsuitable medicine is reduced because of the smallness of dose; the disadvantage of administering the inappropriate medicine is overcome as the smallness of the dose will render it far too weak to resist the natural energy of the body and the swift resistance of the more appropriately selected homoeopathic remedy, in similar smaller dose, will soon remove earlier harm and its beneficial effect will come into play.

Footnote: When I speak of the smallest possible dose in the homoeopathic method of treatment, I cannot put forward in tabular form the weights and

kunde, spreche, so kann ich hier, auch
schon deshalb, weil die Arzneien selbst
an Kraft so verschieden sind, keine Ta-
belle von Maas und Gewicht der Arzneien
hersetzen. Nur anmerken will ich, dafs
die Menschen nach dem Umfange der Kul-
tur ihres Geistes hochst verschiedne Maas-
stabe zur Schatzung der Grofsen und
Kleinheiten haben, dafs Manchem die Zahl
Meilen, von der unsre kleine Erde um-
spannt wird, schon etwas Ungeheures
deuchtet, und dafs man ihm von den Quadrillion und Quintillion Erdmessern, in
denen die zahllosen Sonnen in der unendlichen Schopfung von einander abstehen,
gar nichts vorreden darf. Eben so be-
schränkte Menschen findet man, welche
nichts achtenswerth schatzen, als was die
Faust fullt, und die Dinge nicht nach ihrer wahren inwohnenden Kraft, sondern
nach dem plumpen Handelsgewicht wa-
gen —, deren kleinstes Gewicht bei Arzneien sich nicht unter Einen Gran er-
streckt, wahrend ein Zehntelgran ihnen
schon eine unbedeutende Kleinigkeit zu
seyn deuchtet.

Wie sollte man diesen Menschen mit
so kurzen Maassstäben zumuthen, sich Begriffe zu machen von der nothigen Theilung und Verkleinerung der Arzneigaben

measures of the medicines, because the medicines differ so much in strength. I want only to remark that in accordance with the circumstances of culture of their minds people have very different scales of measurement for estimating the size and the smallness; that to many the number of miles in the circumference of our little earth seems to be something enormous, and that one can hardly say anything before them the quadrillion and quintillion earth-circumferences that separate the innumerable suns in the universe from one another. Persons of such limited intelligence are to be met with who can appreciate nothing that they cannot feel with their hands, and who estimate things not according to their real inherent strength, but by their coarse business weightage. The smallest weight of medicine they will hear of must be not less than 1 grain; a tenth of a grain is for them an unconsidered smallness.

How can one expect from these people, with their restricted standards of measurement, can have an idea of the essential division and diminution of the medicinal doses for homoeopathic purposes into smallest fractions

zu homöopathischer Absicht in die niedrigsten Bruchtheile eines Grans? Vergeblich! ihr beschränkter Geist schwindelt vor Zahlen und Theilungen, die in der Spanne ihres Wirkungskreises nie gehört, nie gedacht worden waren. Und doch ist es nur allzuwahr, dafs in der Unendlichkeit der Schöpfung alles, was wir schwachen Menschen uns als grofs, sehr grofs denken, noch lange nicht grofs — alles was wir uns als möglichst klein denken, noch lange nicht klein zu achten ist. Zerlege, wenn du kannst, die Bestandtheile der Organe des Infusionsthierchens; und du bist kaum zum Anfange der Dinge herabgestiegen, welche in der Schöpfung klein zu nennen sind. Und welche Kraft besitzt nicht jedes der zahllosen Organe, die den Körper des Infusionsthierchens verkurzen, verlängern und seine Bewegung in Flüssigkeiten so gewaltig beschleunigen, aufser was sie sonst noch zu seinem Leben, zu seiner Bestimmung, zu seinen Genüssen und zu seiner Fortpflanzung, uns unwissend, beitragen! Welche unermefslich grofse Energie in diesen nach unsern eingeschränkten Begriffen für so klein geachteten Theilen! Kurzsichtiger wie willst du den wundersamen, fast geistigen Kräften der Arzneien eine Gränze abstecken,

496

of grains? Alas! Their limited intellect turns dizzy at numbers and divisions that do not come within the sphere of their practice, are never even thought of by them. And yet it is all too real that in the infinity of creation all that we weak mortals think large, very large, is still far from being large, and all that we imagine to be the smallest possible is far from being so. Dissect, if you can, the component parts of the organs of the infusorial extent, and you have hardly go down to the commencement of the things which in creation are to be called small. And what *power* possessed by each of the countless organs which shorten and elongate the body of the infusorial animalcule, and enable it to move about quickly in fluids, besides the unknown ways in which it contributes to the operations of life, the purposes, the pleasures and the re-productive work of the minute organism! What immeasurably large amount of energy resides in these parts which our limited faculties deem so small! Myopic vision! how can you assign boundaries to the marvellous, almost spiritual strength of medicines! How with your coarse mechanical scales can you determine the exact weight at which they will cease to be effective!

ihnen ein Gewicht aus deinen alltäglichen Gewichten vorschreiben, unter welchem sie aufhören sollen, etwas Wirksames zu seyn!

Es liegt schon im Begriffe der Theilung, daß kein Theil so klein von uns gemacht werden kann, daß er aufhöre, Etwas zu seyn, und daß er nicht von den sämtlichen Eigenschaften des Ganzen participirte. Wie, wenn nun dieser möglichst kleinste Theil noch so kräftig wäre, als du ihn nur irgend zu deinem Behufe bedarfst; wolltest du ihn dann wider deinen Zweck grösser machen, blos um der Observanz und den Menschen mit den kurzen Maasstäben nicht zu nahe zu treten?

Und was bedarf es beträchtlicher Gewichtsgaben zu arzneilichen Potenzen, wenn sie bei der homöopathischen Anwendungsart schon in der möglichst kleinsten Menge die Krankheiten auf die schnellste und dauerhafteste Art zu besiegen im Stande sind? Wozu Bedenklichkeiten über die Kräftigkeit so kleiner, doch noch immer materieller, obgleich nach dem kleinsten Gewichte zu berechnender Gaben homöopathischer Heilmittel, da gerade die kräftigsten Gegenkrankheitspotenzen völlig unwiegbar sind, und mit ganz impon-

"The doctrine of the *divisibility* of matter teaches us that a part can not be made so small that it shall cease to be *something,* and that it shall not share *all* the characteristic of the whole. If, now, the smallest possible part is powerful enough for the purpose for which you require it, would you employ a greater quantity than you require, in order not to run counter to traditional custom, and out of deference to the prejudices of those whose standard of measurement is imperfect?

And what is the need of larger doses of medicinal powers if the smallest possible quantities given on the homoeopathic principle suffice for the cure of diseases in the most rapid and permanent manner? And why should there be doubts about the strength of such small but still material doses of homoeopathic remedies, though their calculated weight is extremely small, since some of the most powerful counter-disease forces are completely immeasurable, and yet have a great influence on the state of health of men? Who does not know

derabeln Stoßen Einwirkung auf das Befinden des Menschen machen? Wer kennt die arzneilichen Kräfte der Kälte und Wärme nicht? Wer will die der Elektrisität und des Galvanismus miskennen? Wer will die heroischen, oft allzu starken Kräfte des thierischen Einflusses (thierischen Magnetisms) in Umänderung des menschlichen Befindens leugnen? Und was geht über die mächtige Gegenkrankheitspotenz, die der Stahlmagnet nach der vereinigten Beobachtung einer großen Menge scharfsichtiger und redlicher Beobachter in einer Menge von Krankheiten klärlich bewiesen hat? — der Stahlmagnet, dessen unablässig ausströmender, ihponderabler Stoff in keinen unsrer Sinne fällt und dennoch das Befinden selbst des gesundesten Menschen in hohem Grade umändert, wie jeder an sich selbst sich überzeugen kann; wenn er mit dem Nordpole eines größern Magnetstabes, welcher zehn bis zwölfmahl sein eignes Gewicht zu ziehn vermag, nur Eine Stunde lang irgend einen Theil seines Körpers berühren läßt, oder nur bedenkt, was schon die Erfahrungen glaubwürdiger Beobachter an gesunden Personen hierüber gelehrt haben (m. s. *Andry* und *Thouret* Beob. und Unters. üb. d. Gebr. d. Magn. Leipz. 1785. S. 155.)

the medicinal powers of cold and heat? Who does not know the power of electricity and galvanism? Who will deny the heroic, often too great power of animal influence (Animal Magnetism) in altering state of man's health? And what can surpass the counter-disease force which the steel magnet, according to the testimony of many keen and sincere observers, has clearly manifested in a many cases of diseases? — the steel magnet, whose innecessant streaming out of imponderable substances from it is imperceptible to our senses, and inspite of that that it modifies the state of health of men to a great extent of even the most robust man, as any one can convince himself if he lets any part of his body come in contact for one hour with the north pole of a large magnet – capable of lifting ten or twelve times its own weight, as experience of trust-worthy observers on healthy persons have demonstrated (*Andry* and *Thouret, Beob. and Unters. üb. d. Gebr. d. Magn.,* Leipzig. 1785, p. 155)

248

Aus der Thatsache, dafs eine gewisse,
homoopathisch gewahlte Arznei den fur sie
geeigneten Krankheitszustand durch gewohnlich nicht vielmehr als Eine einzige
Gabe uberstimmt und erschopft, und jede
uberflussig starkere Gabe den Körper mehr
als nothig angreift, erklart sich jene wichtige, allgemein gultige Bemerkung; dafs
jede Gaben - Zertheilung (auf mehrere Ein-
nehmungs - Zeiten vertheilt) eine weit starkere Wirkung thut, als die ganze, auf einmahl gereichte Gabe.

Acht Tropfen irgend einer Arzneitink-
tur auf Eine Gabe thun wohl viermal gerin-
gere Wirkung, als eben diese acht Tropfen
auf achtmahl, alle Stunden, oder alle zwei
Stunden zu einem Tropfen gegeben.

Nimmt man nun noch Verdunnung
dazu (wodurch die Gabe eine grofsere Aus-

§ 248

The fact that not more than a single dose of a certain homoeopathically chosen medicine usually overpowers and annihilates the disease-state for which it is suitable, and that every dose which is needlessly stronger affects the body more than is necessary, explains the important observation, which is universally valid that dividing the dose (advantageously administering it at intervals) has a much more powerful effect than giving the total dose all at once.

§ 249

Eight drops of almost any medicinal tincture given in one dose have four times less effect than of the eight drops of the same tincture given eight times, every hour or every two hours, in doses of one drops.

§ 250

If we, now, administer attenuation (whereby the dose gains a greater capability of expansion), an excessive effect

breitungsfahigkeit gewinnt), so kann man den Effekt leicht bis zur Uebermase erhohen; wiewohl auch hierin noch ein nicht geringer Unterschied statt findet, ob die Vermischung mit einer Flussigkeit nur so obenhin,. oder so gleichförmig und innig geschehen ist, dafs der kleinste Theil der Flussigkeit auch einen verhältnifsmasigen Theil der aufgeloseten Arznei in sich aufgenommen hat; denn dann ist erstere weit weniger kraftig als diese.

251.

So wird ein einzelner Tropfen jener Tinktur mit einem Pfunde Wasser durch starkes Umschutteln innig gemischt und alle zwei Stunden zu zwei Unzen eingenommen, wohl viermahl mehr Wirkung thun, als alle acht Tropfen auf einmahl gegeben.

252.

Aus leztern Erfahrungssatze — dafs die Kraft der flussigen Arznei durch das grofsere Volumen Flussigkeit, womit sie

is easily produced; but no minor difference is found in the effects of mixture of a dilution which is, as it were, only superficial and is so uniform and intimate that even the smallest part of the fluid medium has become permeated with proportionate part of the dissolved medicine; the former is far less strong than this one.

§ 251

Thus a single drop of tincture mixed *intimately* with a pound of water and shaken *vigorously*, and two ounce of it be given every two hourly will, no doubt, have four times more effect than when given eight drops of it all at once.

§ 252

By the last mentioned practical-record, the power of a medicine in fluid is considerably enhanced by intimate mixture with a large volume of fluid - it follows undeniably that, in order to make the dose of the homoeopathic remedy as small as possible and is required it must be given in the smallest possible volume, so that when ingested it come in contact with as few nerves as possible.

innig gemischt werden, ansehnlich zu-
nimmt — folgt unleugbar, dafs um die
Gabe des homoopathischen Heilmittels so
klein, als moglich und nothig ist, einzurichten, sie auch in moglichst kleinsten
Volumen gereicht werden musse, damit so
wenig als moglich Nerven von ihr beruhret
werden, wenn sie eingenommen wird.

Anm. Daher auch die Unnothigkeit und
Zweckwidrigkeit des Nachtrinkens auf eine mit Fleifs so klein eingerschlseto Gabe.

253.

So steigert und mindert sich auch die
Wirkung der Gabe nicht in gleicher Pro-
gression mit ihrer intensiven Quantitat.
Acht Tropfen Tinktur von einem Arzneistoffe auf die Gabe wirken nicht viermahl mehr Effekt als zwei Tropfen derselben auf die Gabe, sondern nur etwa
doppelt soviel als zwei Tropfen auf die
Gabe. Eine Mischung von einem einzigen Tropfen der Tinktur mit zehn Tropfen
einer unarzneilichen Flussigkeit gemischt,
wird, zu Einem Tropfen eingenommen,

Foot Note: Therefore, so also the uselessness and uselessness of taking a dose, diligently made so small, after drinking.

§ 253

Moreover, the effect of the dose does not vary with the progressive increase and lessening of the intensive quantity of the same. One dose of *eight* drops of tincture of a medicinal substance do not produce *four times* more the effect of the dose of *two* drops of the same, but only about *double* the effect of the dose of two drops. A mixture of only one drop of a tincture with ten drops of an un-medicated fluid, given in doses of one drop, will not produce *ten times* the effect of drop doses of a mixture ten times as dilute, but *only about* (or about) as stronger the effect *as that of one drop*, and *so on further diminishes following the same law*, so that even a drop of the highest attenuation must possess, and actually manifest, a *very considerable* effect.

nicht zehnmahl grofsere Wirkung thun, als ebenfalls Ein Tropfen einer noch zehnmahl dunnern Mischung, sondern nur etwa (kaum) eine doppelt starkere Wirkung, und so weiter herab nach demselben Gesetze — so dafs ein Tropfen der höchsten Verdunnung immer noch eine sehr beträchtliche Wirkung aufsern mufs, und wirklich aufsert.

Anm. Gesetzt 1 Tropfen einer Mischung, welcher $\frac{1}{10}$ Gran des Arzneistoffs enthält,

thue eine Wirkung $= a$;

so wird 2 Tropfen einer verdunntern Mischung,

welcher $\frac{1}{100}$ Gran des Arzneistoffs enthält, $= \frac{a}{2}$

und wenn er $\frac{1}{1000}$ Gran des Arzneistoffs enthält, $= \frac{a}{4}$ u.s.w.

so dafs, bei gleichem Volumen der Gaben, durch jede (vielleicht mehr als) quadratische Verkleinerung des Arzneigehaltes die Wirkung sich doch nur etwa zur Hälfte mindert.

254.

Die Wirkung der heilenden Gegenkrankheitspotenzen, die man Arzneien

Foot Note: Let us suppose:

1 drop of a mixture which contains 1/10 grain of medicinal substance, has an effect = a;

So, 1 drop of a diluted mixture contains 1/100 grain of medicinal substance =a/2

And, when it contains 1/10000 grain of medicinal substance = a/4 and so forth.

So that, with equal volume of dose through every quadratic attenuation of the medicinal-content effect is somewhat reduced to half.

§ 254

The effect of the remedial counter disease-force upon the living human body which constitutes a medicine is so forceful and spreads widely from sensitive points well supplied with nerves, from sensitive fibres to which medicine is first applied, throughout the whole living individual with such inconceivable promptness and universality that this

nennt, auf den lebenden menschlichen Körper geschieht auf eine so eindringliche Art, verbreitet sich von dem Punkte der mit Nerven begabten, empfindlichen Faser aus, worauf die Arznei zuerst angebracht wird, mit einer so unbegreiflichen Schnelligkeit und Allgemeinheit durch alle Theile des lebenden Individuums, dafs man diese Wirkung fast geistig nennen könnte, fast so geistig als die Vitalität selbst, von welcher ihre Wirkung auf den Organism reflektirt wird; der ihren specifiken Eindruck percipirende, von Reitzbarkeit und Empfindung belebte Körper leiht dieser Wirkung eine Art Leben.

255.

Ieder Theil unsers Körpers, der nur Tastsinn besitzt, ist auch fähig, die Einwirkung der Arzneien aufzunehmen, und die Kraft derselben auf alle übrigen Theile fortzupflanzen.

256.

Am empfänglichsten für die arzneilichen Eindrucke sind freilich Zunge, Mund und Magen, und die an diesen Stellen.

effect must be called spirit-like. It is almost as spirit-like as the action of vitality itself, by which its effect on the organism is reflected; the reactivity to specific impressions, the irritability, and sensitiveness, these effects stimulate the body and lends to it a kind of life.

§ 255

Every part of our bodies that possesses the sense of touch is able to receive the influence of medicine and distribute its force all over the other parts of the organism.

§ 256

The most accessible parts for the medicinal impressions like tongue, mouth and stomach are certainly the parts most sensitive to, and medicines applied to these regions, especially in solution, are absorbed excellently in this form, work with greater power and promptness on all points of the organism.

vorzuglich in aufgeloster Gestalt aufgenom-
menen Arzneien wirken in der vollesten
Mase und mit der grofsten Schnelligkeit
durch sie auf alle Punkte des Organismus
hin.

257.

Indessen ist auch die innere Nase (die
Lungen), die empfindlichsten Stellen der
Zeugungstheile und der Mastdarm nicht
viel weniger empfanglich fur ihre Einwirkung —, so wie hautlose und verwun-
dete oder geschwurige Stellen den Kräften
der aufgelegten Arzneien eine fast eben
so eindringliche Einwirkung auf den ganzen Organismus verstatten, als wenn die
Arznei durch den Mund eingenommen
worden ware.

> Anm. Ia sogar diejenigen Theile, welche
> den ihnen eigenthumlichen Sinn verloren
> haben (z. B. eine Zunge, die den Ge-
> schmack, oder eine Nase, die den Ge-
> ruch verloren hat) theilen die blos auf sie
> zunächst einwirkende Kraft der Arznei in
> nicht geringerer Vollständigkeit der Ge-

§ 257

The inside of the nose (the lungs), genitalia and the rectum, that are not very much susceptible to the its effect, as well as parts devoid of skin, wounded or ulcerating surfaces, permit an action of medicines, even almost an immediate effect, on the whole organism which is nearly as penetrating as if the drugs had been taken by the mouth.

Footnote: Certainly even in those parts which have lost its peculiar senses (e.g. a tongue its taste, or nose which has lost its sense of smell), the effect of power of medicine is almost completely transmitted to all the remaining organs & parts of the body.

samtheit aller Organe und Theile des ubrigen Korpers mit.

258.

Dagegen sind die aufsern mit Haut
und Oberhaut umkleideten Theile des Korpers weit weniger zur Aufnahme der Arzneikraft geschickt, so jedoch, dafs unter
ihnen wiederum diejenigen Stellen, welche die empfindlichsten sind (die Haut des
Unterleibes der Herzgrube, und der innern
Biegungen der Gelenke) auch mehr Eindruck der Arzneien auf die Nerven, und
durch sie auf den ganzen ubrigen Organismus verstatten, obschon weit weniger,
als wenn dieselben Arzneien durch den
Mund eingenommen, oder in den Mastdarm eingespritzt worden waren.

259.

In Fallen also, wo wir gehindert werden, das Nothige durch den Mund einzu-
geben — (wiewohl das Verweilen der passenden homoopathischen Arznei blos im
Munde, und wenn sie auch gar nicht hin-

§ 258

On the contrary, the external surfaces of the body which is covered with skin and the epidermis are less adapted to receive the action of medicines, however, the most sensitive parts (the skin of abdomen, armpits and inner bends of the joints), it is true, allow a certain amount of the effect of medicine to pass to the nerves and from them to the whole body, but far less than the amount that so passes when the medicine is taken by the mouth or injected into the rectum.

§ 259

In some cases, where the necessary medicine cannot be given by the mouth (although, even if it cannot be swallowed, the mere taking of the suitable homoeopathic medicine into the *mouth* cavity often produces the *complete* medicinal effect by delivering it entirely to all the rest of organs), and where it is not appropriate or desirable to give it by the rectum, in such cases, if the patients are most sensitive to medicines, the mere external application of the medicine in solution to the

tergeschluckt werden könnte, doch den vollen Effekt auf die Gesamtheit aller übrigen Organe ausrichtet —) auch wo man sie nicht fuglich durch den After einbringen konnte, oder wollte —, in diesen Fällen kann man durch bloses Auflegen der aufgelösten Arznei auf die empfindlichsten aufsern Theile z. B. auf den Unterleib, die Herzgrube, u. s. w. nicht viel weniger bei empfindlichen Personen ausrichten, als durch das Einnehmen; doch mufs eine kräftigere Arzneiform hiezu gewählt und eine gröfsere Fläche damit belegt, und, wenn die Kraft noch stärker seyn soll, das Einreiben noch mit zu Hülfe genommen, auch wohl die Arznei (in stärkerer Menge) im halben oder ganzen Bade angewendet werden.

Anm. Das Einreiben scheint die Einwirkung der Arzneien nur dadurch zu befördern, in wiefern das Reiben an sich die Haut empfindlicher und so die lebende Faser empfänglicher für die Perception der eigenthümlichen durch sie auf den ganzen Organismus hinstrahlenden Arzneikraft macht. Das vorgängige Reiben der innern Stellen

O

most sensitive external parts, e.g. the abdomen, the armpits, etc., will often achieve a result not much inferior to that obtained when the medicine is given internally. But the medicine must for this purpose be used in a stronger form and spread over a large surface; and, if this strength proves not enough, it should be rubbed in, or applied (in still stronger solution) by means of baths to the whole or part of the body.

Footnote: Rubbing appears to heighten the effect of medicines only in this way that the rubbing makes the skin more sensitive and the living fibres more susceptible to perceive the peculiarity of the medicinal power which is then communicated to the whole organism. The previous employment of friction to the inner side of the thigh makes the mere application of the mercurial ointment afterwards quite as powerfully medicinal as if the ointment itself had been rubbed upon that part.

des Oberschenkels macht die nachgangige blose Auflegung der Quecksilbersalbe eben so heilkraftig, als wenn die Salbe selbst eingerieben worden wäre.

260.

Unter andern Ursachen, welche in der gemeinen Praxis zu den hohen Gaben Anlaſs gegeben haben, ragt vorzuglich die palliative Anwendung der Arzneien hervor.

Anm. Unter andern liegt der ganz entgegen gesetzte Abstand der palliativen von der homoopathischen Heilart mit darin, daſs zu ersterer möglichst groſse, zu letzterer hingegen möglichst kleine Gaben erforderlich sind.

261.

In der palliativen Anwendung der Arzneien, die nur ein Widerschein und das gerade Widerspiel der homoopathischen Heilart ist, suchte man durch einige bekannt gewordene Symptomen der Arzneien

§ 260

Among the other causes which gave rise in general practice to the large doses, the palliative use of medicines is especially preferred.

Footnote: Among other things, the absolute opposition of the palliative to the homoeopathic treatment consists in this, that in the former the largest possible and in the latter the smallest possible doses are required.

§ 261

In the *palliative application* of medicines, which is exactly opposite to the homoeopathic healing method, it was sought to drive-out the exactly opposite fixed symptoms of the disease by means of some well-known symptoms of medicines.

ganz entgegen gesetzte Symptomen der
Krankheit zu vertreiben.

262.

Da hier durch die Arznei nichts Aehnliches vom gegenwärtigen Krankheitszustande (wie in der homöopathischen Heilart),
sondern das gerade Gegentheil desselben im
Organism erregt wird so bemerkt man
auch bei solchen Palliativkuren nicht nur
nicht das Mindeste von anfänglicher (an-
scheinender) Verschlimmerung des Krankheitszustandes wie bei der homöopathischen (§. 132.), sondern im Gegentheile eine fast augenblickliche anscheinende Min-
derung desselben. In der ersten Stunde
nach der Einnahme des Palliativs befindet
sich der Kranke am meisten erleichtert,
welches nach der Einnahme des homöopathischen Heilmittels nie geschieht.

263.

Während in der homöopathischen
Heilart der ganze Krankheitszu-

O 2

§ 262

Then, in this way, the medicine arouses in the organism nothing similar to the existing disease-state (as takes place in the homoeopathic healing method), but its exact opposite, so we perceive in such palliative treatment not only not the slightest trace of initial (apparent) aggravation of the disease-state, as we do in the homoeopathic treatment (§ 132) but, on the contrary, an almost instantaneous apparent improvement. In the first hour after taking the palliative the patient feels himself most relieved, which is never happens after taking the homoeopathic remedy.

§ 263

Whereas in the homoeopathic healing method the entire disease-state is always overpowered, extinguished and annihilated in the organism by the very similar artificial

stand durch die sehr ähnliche künstliche
Gegenkrankheits - Potenz des specifischen
Heilmittels im Organismus in kurzer Zeit
(nur nicht in der ersten Stunde, sondern
allmählig von Stunde zu Stunde immer
mehr) überstimmt, ausgelöscht und vernichtet wird, wird in der Palliation, deren Norm ist: contraria contrariis
curentur — ein einzelnes gegenwär-
tiges Krankheitssymptom durch das
ganz entgegen gesetzte, der Arznei eigne
Symptom schnell nur besänftigt; vielleicht indem sich die Gegensätze durch eine
Art wechselseitiger Ineinander - Schmel-
zung, so zu sagen, dynamisch (aber nur
temporär) neutralisiren, und auf diese Art
ihren Einfluss auf den Organism so lange
verlieren, als die Wirkungsdauer
des opponirten Arzneisymptoms
anhalt.

264.

Das vorige Uebel scheint gleich im Anfange der Palliativkur wie verschwunden;
aber es wird nicht aufgehoben, nicht aus-

counter-disease-force of the specific remedy in a short time (certainly not in the first hour, but always gradually more so from hour to hour), while in the palliative method—whose norm is *contraria contrariis curentur—one single* existing symptom of the disease is merely *soothed*, quickly, by the exactly contrary symptom of the medicine; perhaps because the opposites by a kind of mutual neutralize each another dynamically (though only temporarily), and in this way they loses its influence on the organism *as long as the duration of action of the opposing medicinal symptom lasts.*

§ 264

The original sufferings appears to disappear immediately at the beginning of the palliative treatment; but it is not removed, not extinguished – on the contrary, as soon as the oppositely effecting tendency of the palliative ceases to act

gelöscht — es kehrt, so wie die entgegen
gesetzte Wirkungstendenz des Palliativs zu
wirken nachläfst und ausgewirkt hat, welches in einigen Stunden oder Tagen geschieht, wieder zuruck, nicht nur in gleicher Mase, sondern sogar verstärkt durch
Hinzutritt der Nachwirkungstendenz (Sekundärsymptomen) des Palliativs, die (als
Gegensatz der Primärwirkungen) dem
ursprunglichen Krankheitssymptome sehr
ähnlich ist, und es so, als Zusatz, wesentlich und dauerhaft verschlimmert.

265.

Dem homöopathischen Heilungspro-
cesse ganz entgegengesetzt, befindet sich
in der ersten Stunde des palliativen Arzneigebrauchs der Kranke am meisten erleichtert, in der zweiten Stunde weniger, in der
dritten noch weniger und so fort, bis nach
Verfluss der opponirten Primärwirkung der
Arznei, die Tendenz der Sekundarwirkung
hinzutritt und dann befindet sich der Kranke schlechter, als vor der Einnahme des
Palliativs.

and has exhausted its action, which takes place in a few hours or days, it returns not merely in the same degree but even in increased intensity by the appearance of the after-effect tendency (secondary symptoms) of the palliative, which (as the opposite of the primary effect) is very similar to the original disease symptoms, and thus, as an addition to it, seriously and permanently aggravates it.

§ 265

Completely opposite to the homoeopathic healing process, the patient feels most relieved in the first hour of the application of the palliative medicine, less in the second hour, still less in the third, and so on, until when the opposite primary action of medicine has ceased, the tendency of the secondary action appears, and then the patient becomes worse than he was before the palliative was administered.

Anm. Da der Zutritt einer neuen Krankheit
zu einer schon vorhandnen ganz die Natur
einer Arznei besitzt, und man sich einer solchen Krankheit, wenn diese neue der ältern
an Symptomen ähnlich ist, als eines vollkommen homoopathischen Heilmittels bedienen und die ältere Krankheit damit vernichten und auslöschen kann (§. 28. 30.
36.); so kann man sich auch der Krankheiten fehlerhaft als Palliative bedienen, wie
auch schon geschehen ist.

So glaubte *Leroy*, der diesen Unterschied und seine Bedeutung nicht kannte
(Heilk. für Mütter, S. 383.) die skrophulö-
sen Drüsenverhartungen des ganzen Körpers bei einem Kinde durch Einimpfung
der Menschenpocken heben zu können.
Beim Ausbruche der Pocken waren auch
alle Drüsenverhartungen gleich wie verschwunden; aber sechs Wochen hernach
— langer dauerte die palliative Suspension
des alten Uebels nicht — erschienen die
Drüsenverhartungen alle wieder —
ganz naturlich, da die Drüsenverhartungen, welche auf Menschenpocken zu pflegen, nicht in ihrer Primärwirkung, das
ist, nicht in ihrem akuten Stadium, sondern in ihrer Nachkrankheit (Sekundärwir-
kung) enthalten sind, folglich schon am

Foot Note: As a new disease approaching the system where there is one already present possess the nature of a medicine and one can make use of such a disease when the symptoms of this new one and the older one are similar, as a perfect homoeopathic remedy, and by means of it annihilate and extinguish the older diseases (§§ 28, 30, 36), so also diseases may be improperly used as palliatives, as has already been done.

So, Leroy, who did not know this difference and its importance (Heilkunde für Mütter, p. 383 **(Translator's Note:** The Therapy for the Mother, p. 383]), believed that he could remove the scrofulous glandular indurations all over the body of a child by inoculation of smallpox. When the smallpox broke out all the indurated glands immediately disappeared; but six weeks later - the palliative suppression of the old illness did not last longer - all the glandular indurations appeared all over again, as was quite natural, because the indurated glands that come on after smallpox do not belong to its primary action, that is not to its acute stage, but to its after-disease (secondary action), consequently the existing glandular induration on the body cannot be cured homoeopathically, removed and annihilated.

Körper vorhandne Drüsenverhärtungen
nicht homöopathisch heilen, aufheben und
vernichten können.

266.

Um nun die schmeichelhafte Erleichterung zu erneuern, ist man genöthigt, das
Palliativ in jedesmahl verstärkten, oft ansehnlich verstärkten Gaben zu reichen, weil
jede Gabe außer dem zu bestreitenden
Krankheitssymptome, auch noch die durch
die Sekundärsymptomen der vorigen Gabe
erzeugte Verschlimmerung des Krankheitszustandes mit zu verdecken hat.*)

267.

Ohne Verstärkung der Gabe des Palliativs wird die (temporäre) Erleichterung immer geringer, zuletzt unbemerklich und zu
Nichts (und dann erfolgt eine desto stärke-

----

*) Ein starkes Beispiel dieser Art sehe man in *J. H.
Schulze*, Diss. qua corporis humani momentanearum alterationum specimina quaedam expenduntur, Halae, 1741. §. 28.

§ 266

Now, in order to renew the flattering improvement, it is necessary to increase the palliative every time, often to increase its dose considerably, because every dose has to cover not only the disease-symptoms itself, but also the aggravation of the disease-state caused by the secondary symptoms of the previous dose.

Foot Note: One sees a striking example of this type in J. H. Schulze's Diss. *qua corporis humani momentanearum alterationum specimina quaedam expenduntur*, Halae, 1741, § 28.

§ 267

Without increasing the dose of the palliative, the (temporary) relief become gradually less, at length unobservable and none (and there then ensues an increased aggravation of the disease-state).

e Verschlimmerung des Krankheitszustan-
es hinterdrein)

268.

Iede blos in immer verstarkter Gabe
rleichternde (in ihrer Wirkung einem
Hauptsymptome der Krankheit antiloge
nd opponirte) Arznei, ist ein Palliativ.

Anm. Das Irrationelle der palliativen Ver-
fahrungsart leuchtet von selbst ein, da der
Kranke ja nicht eine täuschende, temporäre Erleichterung, welche im
Erfolge das Uebel verstarkt, sondern grundliche Heilung bedarf, und sie
ist auch schon deshalb fehlerhaft, weil
man nur ein einzelnes Symptom — oft nur
den zwanzigsten Theil der Krankheit und
ihres Symptomeninbegriffs dadurch zu bestreiten vermag, das ist, nur symptoma-
tisch, und dennoch nicht hulfreich ver-
ahrt.

Doch war es noch ein Gluck, dafs man
die den Arzneien eignen Symptome zu wenig kannte, als dafs man zur Bestreitung
gegenseitiger Zustande gar zu häufig von
ihnen hätte Misbrauch machen können.

§ 268

Every medicine, (antagonistic and opposite in its action to one chief symptom of the disease) when it can only relieve in always increasing doses, is a palliative.

Footnote: The irrational character of palliative treatment is self-evident, for the patient requires a radical cure, not a *temporary relief, which ends in an aggravation* of the original disease and such treatment is also fallacious, because by it only one symptom is attacked - often only the twentieth part of the disease and thereby its symptom totality is denied, that is, is only symptomatic and nevertheless is not helpful.

Anyway, it was fortunate that so little was known of the individual symptoms of medicines; otherwise too frequent an application might have been made of them for the purpose of combating opposite conditions. There remained but few operations of this kind available: Coffee was given for a tendency to drowsiness; for chronic diarrhoea, the primary action of opium to constipate was employed; its action in causing a heavy stupefying sleep was

Es blieb nur bei einigen Operationen dieser
Art: habitueller Neigung zur Schlafrigkeit
setzte man Kaffee — den, selbst chronischen
Durchfällen die Leib verstopfende primäre
Kraft des Mohnsafts, die betäubten, dum-
men Schlaf machende Wirkung desselben
der, oft langwierigen Nachtmunterkeit,
und allen erdenklichen Arten Schmerzen
den Stupor und die Fühllosigkeit entgegen,
welche diese Substanz über das ganze Sensorium verbreitet —; mit den in starker
Gabe die Därme zu häufiger Ausleerung
reitzenden Purgirarzneien und Laxirsalzen
wollte man die Neigung zur Leibesverstopfung aufheben, durch erhitzende Gewürze und geistige Getränke dem Mangel an
Blutwärme, und der sogenannten Magen-
schwäche abhelfen, durch Niesemittel
langwierigen Stockschnupfen heilen, mit
kühlenden Dingen der Verbrennungs - Entzündung steuern, mit Blutausleerung jede
Hitze mindern, mit den die Harnauslee-
rung so mächtig aufreitzenden Kanthariden
die fast vollendete Blasenlähmung selbst in
chronischen Fällen zur Thätigkeit erwe-
cken, alte Lähmungen verschiedner Art
mit der in der Primärwirkung die Muskeln
in Bewegung setzenden Elektrisität und
galvanischen Kraft vertreiben, u. s. w.

used for chronic wakefulness, and the state of stupor and insensibility which this substance can extend over the whole sensorium was utilised to relieve every imaginable kind of pain; the tendency to constipation was sought to be treated with large doses of irritating purgative medicines and laxative salts that caused frequent evacuations; a deficiency of body-heat and so-called weakness of the stomach were remedied by stimulating spices and spirituous drinks; chronic stuffed nose by sternutative remedies; inflammation by cooling things; heat of the body by blood-letting; even chronic cases of almost complete paralysis of the bladder were sought to be activated by cantharides which has such a powerfully irritating action on the urinary system; old paralyses of various kinds were treated with electricity and galvanism, which in their primary action set the muscles in movement, etc. Often too late, but experience proved that how rarely health was thereby restored, and how frequently disease aggravation or even something worse ensued.

Wie selten man aber Gesundheit, wie oft
man verstärkte Krankheit und noch etwas
Schlimmeres damit erreichte, lehrte die
oft zu späte Ueberzeugerin, Erfahrung.

269.

Blos bei höchst dringenden Gefahren
bei Asphyxien und dem Scheintode
Blitze, vom Ersticken, Erfrieren, u.
. ist es erlaubt und zweckmäsig, durch
Palliativ. z. B. durch gelinde elektrische
hütterungen, durch starken Kaffee,
h ein excitirendes Riechmittel u. s. w.
rst wenigstens die Empfindung und
zbarkeit (das physische Leben) wieder
ang zu bringen, bis man weiter, wo
ig, homöopathisch verfahren kann.
er gehören auch verschiedne Antidote
ger Vergiftungen.

270.

Auch ist eine homöopathische Arznei
eilung der Krankheiten deshalb noch
unpassend gewählt, wenn einige
eisymptonien einigen mittlern und klei-

§ 269

Only in the most urgent emergencies, *e. g.* asphyxia, apparent death from lightning, from suffocation, freezing to death, and so forth, is it permissible and practical to restore, at least as a preliminary measure for the time being, the sensibility and irritability (the physical life) by a palliative, e.g. by mild electrical shocks, by strong coffee, or, with a stimulating odour, etc. to gain time until, if needed, homoeopathy can act. To this category belong also the different antidotes to acute poisonings.

§ 270

Similarly, a homoeopathic medicine is not to be regarded as unsuitably chosen for curing diseases if a few of the medicinal symptoms are only palliatives to some of the less important and minor symptoms of the disease, provided only that the other, and especially the stronger, peculiar and characteristic chief symptoms of the disease are countered and covered by the same remedy homoeopathically, (with similarity of symptoms).

nern Krankheitssymptomen nur palliativ
entsprechen, wenn nur die übrigen, vorzüglich die stärkern, besondern und charakteristischen Hauptsymptomen der Krankheit durch dasselbe Arzneimittel homöopathisch (durch Symptomenähnlichkeit) gedeckt und befriedigt werden.

271.

Es erfolgt in diesem Falle nichts von
den Nachtheilen der gewöhnlichen einseitigen Palliation eines einzelnen Krankheits-
symptoms; es erfolgt vollständige Heilung
ohne Nebenbeschwerden oder Nachwehen,
doch so, dafs die Symptomen, welche hier
nur durch entgegengesetzte, in der Kraft
der Arzneisubstanz liegende Symptomen
(palliativ) bestritten werden, gewöhnlich
nicht eher vergehen, als nach gänzlich
vollendeter Wirkungsdauer des Medikaments.

Anm. 1. Eine andre, sehr häufige Methode,
   Arzneien in der niedern Praxis anzuwenden, welche den Wahn von der Nöthigkeit

536

§ 271

In this case, none of the ill consequences of the common one-sided palliation of a single disease-symptom are seen; there follows a complete cure without accessory sufferings or after-pains effects, but in such a way that those symptoms which were here attacked only by the opposite (palliative) symptoms of action of the medicinal substance, usually do not disappear until the duration of action of the medicine is entirely finished.

Footnote No. 1: Another more frequently used but inferior practice of administering medicine selected on some illusion that large medicinal doses

großer Arzneigaben hervorgebracht und unterhalten hat, ist die, durch heftige Arzneien einen (weder analogen, noch opponirten, sondern) andersartigen Reitz im Organismus anzubringen, um, so zu sagen, die Krankheit durch die Starke des Arzneisturms zu uberwältigen. Während nun so die andersartig reitzenden Mittel den Organism, oder vorzüglich den einen Theil desselben in einer stärkern, andersartigen Krankheitsstimmung erhalten, schweigt indefs die ursprungliche Krankheit, kömmt aber sogleich wieder, wenn der Kranke solche Arzneien zu nehmen aufhört. Die meisten sogenannten Revulsionen gehören in diese Kategorie.

So wenn der gemeine Praktiker z. B. die Krätze mit Purgirmitteln zu besturmen anfängt, fängt auch die Krätze an, von der Haut zu verschwinden, verläfst, wenn mit den Purganzen gestiegen wird, die Haut fast ganz, und bleibt so lange fast ganz weg, als der Darmkanal durch die Purgirmittel recht krank und kränker erhalten wird, als die Krätze die Haut zu machen pflegte. Mufs aber der Praktiker endlich dennoch mit den Purganzen nachlassen, so kömmt der Ausschlag in voller Mase wieder auf die Haut — weil von einem andersartigen

of violent medicine (neither analogous, nor opposite) produces a different stimulus in the organism, in order to, so to say, the force of the medicinal strength overpowers the disease. Due to this differently stimulated remedy, the organism gets a stronger, different disease disposition, in the meanwhile the original disease is silenced which comes back immediately when the patients stops taking such a medicine. Most of the so-called revolutions belongs to this category.

So when the common practitioner for example begins to assail scabies with purgative medicine, it disappears completely from the skin and while the purgative continues its action on the intestinal canal making it sick and worse, the skin so long remains nearly completely free though the scabies of the skin is being maintained. Finally when the practitioner stops the purgatives and

Krankheitsreitze keine Krankheit geheilt,
sondern nur (fast wie bei Palliativen; nur
nicht so schnell und mit noch angreifende-
rer Heftigkeit) suspendirt und die Zeit über,
als die Uebermacht des künstlichen unpassenden Reitzes anhält, nur zum Schwei-
gen gebracht wird (§. 22. 24. 26. 27.).
So wirken die Haarseile, die Fontanelle,
die Exutorien, u. s. w.

Anm. 2. Neben der homöopathischen Heilart
wird der rationelle Arzt höchst selten Ursache finden, jene revolutionirende Methode, Ausleerungsmittel von oben oder unten,
anzuwenden, aufser wenn ganz unverdau-
liche oder fremdartige, sehr schädliche
Substanzen in den Magen oder in die Ge-
därme gerathen sind.

Aufserdem findet zuweilen die Anwendung einiger undynamischen Mittel statt.
Da hat man Fette, welche den Zusammen-
hang der Faser und ihre Dichtigkeit gleichsam mechanisch oder physisch auflockern
— Gerbestoff, welcher die lebende Faser,
fast eben so wie die todte, verdich-
tet — Holzkohle, welche den übeln Geruch ungesunder Stellen am lebenden Körper mindert, wie sie ihn von leblosen Dingen hinwegnimmt — Kalkerde, Laugen-

540

its effect fades away, rash of the full veins reappears on the skin, - because stimulation from a different disease can not cure a disease but can only suspend it (nearly palliates them, attacks with more severity but not so quick) and till the time the stronger artificial stimulation stops, the intercurrent measures brought in continues (§§22, 24, 26, 27). So works the setons, the fontanelles, the exutorien, etc.

Footnote No. 2: Besides the homoeopathic healing method, the rational physician will very rarely have a reason to employ that revolutionary method of evacuations upwards and downwards, except when highly indigestible or foreign or harmful substances have been taken into the stomach or bowels.

At times, the use of some undynamic remedies becomes necessary. Such as fatty matters, which mechanically or physically loosen the connection and

salze, Seife und Schwefel, welche die atzenden Sauren und Metallsalze in oder an dem menschlichen Körper chemisch zu zersetzen, zu neutralisiren und unschädlicher zu machen im Stande sind und Sauren und Laugensalze, welche die verschiedenartigen Harnsteine in der Blase aufzulösen vermogen — so das physisch zerstorende glühende Eisen, die chemisch wegätzenden Dinge mancher Art, u. s. w. — des blos minorativen, selten rationell anzuwendenden Blutlassens, der Blutigel, u. s. w. hier nicht zu erwähnen,

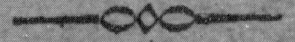

compactness of the fibres; tannin, which thickens the living fibres almost as much as it does the dead ones; charcoal, which diminishes the bad odour of unhealthy parts in the living body, just as it destroys that of dead things; chalk, alkaline salt, soap and sulphur, which can chemically decompose, neutralize and render harmless the corrosive acids and metallic salts in or on the human body; acids and alkaline salts which are able to dissolve different kinds of urinary calculi in the bladder; the actual physically cautery, chemical caustics of various kinds, etc. Blood-letting, leeches, etc. which are less used and only rarely rationally indicated are not required to be mentioned here.

Verbesserungen.

S. 40 Z. 3 l. einleuchtendem st. einleuchtenden

- 40 - 3 l. wahrem st. wahren
- 40 - 18 l. den st. der
- 55 - 15 l. schon st. sehr
- 199 - 23 24 l. Genüßen st. Gemüssen.

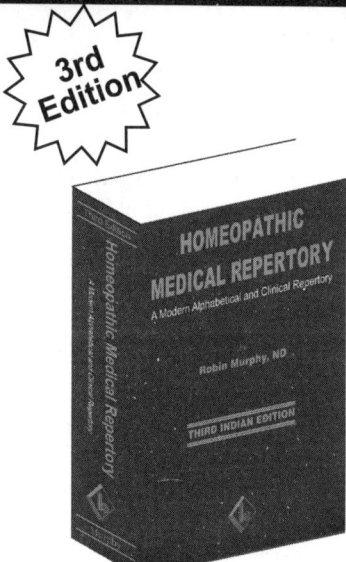
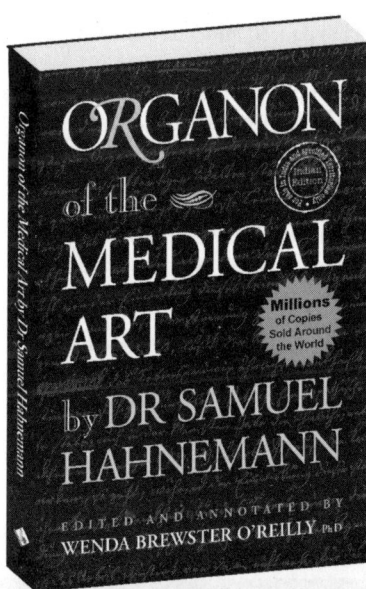

Fundamentals of Prescribing

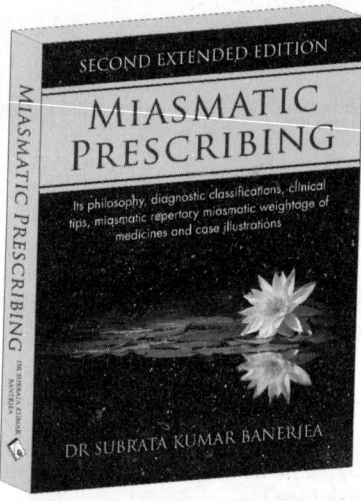
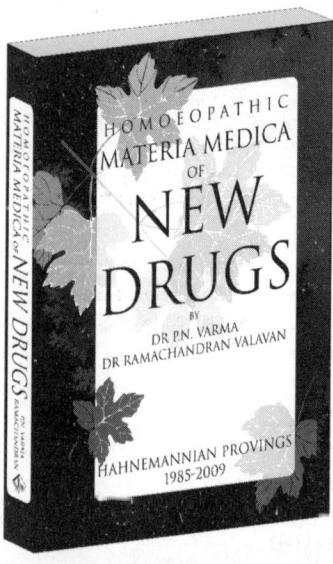

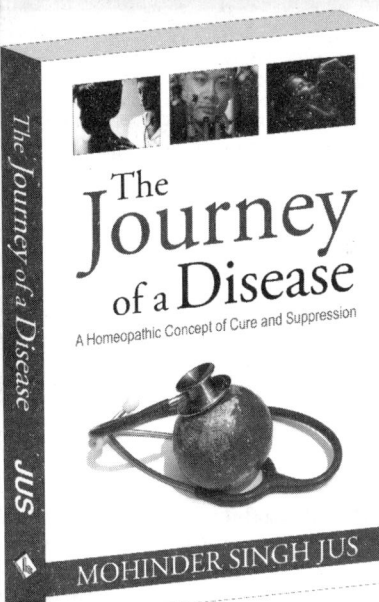
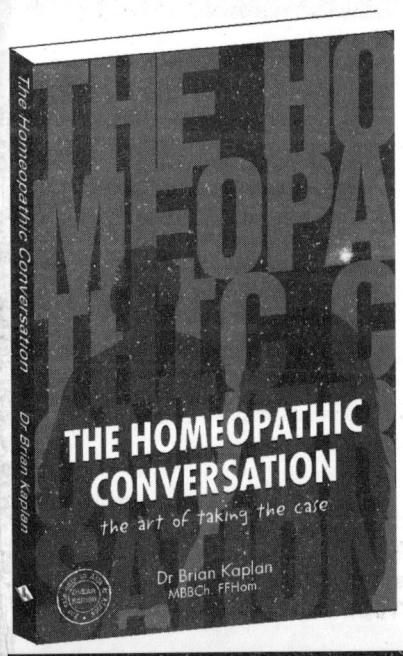

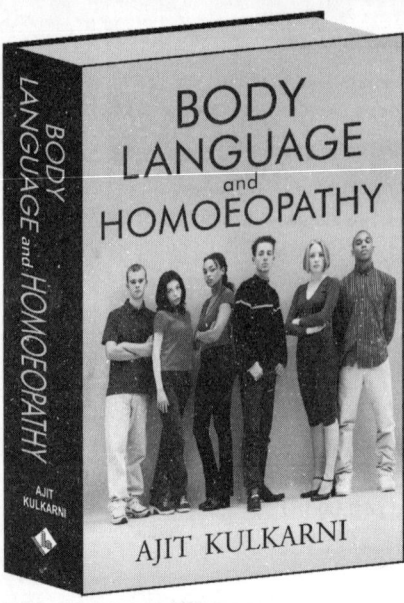
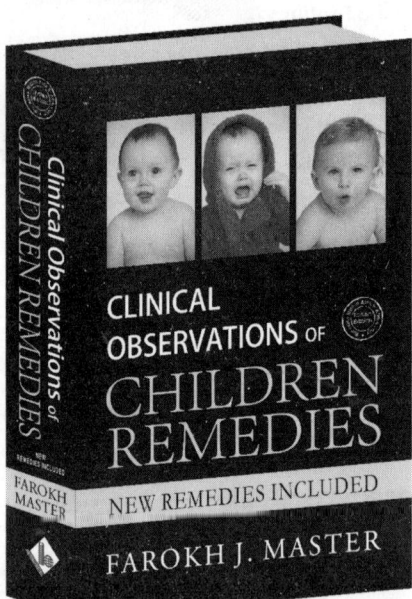